Allergies

SOURCEBOOK

Sixth Edition

Health Reference Series

Sixth Edition

Allergies
SOURCEBOOK

Basic Consumer Health Information about the Immune System and Allergic Disorders, Including Rhinitis (Hay Fever), Sinusitis, Conjunctivitis, Asthma, Atopic Dermatitis, and Anaphylaxis, and Allergy Triggers Such As Pollen, Mold, Dust Mites, Animal Dander, Chemicals, Foods and Additives, and Medications

Along with Facts about Allergy Diagnosis and Treatment, Tips on Avoiding Triggers and Preventing Symptoms, a Glossary of Related Terms, and Directories of Resources for Additional Help and Information

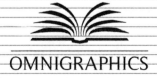

OMNIGRAPHICS

615 Griswold, Ste. 901, Detroit, MI 48226

Bibliographic Note
Because this page cannot legibly accommodate all the copyright notices, the Bibliographic Note portion of the Preface constitutes an extension of the copyright notice.

* * *

OMNIGRAPHICS
Angela L. Williams, *Managing Editor*
***

Copyright © 2018 Omnigraphics
ISBN 978-0-7808-1646-6
E-ISBN 978-0-7808-1647-3

Library of Congress Cataloging-in-Publication Data

Names: Omnigraphics, Inc., issuing body.

Title: Allergies sourcebook: basic consumer health information about the immune system and allergic disorders, including rhinitis (hay fever), sinusitis, conjunctivitis, asthma, atopic dermatitis, and anaphylaxis, and allergy triggers such as pollen, mold, dust mites, animal dander, chemicals, foods and additives, and medications; along with facts about allergy diagnosis and treatment, tips on avoiding triggers and preventing symptoms, a glossary of related terms, and directories of resources for additional help.

Description: Sixth edition. | Detroit, MI: Omnigraphics, Inc., [2019] | Includes bibliographical references and index.

Identifiers: LCCN 2018034650 (print) | LCCN 2018035335 (ebook) | ISBN 9780780816473 (ebook) | ISBN 9780780816466 (hard cover: alk. paper) | ISBN 9780780816473 (ebook)

Subjects: LCSH: Allergy--Popular works.

Classification: LCC RC584 (ebook) | LCC RC584.A3443 2019 (print) | DDC 616.97/3--dc23

LC record available at https://lccn.loc.gov/2018034650

Table of Contents

v

Part II: Types of Allergic Reactions

Part IV: Airborne, Chemical, and Other Environmental Allergy Triggers

Part V: Diagnosing and Treating Allergies

Part VI: Avoiding Allergy Triggers and Preventing Symptoms

Part VII: Additional Help and Information

Preface

About This Book

Allergies are the sixth leading cause of chronic disease in the United States, and according to the National Institute of Allergy and Infectious Diseases (NIAID), "About half of all Americans test positive for at least one of the ten most common allergens: Ragweed, Bermuda grass, ryegrass, white oak, Russian thistle, Alternaria mold, cat, house dust mite, German cockroach, and peanut." Symptoms associated with allergic reactions can range from mild annoyances to anaphylaxis, a life-threatening emergency. Combined, allergies cost the U.S. healthcare system an estimated $18 billion annually according to Centers for Disease Control and Prevention (CDC).

Despite their widespread occurrence, however, many people do not understand the basic biological processes involved in allergic reactions and the role the immune system plays in causing common symptoms. Furthermore, medical science has yet to identify the specific genetic and environmental interactions that lead to the development of allergies or to fully understand why the prevalence of allergic diseases is increasing.

Allergies Sourcebook, Sixth Edition provides updated information about the causes, triggers, treatments, and prevalence of common allergic disorders, including rhinitis, sinusitis, conjunctivitis, allergic asthma, dermatitis, eczema, hives, and anaphylaxis. It discusses the immune system and its role in the development of allergic disorders and describes such commonly encountered allergens as pollen, mold, dust mites, and animal dander. Facts about allergies to foods and food additives, medications, and chemicals are also included, along with information about allergy diagnosis, treatments, coping strategies, and prevention efforts. The book concludes with a glossary of related terms and directories of resources for additional help and information.

How to Use This Book

This book is divided into parts and chapters. Parts focus on broad areas of interest. Chapters are devoted to single topics within a part.

Part I: Introduction to Allergies and the Immune System discusses the components and functions of the immune system and explains the link between genes, environment, and allergy development. Facts about how allergies affect breathing and allergies in children are also included.

Part II: Types of Allergic Reactions identifies the signs and symptoms of common allergic reactions, including rhinitis (hay fever), sinusitis, conjunctivitis (eye allergies), asthma, atopic dermatitis (eczema), rashes, hives, and life-threatening anaphylaxis.

Part III: Foods and Food Additives That Trigger Allergic Reactions provides information about the most common food allergens, including milk, egg, fish and shellfish, peanut and tree nut, wheat, and soy. Information about food additives and ingredients that trigger reactions, food intolerances, tips on living with a food allergy, and advice for consumers about food labels are also included.

Part IV: Airborne, Chemical, and Other Environmental Allergy Triggers discusses symptoms of allergies to pollen and ragweed, mold, dust mites, cockroaches, insect sting, animal dander, and medications. The part also talks about how tobacco smoke, air quality, climate change, multiple chemical sensitivity can have an impact on health. Lanolin allergy and sick building syndrome are also included.

Part V: Diagnosing and Treating Allergies identifies tests, therapies, and medications that alleviate allergy symptoms, including antihistamines, decongestants, nasal sprays, and allergy shots. It also provides tips on choosing an allergist and complementary and alternative medicine for allergies.

Part VI: Avoiding Allergy Triggers and Preventing Symptoms provides information about reducing indoor allergy triggers, environmental triggers, and improving air quality. This part also offers strategies for preventing allergy symptoms during travel and pregnancy, finding an allergy support group, and remaining free of symptoms at school. Health insurance issues for people affected with allergies are also included in this part.

Part VII: Additional Help and Information provides a glossary of important terms related to allergies and the immune system. A directory of organizations that provide health information about allergies and asthma is also included, along with a list of cookbooks, websites, and companies that market allergy-free products for people with food allergies.

Bibliographic Note

This volume contains documents and excerpts from publications issued by the following government agencies: Agency for Healthcare Research and Quality (AHRQ); Centers for Disease Control and Prevention (CDC); Centers for Medicare & Medicaid Services (CMS); Genetic and Rare Diseases Information Center (GARD); Genetics Home Reference (GHR); National Center for Complementary and Integrative Health (NCCIH); National Eye Institute (NEI); National Heart, Lung, and Blood Institute (NHLBI); National Human Genome Research Institute (NHGRI); National Institute of Allergy and Infectious Diseases (NIAID); National Institute of Arthritis and Musculoskeletal and Skin Diseases (NIAMS); National Institute of Diabetes and Digestive and Kidney Diseases (NIDDK); National Institute of Environmental Health Sciences (NIEHS); National Institutes of Health (NIH); National Oceanic and Atmospheric Administration (NOAA); *NIH News in Health*; Occupational Safety and Health Administration (OSHA); Office of Disease Prevention and Health Promotion (ODPHP); Office on Women's Health (OWH); U.S. Access Board; U.S. Department of Agriculture (USDA); U.S. Department of Health and Human Services (HHS); U.S. Department of Veterans Affairs (VA); U.S. Environmental Protection Agency (EPA); U.S. Food and Drug Administration (FDA); and U.S. Global Change Research Program (USGCRP).

It may also contain original material produced by Omnigraphics and reviewed by medical consultants.

About the Health Reference Series

The *Health Reference Series* is designed to provide basic medical information for patients, families, caregivers, and the general public.

Each volume takes a particular topic and provides comprehensive coverage. This is especially important for people who may be dealing with a newly diagnosed disease or a chronic disorder in themselves or in a family member. People looking for preventive guidance, information about disease warning signs, medical statistics, and risk factors for health problems will also find answers to their questions in the *Health Reference Series*. The *Series*, however, is not intended to serve as a tool for diagnosing illness, in prescribing treatments, or as a substitute for the physician/patient relationship. All people concerned about medical symptoms or the possibility of disease are encouraged to seek professional care from an appropriate healthcare provider.

A Note about Spelling and Style

Health Reference Series editors use *Stedman's Medical Dictionary* as an authority for questions related to the spelling of medical terms and the *Chicago Manual of Style* for questions related to grammatical structures, punctuation, and other editorial concerns. Consistent adherence is not always possible, however, because the individual volumes within the *Series* include many documents from a wide variety of different producers, and the editor's primary goal is to present material from each source as accurately as is possible. This sometimes means that information in different chapters or sections may follow other guidelines and alternate spelling authorities. For example, occasionally a copyright holder may require that eponymous terms be shown in possessive forms (Crohn's disease vs. Crohn disease) or that British spelling norms be retained (leukaemia vs. leukemia).

Medical Review

Omnigraphics contracts with a team of qualified, senior medical professionals who serve as medical consultants for the *Health Reference Series*. As necessary, medical consultants review reprinted and originally written material for currency and accuracy. Citations including the phrase, "Reviewed (month, year)" indicate material reviewed by this team. Medical consultation services are provided to the *Health Reference Series* editors by:

Dr. Vijayalakshmi, MBBS, DGO, MD
Dr. Senthil Selvan, MBBS, DCH, MD
Dr. K. Sivanandham, MBBS, DCH, MS (Research), PhD

Our Advisory Board

We would like to thank the following board members for providing initial guidance on the development of this series:

- Dr. Lynda Baker, Associate Professor of Library and Information Science, Wayne State University, Detroit, MI

- Nancy Bulgarelli, William Beaumont Hospital Library, Royal Oak, MI

- Karen Imarisio, Bloomfield Township Public Library, Bloomfield Township, MI

- Karen Morgan, Mardigian Library, University of Michigan-Dearborn, Dearborn, MI

- Rosemary Orlando, St. Clair Shores Public Library, St. Clair Shores, MI

Health Reference Series *Update Policy*

The inaugural book in the *Health Reference Series* was the first edition of *Cancer Sourcebook* published in 1989. Since then, the *Series* has been enthusiastically received by librarians and in the medical community. In order to maintain the standard of providing high-quality health information for the layperson the editorial staff at Omnigraphics felt it was necessary to implement a policy of updating volumes when warranted.

Medical researchers have been making tremendous strides, and it is the purpose of the *Health Reference Series* to stay current with the most recent advances. Each decision to update a volume is made on an individual basis. Some of the considerations include how much new information is available and the feedback we receive from people who use the books. If there is a topic you would like to see added to the update list, or an area of medical concern you feel has not been adequately addressed, please write to:

Managing Editor
Health Reference Series
Omnigraphics
615 Griswold, Ste. 901
Detroit, MI 48226

Part One

Introduction to Allergies and the Immune System

Chapter 1

Understanding the Immune System and Allergic Reactions

The Immune System

Function

The overall function of the immune system is to prevent or limit infection. An example of this principle is found in immune-compromised people, including those with genetic immune disorders, immune-debilitating infections like human immunodeficiency virus (HIV), and even pregnant women, who are susceptible to a range of microbes that typically do not cause infection in healthy individuals.

The immune system can distinguish between normal, healthy cells and unhealthy cells by recognizing a variety of "danger" cues called danger-associated molecular patterns (DAMPs). Cells may be unhealthy because of infection or because of cellular damage caused by noninfectious agents like sunburn or cancer. Infectious microbes such as viruses and bacteria release another set of signals recognized by the immune system called pathogen-associated molecular patterns (PAMPs).

This chapter includes text excerpted from "Overview of the Immune System," National Institute of Allergy and Infectious Diseases (NIAID), December 30, 2013. Reviewed August 2018.

3

When the immune system first recognizes these signals, it responds to address the problem. If an immune response cannot be activated when there is sufficient need, problems arise, like infection. On the other hand, when an immune response is activated without a real threat or is not turned off once the danger passes, different problems arise, such as allergic reactions and autoimmune disease.

The immune system is complex and pervasive. There are numerous cell types that either circulate throughout the body or reside in a particular tissue. Each cell type plays a unique role, with different ways of recognizing problems, communicating with other cells, and performing their functions. By understanding all the details behind this network, researchers may optimize immune responses to confront specific issues, ranging from infections to cancer.

Location

All immune cells come from precursors in the bone marrow and develop into mature cells through a series of changes that can occur in different parts of the body.

- **Skin:** The skin is usually the first line of defense against microbes. Skin cells produce and secrete important antimicrobial proteins, and immune cells can be found in specific layers of skin.

- **Bone marrow:** The bone marrow contains stems cells that can develop into a variety of cell types. The common myeloid progenitor stem cell in the bone marrow is the precursor to innate immune cells—neutrophils, eosinophils, basophils, mast cells, monocytes, dendritic cells, and macrophages—that are important first-line responders to infection.

The common lymphoid progenitor stem cell leads to adaptive immune cells—B cells and T-cells—that are responsible for mounting responses to specific microbes based on previous encounters (immunological memory). Natural killer (NK) cells also are derived from the common lymphoid progenitor and share features of both innate and adaptive immune cells, as they provide immediate defenses like innate cells but also may be retained as memory cells like adaptive cells. B, T, and NK cells also are called lymphocytes.

- **Bloodstream:** Immune cells constantly circulate throughout the bloodstream, patrolling for problems. When blood tests are used to monitor white blood cells (WBCs), another term for immune cells, a snapshot of the immune system is taken. If a cell type is either scarce or overabundant in the bloodstream, this may reflect a problem.

- **Thymus:** T-cells mature in the thymus, a small organ located in the upper chest.

- **Lymphatic system:** The lymphatic system is a network of vessels and tissues composed of lymph, an extracellular fluid, and lymphoid organs, such as lymph nodes. The lymphatic system is a conduit for travel and communication between tissues and the bloodstream. Immune cells are carried through the lymphatic system and converge in lymph nodes, which are found throughout the body.

- **Lymph nodes:** Lymph nodes are a communication hub where immune cells sample information brought in from the body. For instance, if adaptive immune cells in the lymph node recognize pieces of a microbe brought in from a distant area, they will activate, replicate, and leave the lymph node to circulate and address the pathogen. Thus, doctors may check patients for swollen lymph nodes, which may indicate an active immune response.

- **Spleen:** The spleen is an organ located behind the stomach. While it is not directly connected to the lymphatic system, it is important for processing information from the bloodstream. Immune cells are enriched in specific areas of the spleen, and upon recognizing bloodborne pathogens (BBPs), they will activate and respond accordingly.

- **Mucosal tissue:** Mucosal surfaces are prime entry points for pathogens, and specialized immune hubs are strategically located in mucosal tissues like the respiratory tract and gut. For instance, Peyer's patches are important areas in the small intestine where immune cells can access samples from the gastrointestinal tract.

Features of an Immune Response

An immune response is generally divided into innate and adaptive immunity. Innate immunity occurs immediately, when circulating innate cells recognize a problem. Adaptive immunity occurs later, as it relies on the coordination and expansion of specific adaptive immune cells. Immune memory follows the adaptive response, when mature adaptive cells, highly specific to the original pathogen, are retained for later use.

Innate Immunity

Innate immune cells express genetically encoded receptors, called Toll-like receptors (TLRs), which recognize general danger- or pathogen-associated patterns. Collectively, these receptors can broadly recognize viruses, bacteria, fungi, and even noninfectious problems. However, they cannot distinguish between specific strains of bacteria or viruses.

There are numerous types of innate immune cells with specialized functions. They include neutrophils, eosinophils, basophils, mast cells, monocytes, dendritic cells, and macrophages. Their main feature is the ability to respond quickly and broadly when a problem arises, typically leading to inflammation. Innate immune cells also are important for activating adaptive immunity. Innate cells are critical for host defense, and disorders in innate cell function may cause chronic susceptibility to infection.

Adaptive Immunity

Adaptive immune cells are more specialized, with each adaptive B or T cell bearing unique receptors, B-cell receptors (BCRs) and T-cell receptors (TCRs), that recognize specific signals rather than general patterns. Each receptor recognizes an antigen, which is simply any molecule that may bind to a BCR or TCR. Antigens are derived from a variety of sources including pathogens, host cells, and allergens. Antigens are typically processed by innate immune cells and presented to adaptive cells in the lymph nodes.

The genes for BCRs and TCRs are randomly rearranged at specific cell maturation stages, resulting in unique receptors that may potentially recognize anything. Random generation of receptors allows the immune system to respond to new or unforeseen problems. This concept is especially important because environments may frequently change, for instance, when seasons change or a person relocates, and pathogens are constantly evolving to survive. Because BCRs and TCRs are so specific, adaptive cells may only recognize one strain of a particular pathogen, unlike innate cells, which recognize broad classes of pathogens. In fact, a group of adaptive cells that recognize the same strain will likely recognize different areas of that pathogen.

If a B or T cell has a receptor that recognizes an antigen from a pathogen and also receives cues from innate cells that something is wrong, the B or T cell will activate, divide, and disperse to address the problem. B cells make antibodies, which neutralize pathogens, rendering them harmless. T-cells carry out multiple functions, including killing infected cells and activating or recruiting other immune cells. The adaptive response has a system of checks and balances to prevent unnecessary activation that could cause damage to the host. If a B or T cell is autoreactive, meaning its receptor recognizes antigens from the body's own cells, the cell will be deleted. Also, if a B or T cell does not receive signals from innate cells, it will not be optimally activated.

Immune memory is a feature of the adaptive immune response. After B or T-cells are activated, they expand rapidly. As the problem resolves, cells stop dividing and are retained in the body as memory cells. The next time this same pathogen enters the body, a memory cell is already poised to react and can clear away the pathogen before it establishes itself.

Vaccination

Vaccination, or immunization, is a way to train your immune system against a specific pathogen. Vaccination achieves immune memory without an actual infection, so the body is prepared when the virus or bacterium enters. Saving time is important to prevent a pathogen from establishing itself and infecting more cells in the body.

An effective vaccine will optimally activate both the innate and adaptive response. An immunogen is used to activate the adaptive immune response so that specific memory cells are generated. Because BCRs and TCRs are unique, some memory cells are simply better at eliminating the pathogen. The goal of vaccine design is to select immunogens that will generate the most effective and efficient memory response against a particular pathogen. Adjuvants, which are important for activating innate immunity, can be added to vaccines to optimize the immune response. Innate immunity recognizes broad patterns, and without innate responses, adaptive immunity cannot be optimally achieved.

Immune Cells

Granulocytes include basophils, eosinophils, and neutrophils. Basophils and eosinophils are important for host defense against parasites. They also are involved in allergic reactions. Neutrophils, the most numerous innate immune cell, patrol for problems by circulating in the bloodstream. They can phagocytose, or ingest, bacteria, degrading them inside special compartments called vesicles.

Mast cells also are important for defense against parasites. Mast cells are found in tissues and can mediate allergic reactions by releasing inflammatory chemicals like histamine.

Monocytes, which develop into macrophages, also patrol and respond to problems. They are found in the bloodstream and in tissues. Macrophages, "big eater" in Greek, are named for their ability to ingest and degrade bacteria. Upon activation, monocytes and macrophages coordinate an immune response by notifying other immune cells of the problem. Macrophages also have important nonimmune functions, such as recycling dead cells, like red blood cells (RBCs), and clearing away cellular debris. These "housekeeping" functions occur without activation of an immune response.

Neutrophils accumulate within minutes at sites of local tissue injury. They then communicate with each other using lipid and other secreted mediators to form cellular "swarms." Their coordinated movement and exchange of signals then instructs other innate immune cells called macrophages and monocytes to surround the neutrophil cluster and form a tight wound seal.

Dendritic cells (DC) are an important antigen-presenting cell (APC), and they also can develop from monocytes. Antigens are molecules from pathogens, host cells, and allergens that may be recognized by adaptive immune cells. APCs like DCs are responsible for processing large molecules into "readable" fragments (antigens) recognized by adaptive B or T-cells. However, antigens alone cannot activate T-cells. They must be presented with the appropriate major histocompatibility complex (MHC) expressed on the APC. MHC provides a checkpoint and helps immune cells distinguish between host and foreign cells.

Natural killer (NK) cells have features of both innate and adaptive immunity. They are important for recognizing and killing virus-infected cells or tumor cells. They contain intracellular compartments called granules, which are filled with proteins that can form holes in the target cell and also cause apoptosis, the process for programmed cell death. It is important to distinguish between apoptosis and other forms of cell death like necrosis. Apoptosis, unlike necrosis, does not release danger signals that can lead to greater immune activation and inflammation. Through apoptosis, immune cells can discreetly remove infected cells and limit bystander damage. Researchers have shown in mouse models that NK cells, like adaptive cells, can be retained as memory cells and respond to subsequent infections by the same pathogen.

Adaptive Cells

B cells have two major functions: They present antigens to T-cells, and more importantly, they produce antibodies to neutralize infectious microbes. Antibodies coat the surface of a pathogen and serve three major roles: neutralization, opsonization, and complement activation.

Neutralization occurs when the pathogen, because it is covered in antibodies, is unable to bind and infect host cells. In opsonization, an antibody-bound pathogen serves as a red flag to alert immune cells like neutrophils and macrophages, to engulf and digest the pathogen. Complement is a process for directly destroying, or lysing, bacteria.

Antibodies are expressed in two ways. The B-cell receptor (BCR), which sits on the surface of a B cell, is actually an antibody. B cells also secrete antibodies to diffuse and bind to pathogens. This dual expression is important because the initial problem, for instance, a bacterium is recognized by a unique BCR and activates the B cell. The activated B cell responds by secreting antibodies, essentially the BCR but in soluble form. This ensures that the response is specific against the bacterium that started the whole process.

Every antibody is unique, but they fall under general categories: IgM, IgD, IgG, IgA, and IgE. (Ig is short for immunoglobulin, which is another word for antibody.) While they have overlapping roles, IgM generally is important for complement activation; IgD is involved in activating basophils; IgG is important for neutralization, opsonization, and complement activation; IgA is essential for neutralization in the gastrointestinal tract; and IgE is necessary for activating mast cells in parasitic and allergic responses.

T-cells have a variety of roles and are classified by subsets. T-cells are divided into two broad categories: CD8+ T-cells or CD4+ T-cells, based on which protein is present on the cell's surface. T-cells carry out multiple functions, including killing infected cells and activating or recruiting other immune cells.

CD8+ T-cells also are called cytotoxic T-cells or cytotoxic lymphocytes (CTLs). They are crucial for recognizing and removing virus-infected cells and cancer cells. CTLs have specialized compartments, or granules, containing cytotoxins that cause apoptosis, i.e., programmed cell death. Because of its potency, the release of granules is tightly regulated by the immune system.

The four major CD4+ T-cell subsets are TH1, TH2, TH17, and Treg, with "TH" referring to "T helper cell." TH1 cells are critical for coordinating immune responses against intracellular microbes, especially bacteria. They produce and secrete molecules that alert and activate other immune cells, like bacteria-ingesting macrophages. TH2 cells are important for coordinating immune responses against extracellular pathogens, like helminths (parasitic worms), by alerting B cells, granulocytes, and mast cells. TH17 cells are named for their ability to produce interleukin 17 (IL-17), a signaling molecule that activates immune and nonimmune cells. TH17 cells are important for recruiting neutrophils.

Regulatory T-cells (Tregs), as the name suggests, monitor and inhibit the activity of other T-cells. They prevent adverse immune activation and maintain tolerance, or the prevention of immune responses against the body's own cells and antigens.

Communication

Immune cells communicate in a number of ways, either by cell-to-cell contact or through secreted signaling molecules. Receptors and ligands are fundamental for cellular communication. Receptors are protein structures that may be expressed on the surface of a cell or in intracellular compartments. The molecules that activate receptors are called ligands, which may be free-floating or membrane-bound.

Ligand-receptor interaction leads to a series of events inside the cell involving networks of intracellular molecules that relay the message. By altering the expression and density of various receptors and ligands, immune cells can dispatch specific instructions tailored to the situation at hand.

Cytokines are small proteins with diverse functions. In immunity, there are several categories of cytokines important for immune cell growth, activation, and function.

- Colony-stimulating factors are essential for cell development and differentiation.

- Interferons are necessary for immune-cell activation. Type I interferons mediate antiviral immune responses, and type II interferon is important for antibacterial responses.

- Interleukins, which come in over 30 varieties, provide context-specific instructions, with activating or inhibitory responses.

- Chemokines are made in specific locations of the body or at a site of infection to attract immune cells. Different chemokines will recruit different immune cells to the site needed.

- The tumor necrosis factor (TNF) family of cytokines stimulates immune-cell proliferation and activation. They are critical for activating inflammatory responses, and as such, TNF blockers are used to treat a variety of disorders, including some autoimmune diseases.

Toll-like receptors (TLRs) are expressed on innate immune cells, like macrophages and dendritic cells. They are located on the cell surface or in intracellular compartments because microbes may be found in the body or inside infected cells. TLRs recognize general microbial patterns, and they are essential for innate immune-cell activation and inflammatory responses.

B-cell receptors (BCRs) and T-cell receptors (TCRs) are expressed on adaptive immune cells. They are both found on the cell surface, but BCRs also are secreted as antibodies to neutralize pathogens. The genes for BCRs and TCRs are randomly rearranged at specific cell-maturation stages, resulting in unique receptors that may potentially recognize anything. Random generation of receptors allows the immune system to respond to unforeseen problems. They also explain why memory B or T-cells are highly specific and, upon re-encountering their specific pathogen, can immediately induce a neutralizing immune response.

Major histocompatibility complex (MHC), or human leukocyte antigen (HLA), proteins serve two general roles.

MHC proteins function as carriers to present antigens on cell surfaces. MHC class I proteins are essential for presenting viral antigens and are expressed by nearly all cell types, except red blood cells. Any cell infected by a virus has the ability to signal the problem through MHC class I proteins. In response, CD8+ T-cells (also called CTLs) will recognize and kill infected cells. MHC class II proteins are generally only expressed by antigen-presenting cells like dendritic cells and macrophages. MHC class II proteins are important for presenting antigens to CD4+ T-cells. MHC class II antigens are varied and include both pathogen- and host-derived molecules.

MHC proteins also signal whether a cell is a host cell or a foreign cell. They are very diverse, and every person has a unique set of MHC proteins inherited from his or her parents. As such, there are similarities in MHC proteins between family members. Immune cells use MHC to determine whether or not a cell is friendly. In organ transplantation, the MHC or HLA proteins of donors and recipients are matched to lower the risk of transplant rejection, which occurs when the recipient's immune system attacks the donor tissue or organ. In stem cell or bone marrow transplantation, improper MHC or HLA matching can result in graft-versus-host disease (GVHD), which occurs when the donor cells attack the recipient's body.

Complement refers to a unique process that clears away pathogens or dying cells and also activates immune cells. Complement consists of a series of proteins found in the blood that form a membrane-attack complex. Complement proteins are only activated by enzymes when a problem, like an infection, occurs. Activated complement proteins stick to a pathogen, recruiting and activating additional complement proteins, which assemble in a specific order to form a round pore or hole. Complement literally punches small holes into the pathogen, creating leaks that lead to cell death. Complement proteins also serve as signaling molecules that alert immune cells and recruit them to the problem area.

Immune Tolerance

Tolerance is the prevention of an immune response against a particular antigen. For instance, the immune system is generally tolerant of self-antigens, so it does not usually attack the body's own cells, tissues, and organs. However, when tolerance is lost, disorders like autoimmune disease or food allergy may occur. Tolerance is maintained in a number of ways:

- When adaptive immune cells mature, there are several checkpoints in place to eliminate autoreactive cells. If a B cell produces antibodies that strongly recognize host cells, or if a T-cell strongly recognizes self-antigen, they are deleted.

- Nevertheless, there are autoreactive immune cells present in healthy individuals. Autoreactive immune cells are kept in a nonreactive, or anergic, state. Even though they recognize the body's own cells, they do not have the ability to react and cannot cause host damage.

- Regulatory immune cells circulate throughout the body to maintain tolerance. Besides limiting autoreactive cells, regulatory cells are important for turning an immune response off after the problem is resolved. They can act as drains, depleting areas of essential nutrients that surrounding immune cells need for activation or survival.

- Some locations in the body are called immunologically privileged sites. These areas, like the eye and brain, do not typically elicit strong immune responses. Part of this is because of physical barriers, like the blood–brain barrier (BBB), that limit the degree to which immune cells may enter. These areas also may express higher levels of suppressive cytokines to prevent a robust immune response.

Fetomaternal tolerance is the prevention of a maternal immune response against a developing fetus. Major histocompatibility complex (MHC) proteins help the immune system distinguish between host and foreign cells. MHC also is called human leukocyte antigen (HLA). By expressing paternal MHC or HLA proteins and paternal antigens, a fetus can potentially trigger the mother's immune system. However, there are several barriers that may prevent this from occurring: The placenta reduces the exposure of the fetus to maternal immune cells, the proteins expressed on the outer layer of the placenta may limit immune recognition, and regulatory cells and suppressive signals may play a role.

Transplantation of a donor tissue or organ requires appropriate MHC or HLA matching to limit the risk of rejection. Because MHC or HLA matching is rarely complete, transplant recipients must continuously take immunosuppressive drugs, which can cause complications like higher susceptibility to infection and some cancers. Researchers are developing more targeted ways to induce tolerance to transplanted tissues and organs while leaving protective immune responses intact.

Disorders of the Immune System

Complications arise when the immune system does not function properly. Some issues are less pervasive, such as pollen allergy, while others are extensive, such as genetic disorders that wipe out the presence or function of an entire set of immune cells.

Allergy

Allergies are a form of hypersensitivity reaction, typically in response to harmless environmental allergens like pollen or food. Hypersensitivity reactions are divided into four classes. Class I, II, and III are caused by antibodies, IgE or IgG, which are produced by B cells in response to an allergen. Overproduction of these antibodies activates immune cells like basophils and mast cells, which respond by releasing inflammatory chemicals like histamine. Class IV reactions are caused by T-cells, which may either directly cause damage themselves or activate macrophages and eosinophils that damage host cells.

Immune Deficiencies

Immune deficiencies may be temporary or permanent. Temporary immune deficiency can be caused by a variety of sources that weaken the immune system. Common infections, including influenza and mononucleosis, can suppress the immune system.

When immune cells are the target of infection, severe immune suppression can occur. For example, human immunodeficiency virus (HIV) specifically infects T-cells, and their elimination allows for secondary infections by other pathogens. Patients receiving chemotherapy, bone marrow transplants, or immunosuppressive drugs experience weakened immune systems until immune cell levels are restored. Pregnancy also suppresses the maternal immune system, increasing susceptibility to infections by common microbes.

Primary immune deficiency diseases (PIDDs) are inherited genetic disorders and tend to cause chronic susceptibility to infection. There are over 150 PIDDs, and almost all are considered rare (affecting fewer than 200,000 people in the United States). They may result from altered immune signaling molecules or the complete absence of mature immune cells. For instance, X-linked severe combined immunodeficiency (SCID) is caused by a mutation in a signaling receptor gene, rendering immune cells insensitive to multiple cytokines. Without the growth and activation signals delivered by cytokines, immune cell subsets, particularly T and natural killer cells, fail to develop normally. The National Institute of Allergy and Infectious Diseases (NIAID) Primary Immune Deficiency (PID) clinic was established with the goal of accepting all PIDD patients for examination to provide a disease diagnosis and better treatment recommendations.

Autoimmune Diseases

Autoimmune diseases occur when self-tolerance is broken. Self-tolerance breaks when adaptive immune cells that recognize host cells persist unchecked. B cells may produce antibodies targeting host cells, and active T-cells may recognize self-antigen. This amplifies when they recruit and activate other immune cells.

Autoimmunity is either organ-specific or systemic, meaning it affects the whole body. For instance, type I diabetes is organ-specific and caused by immune cells erroneously recognizing insulin-producing pancreatic β cells as foreign. However, systemic lupus erythematosus (SLE), commonly called lupus, can result from antibodies that recognize antigens expressed by nearly all healthy cells. Autoimmune diseases have a strong genetic component, and with advances in gene sequencing tools, researchers have a better understanding of what may contribute to specific diseases.

Sepsis

Sepsis may refer to an infection of the bloodstream, or it can refer to a systemic inflammatory state caused by the uncontrolled, broad release of cytokines that quickly activate immune cells throughout the body. Sepsis is an extremely serious condition and is typically triggered by an infection. However, the damage itself is caused by cytokines (the adverse response is sometimes referred to as a "cytokine storm"). The systemic release of cytokines may lead to loss of blood pressure, resulting in septic shock and possible multi-organ failure.

Cancer

Some forms of cancer are directly caused by the uncontrolled growth of immune cells. Leukemia is cancer caused by white blood cells, which is another term for immune cells. Lymphoma is cancer caused by lymphocytes, which is another term for adaptive B or T-cells. Myeloma is cancer caused by plasma cells, which are mature B cells. Unrestricted growth of any of these cell types causes cancer. In addition, an emerging concept is that cancer progression may partially result from the ability of cancer cells to avoid immune detection. The immune system is capable of removing infectious pathogens and dangerous host cells like tumors. Cancer researchers are studying how the tumor microenvironment may allow cancer cells to evade immune cells. Immune evasion may result from the abundance of suppressive, regulatory immune cells, excessive inhibitory cytokines, and other features that are not well understood.

Chapter 2

How Allergies Develop

Chapter Contents

Section 2.1

Genetic Connections

This section contains text excerpted from the following sources:
Text in this section begins with excerpts from "Genetic Finding
Suggests Alternative Treatment Strategy for Common, Complex
Skin Disorders and Asthma," National Human Genome Research
Institute (NHGRI), April 25, 2006. Reviewed August 2018; Text
under the heading "Allergic Asthma and Genes" is excerpted from
"Allergic Asthma," Genetics Home Reference (GHR), National
Institutes of Health (NIH), August 21, 2018.

A genetic finding by researchers at the National Institutes of Health (NIH) provides new insight into the cause of a series of related, common and complex illnesses—including hay fever and asthma as well as the skin disorders eczema and psoriasis—and suggests a novel therapeutic approach. All of these illnesses are essentially inflammatory disorders of the tissues that separate the inside of the body from the outside world, such as the skin and the linings of the throat and lungs.

In one of the issues of *The Journal of Clinical Investigation* (JCI), researchers from the National Human Genome Research Institute (NHGRI), the National Eye Institute (NEI), and the *Eunice Kennedy Shriver* National Institute of Child Health and Human Development (NICHD), all part of the NIH report, that excessive production of a specific protein disrupts the protective properties of the skin barrier. Once the skin barrier is compromised, immune-system-stimulating chemicals—allergens—can enter the body and cause an inflammatory reaction that, in turn, stimulates skin cells to grow rapidly, further diminishing the protective function of the skin. The compromised barrier, in turn, becomes more porous to allergens that then stimulate more inflammation in a cycle that eventually produces common skin conditions such as psoriasis and eczema.

It may, however, be possible to break the cycle by creating a temporary, artificial barrier on the skin that blocks incoming allergens. The solution could be as simple as developing a lotion that effectively blocks allergens from getting through damaged skin. Keeping allergens out of the skin would keep the immune system from over-stimulating cell growth, giving the skin time to recreate a normal barrier. Therapies for these skin conditions principally focus on suppressing the immune system, but the medicines used can produce undesired side-effects.

"The human body is an incredibly complex system," said Elias A. Zerhouni, M.D., director of the National Institutes of Health. "Only by conducting this kind of basic research can we hope to understand the causes of complex diseases. And only by understanding disease can we produce a future in which we can predict who is at risk, preempt the illness from ever occurring and personalize the treatment when it does."

Several studies have suggested that defects in the skin barrier may be as important to eczema and psoriasis as the hyperactive response of the immune system. In addition, doctors have observed that individuals with eczema are also likely to develop hay fever and asthma, suggesting a common mechanism for both disorders. The other risk factor for these conditions is having a relative with the disorder, suggesting a genetic connection.

To test whether a defective skin barrier can produce these diseases, a team of NIH researchers focused on a specific gene called connexin 26, which makes a protein that forms connections between skin cells that create the normal barrier. When the skin is intact, the production of connexin 26 is turned off once there is enough to hook all the skin cells together. When skin is damaged by a cut or a scrape, connexin 26 is produced while new skin cells reproduce and heal the wound. Researchers have shown that connexin 26 production is turned on in the sore skin of people with psoriasis, but it wasn't clear what role connexin 26 played in the disorder.

To determine connexin 26's role in psoriasis, NIH researchers created a line of transgenic mice that over-produce connexin 26. The resulting mice develop psoriatic-type skin sores, just like humans with psoriasis.

"This discovery demonstrates the power of animal models to unravel complex conditions of medical importance," said Eric D. Green, M.D., Ph.D., NHGRI's scientific director and the director of the institute's Division of Intramural Research, where the research was conducted. "Our current abilities to rapidly create new genetically altered animal models allow researchers to move from conception of an idea to its implementation at an incredible pace."

The discovery broadens the basic understanding of the causes of skin disorders such as psoriasis and eczema, and may well contribute to the basic understanding of asthma and hay fever, conditions that arise when allergens penetrate the tissue barrier in the lungs and nose, respectively.

"Hopefully, this will help us understand the complex genetics of psoriasis," said Julie A. Segre, Ph.D., an investigator in National Human

Genome Research Institute (NHGRI) Genetics and Molecular Branch and the senior author on the paper. "Previous genetic studies have focused on the genes that regulate immune response. We are now examining the effect of genes that are involved in both regulating the growth of skin cells and signaling to the immune cells."

The problem causing these related disorders may simply be the body overreacting to an allergen getting through the barrier that is supposed to block it. "The skin goes into a stress response and overcompensates by trying to rebuild the barrier too fast, actually becoming less effective," Dr. Segre said. "The skin cells grow so fast that they fail to make a normal barrier, and the body is stimulating the immune response because of material (chemicals and allergens) coming through the barrier."

Understanding the genetics of skin disorders may well have important implications for other serious illnesses, such as asthma. It is not uncommon for a family doctor to face the dilemma of a child who has eczema and then having to decide how aggressively to treat the disease. Eczema is not particularly dangerous, but children presenting with eczema commonly go on to develop asthma, which severely compromises quality of life and in rare cases can be lethal. Treating eczema with immune-suppressing drugs, which may also prevent asthma from developing, may cause undesirable side effects.

The genetic studies suggest that researchers now need to focus on both turning down the immune response, as well as restoring a normal skin barrier to keep the outside world out of the body.

"The barrier function of epithelial surfaces is important in all tissues that have contact with the outside world. In addition to the skin and respiratory tract, it includes the gastrointestinal tract, and the ocular surface," said Ali Djalilian, M.D., formerly a research fellow and medical officer at the National Eye Institute (NEI) but now at the University of Illinois in Chicago, and the lead author of the paper. "These findings underline the importance of this barrier function and suggests a new strategy for restoring it in human diseases."

The National Human Genome Research Institute (NHGRI), the National Eye Institute and the *Eunice Kennedy Shriver* National Institute of Child Health and Human Development (NICHD) are among the 27 institutes and centers that make up the National Institutes of Health (NIH)—The Nation's Medical Research Agency. NIH is a component of the U. S. Department of Health and Human Services (HHS). It is the primary federal agency for conducting and supporting basic, clinical, and translational medical research, and it investigates the causes, treatments, and cures for both common and rare diseases.

Allergic Asthma and Genes

The cause of allergic asthma is complex. It is likely that a combination of multiple genetic and environmental factors contribute to development of the condition. Doctors believe genes are involved because having a family member with allergic asthma or another allergic disorder increases a person's risk of developing asthma.

Studies suggest that more than 100 genes may be associated with allergic asthma, but each seems to be a factor in only one or a few populations. Many of the associated genes are involved in the body's immune response. Others play a role in lung and airway function.

There is evidence that an unbalanced immune response underlies allergic asthma. While there is normally a balance between type 1 (or Th1) and type 2 (or Th2) immune reactions in the body, many individuals with allergic asthma predominantly have type 2 reactions. Type 2 reactions lead to the production of immune proteins called IgE antibodies and the generation of other factors that predispose to bronchial hyperresponsiveness. Normally, the body produces IgE antibodies in response to foreign invaders, particularly parasitic worms. For unknown reasons, in susceptible individuals, the body reacts to an allergen as if it is harmful, producing IgE antibodies specific to it. Upon later encounters with the allergen, IgE antibodies recognize it, which stimulates an immune response, causing bronchoconstriction, airway swelling, and mucus production.

Not everyone with a variation in one of the allergic asthma-associated genes develops the condition; exposure to certain environmental factors also contributes to its development. Studies suggest that these exposures trigger epigenetic changes to the deoxyribonucleic acid (DNA). Epigenetic changes modify DNA without changing the DNA sequence. They can affect gene activity and regulate the production of proteins, which may influence the development of allergies in susceptible individuals.

Section 2.2

Breastfeeding and Allergic Disease Development

This section includes text excerpted from documents published by two public domain sources. Text under the headings marked 1 are excerpted from "Gateway to Health Communication and Social Marketing Practice—Breastfeeding," Centers for Disease Control and Prevention (CDC), September 15, 2017; Text under the heading marked 2 is excerpted from "Women Veterans Healthcare—Breastfeeding," U.S. Department of Veterans Affairs (VA), May 30, 2018.May 30, 2018.

Who's at Risk?[1]

Any baby who is not breastfed faces higher risk of health problems, including long-term (chronic) problems such as allergies, asthma, and obesity and short-term (acute) infections such as diarrhea, ear, and respiratory infections. Babies who are premature, who are sick when they are born, or who attend group day care are at highest risk for health problems if they are not breastfed.

Mothers who work, have only a high school education, are unmarried, are not Caucasian, or do not have a lot of money are at highest risk for not breastfeeding. Many people mistakenly think that in order to breastfeed, mothers need to make many changes to their lives such as eat a very healthy diet or always be home with their babies.

Can It Be Prevented?[1]

The 'problem' to be prevented isn't a disease, per se, instead, it is the lack of breastfeeding.

Mothers and babies often need some help in order to breastfeed. They need:

- Accurate breastfeeding education. This education can happen during prenatal visits, during routine nursing care in the hospital, and during pediatrician visits.

- Help in the hospital. This help includes keeping mothers and babies together in the same room in the hospital, not giving the baby bottles or pacifiers in the hospital, and having someone on staff who is a breastfeeding expert help mothers with breastfeeding.

- Support from fathers, grandmothers, bosses, store owners, religious leaders, coworkers, and friends. This includes encouragement and help with breastfeeding and other daily tasks and refraining from teasing, making jokes, or harassing mothers for breastfeeding.

Breastfeeding[2]

Breastfeeding has many positive benefits for moms and their babies and is the ideal method of feeding and nurturing infants. Human breast milk is the most complete form of nutrition for infants and protects them from a wide array of infections and other health problems. If you are thinking about breastfeeding, consider the following benefits both for you and your child.

Breastfeeding is important for babies.

- Protects your baby from infection—even the milk produced during the first few days after birth is packed with antibodies that fight infection.

- Reduces your baby's risk of severe chest infections like pneumonia, ear infections, and stomach issues.

- Helps your baby's immune system develop and lowers the risk of asthma, allergies, type 1 diabetes, and childhood leukemia.

- Reduces the risk of sudden infant death syndrome (SIDS).

- Reduces your child's risk for obesity.

- Improves your child's ability to learn and process information.

Breastfeeding is important for moms.

- Helps your body recover from pregnancy. For instance, breastfeeding helps with postpartum weight loss.

- May reduce your risk of ovarian, endometrial, and breast cancer.

- May reduce your risk for osteoporosis later in life.

- Mothers who don't breastfeed may face higher risks of hypertension, type 2 diabetes, and heart disease.

- Reduces costs since breastfeeding is cheaper than formula feeding.

- Releases hormones that not only help the milk flow, but increases a mother's sense of calm and well-being. These hormonal changes may reduce your risk for postpartum depression.

Bottom Line[1]

Breastfeeding is important for mothers' and babies' health. Unfortunately, many people mistakenly think breastfeeding is simply an alternative method to feed babies and just a personal choice. With education and support, many more mothers would be able to breastfeed, preventing many deaths and illnesses every year. Breastfeeding mothers need education, support, help, and encouragement.

Section 2.3

The Hygiene Hypothesis

This section includes text excerpted from "Asthma: The Hygiene Hypothesis," U.S. Food and Drug Administration (FDA), March 27, 2018.

What Do Clean Houses Have in Common with Childhood Infections?

One of the many explanations for asthma being the most common chronic disease in the developed world is the "hygiene hypothesis." This hypothesis suggests that the critical postnatal period of immune response is derailed by the extremely clean household environments often found in the developed world. In other words, the young child's environment can be "too clean" to pose an effective challenge to a maturing immune system.

According to the "hygiene hypothesis," the problem with extremely clean environments is that they fail to provide the necessary exposure to germs required to "educate" the immune system so it can learn to launch its defense responses to infectious organisms. Instead, its defense responses end up being so inadequate that they actually contribute to the development of asthma.

Scientists based this hypothesis in part on the observation that, before birth, the fetal immune system's "default setting" is suppressed to prevent it from rejecting maternal tissue. Such a low default setting is necessary before birth—when the mother is providing the fetus with her own antibodies. But in the period immediately after birth the child's own immune system must take over and learn how to fend for itself.

The "hygiene hypothesis" is supported by epidemiologic studies demonstrating that allergic diseases and asthma are more likely to occur when the incidence and levels of endotoxin (bacterial lipopolysaccharide, or LPS) in the home are low. LPS is a bacterial molecule that stimulates and educates the immune system by triggering signals through a molecular "switch" called Toll-like receptor 4 (TLR4), which is found on certain immune system cells.

The Science behind the Hygiene Hypothesis

The Inflammatory Mechanisms Section of the Laboratory of Immunobiochemistry (LIB) is working to better understand the hygiene hypothesis, by looking at the relationship between respiratory viruses and allergic diseases and asthma, and by studying the respiratory syncytial virus (RSV) in particular.

What Does Respiratory Syncytial Virus Have to Do with the Hygiene Hypothesis?

- RSV is often the first viral pathogen encountered by infants.

- RSV pneumonia puts infants at higher risk for developing childhood asthma. (Although children may outgrow this type of asthma, it can account for clinic visits and missed school days.)

- RSV carries a molecule on its surface called the F protein, which flips the same immune system "switch" toll-like receptors 4 (TLR4) as do bacterial endotoxins.

It may seem obvious that, since both the RSV F protein and LPS signal through the same toll-like receptors 4 (TLR4) "switch," they both would educate the infant's immune system in the same beneficial way. But that may not be the case.

The large population of bacteria that normally lives inside humans educates the growing immune system to respond using the TLR4 switch. When this education is lacking or weak, the response to RSV

25

by some critical cells in the immune system's defense against infections—called "T-cells"—might inadvertently trigger asthma instead of protecting the infant and clearing the infection. How this happens is a mystery.

In order to determine RSV's role in triggering asthma, the laboratory studied how RSV blocks T-cell proliferation.

Studying the effect of RSV on T-cells in the laboratory, however, has been very difficult. That's because when RSV is put into the same culture as T-cells, it blocks them from multiplying as they would naturally do when they are stimulated. To get past this problem, most researchers kill RSV with ultraviolet light before adding the virus to T-cell cultures. The first major discovery was that RSV causes the release from certain immune system cells of signaling molecules called Type I and Type III interferons that can suppress T-cell proliferation.

The hygiene hypothesis suggests that a newborn baby's immune system must be educated so it will function properly during infancy and the rest of life. One of the key elements of this education is a switch on T-cells called TLR4. The bacterial protein LPS normally plays a key role by flipping that switch into the "on" position.

Prior research suggested that since RSV flips the TLR4 switch, RSV should "educate" the child's immune system to defend against infections just like LPS does.

But it turns out that RSV does not flip the TLR switch in the same way as LPS. This difference in switching on TLR, combined with other characteristics of RSV, can prevent the proper education of the immune system.

One difference in the way that RSV flips the TLR4 switch may be through the release of interferons, which suppresses the proliferation of T-cells. It's still not known whether these interferons are part of the reason the immune system is not properly educated or simply an indicator of the problem.

Chapter 3

Allergens and Breathing Problems

Chapter Contents

Section 3.1

When Breathing Becomes Bothersome

This section includes text excerpted from "Seeking Allergy Relief,"
NIH News in Health, National Institutes of Health (NIH), June 2016.

A change in season can brighten your days with vibrant new colors. But blooming flowers and falling leaves can usher in more than beautiful backdrops. Airborne substances that irritate your nose can blow in with the weather. When sneezing, itchy eyes, or a runny nose suddenly appears, allergies may be to blame.

Allergies arise when the body's immune system overreacts to substances, called allergens, that are normally harmless. When a person with allergies breathes in allergens—such as pollen, mold, pet dander, or dust mites—the resulting allergic reactions in the nose are called allergic rhinitis, or hay fever.

Allergy is one of the most common long-term health conditions. "Over the past several decades, the prevalence of allergies has been increasing," says Dr. Paivi Salo, an allergy expert at National Institutes of Health (NIH). "Currently, airborne allergies affect approximately 10–30 percent of adults and 40 percent of children."

Avoiding your allergy triggers is the best way to control your symptoms. But triggers aren't always easy to identify. Notice when and where your symptoms occur. This can help you figure out the cause.

"Most people with allergies are sensitive to more than one allergen," Salo explains. "Grass, weed, and tree pollens are the most common causes of outdoor allergies." Pollen is often the source if your symptoms are seasonal. Indoor allergens usually trigger symptoms that last all year. If your symptoms become persistent and bothersome, visit your family physician or an allergist. They can test for allergy sensitivities by using a skin or blood test. The test results, along with a medical exam and information about when and where your symptoms occur, will help your doctor determine the cause.

Even when you know your triggers, avoiding allergens can be difficult. When pollen counts are high, stay inside with the windows closed and use the air conditioning. Avoid bringing pollen indoors. "If you go outside, wash your hair and clothing," Salo says. Pets can also bring in pollen, so clean them too.

For indoor allergens, keep humidity levels low in the home to keep dust mites and mold under control. Avoid upholstered furniture and carpets because they harbor allergens. Wash your bedding in hot water, and vacuum the floors once a week.

Allergies run in families. Your children's chances of developing allergies are higher if you have them. While there's no "magic bullet" to prevent allergies, experts recommend breastfeeding early in life. "Breast milk is the least likely to trigger allergic reactions, it's easy to digest, and it strengthens an infant's immune system," Salo says.

Sometimes, avoiding allergens isn't possible or isn't enough. Untreated allergies are associated with chronic conditions like sinus infections and asthma. Over-the-counter (OTC) antihistamines, nasal sprays, and decongestants can often ease mild symptoms. Prescription medications and allergy shots are sometimes needed for more severe allergies. Talk with your doctor about treatment options. Allergy relief can help clear up more than just itchy, watery eyes. It can allow you to breathe easy again and brighten your outlook on seasonal changes.

Section 3.2

Biological Pollutants' and Indoor Air Quality

This section includes text excerpted from "Biological Pollutants'
Impact on Indoor Air Quality," U.S. Environmental Protection
Agency (EPA), November 6, 2017.

Biological contaminants include bacteria, viruses, animal dander and cat saliva, house dust, mites, cockroaches, and pollen. There are many sources of these pollutants. By controlling the relative humidity level in a home, the growth of some sources of biologicals can be minimized. A relative humidity of 30–50 percent is generally recommended for homes. Standing water, water-damaged materials or wet surfaces also serve as a breeding ground for molds, mildews, bacteria, and insects. House dust mites, the source of one of the most powerful biological allergens, grow in damp, warm environments.

Sources

Sources for these contaminants include:

- Pollens, which originate from plants
- Viruses, which are transmitted by people and animals
- Molds
- Bacterias, which are carried by people, animals, and soil and plant debris
- Household pets, which are sources of saliva and animal dander (skin flakes)
- Droppings and body parts from cockroaches, rodents and other pests or insects
- Viruses and bacteria
- The protein in urine from rats and mice is a potent allergen. When it dries, it can become airborne.
- Contaminated central air handling systems can become breeding grounds for mold, mildew and other sources of biological contaminants and can then distribute these contaminants through the home

Many of these biological contaminants are small enough to be inhaled.

Biological contaminants are, or are produced by, living things. Biological contaminants are often found in areas that provide food and moisture or water. For example:

- Damp or wet areas such as cooling coils, humidifiers, condensate pans or unvented bathrooms can be moldy
- Draperies, bedding, carpet, and other areas where dust collects may accumulate biological contaminants

Health Effects from Biological Contaminants

Some biological contaminants trigger allergic reactions, including:

- Hypersensitivity pneumonitis
- Allergic rhinitis
- Some types of asthma

Infectious illnesses, such as influenza, measles, and chickenpox are transmitted through the air. Molds and mildews release disease-causing toxins. Symptoms of health problems caused by biological pollutants include:

- Sneezing

- Watery eyes

- Coughing

- Shortness of breath

- Dizziness

- Lethargy

- Fever

- Digestive problems

Allergic reactions occur only after repeated exposure to a specific biological allergen. However, that reaction may occur immediately upon reexposure or after multiple exposures over time. As a result, people who have noticed only mild allergic reactions, or no reactions at all, may suddenly find themselves very sensitive to particular allergens.

Some diseases, like humidifier fever, are associated with exposure to toxins from microorganisms that can grow in large building ventilation systems. However, these diseases can also be traced to microorganisms that grow in home heating and cooling systems and humidifiers.

Children, elderly people and people with breathing problems, allergies, and lung diseases are particularly susceptible to disease-causing biological agents in the indoor air.

Mold, dust mites, pet dander, and pest droppings or body parts can trigger asthma. Biological contaminants, including molds and pollens, can cause allergic reactions for a significant portion of the population. Tuberculosis (TB), measles, staphylococcus infections, *Legionella,* and influenza are known to be transmitted by air.

Reducing Exposure to Biological Contaminants

General good housekeeping, and maintenance of heating and air conditioning equipment, are very important. Adequate ventilation and good air distribution also help. The key to mold control is moisture control. If mold is a problem, clean up the mold and get rid of excess water or moisture. Maintaining the relative humidity between 30–60 percent will help control mold, dust mites, and cockroaches. Employ integrated pest management to control insect and animal allergens. Cooling tower treatment procedures exist to reduce levels of *Legionella* and other organisms.

- Install and use exhaust fans that are vented to the outdoors in kitchens and bathrooms and vent clothes dryers outdoors. These actions can eliminate much of the moisture that builds up from everyday activities. There are exhaust fans on the market that produce little noise, an important consideration for some people. Another benefit to using kitchen and bathroom exhaust fans is that they can reduce levels of organic pollutants that vaporize from hot water used in showers and dishwashers.

- Ventilate the attic and crawl spaces to prevent moisture buildup. Keeping humidity levels in these areas below 50 percent can prevent water condensation on building materials.

- If using cool mist or ultrasonic humidifiers, clean appliances according to manufacturer's instructions and refill with fresh water daily. Because these humidifiers can become breeding grounds for biological contaminants, they have the potential for causing diseases such as hypersensitivity pneumonitis (HP) and humidifier fever. Evaporation trays in air conditioners, dehumidifiers, and refrigerators should also be cleaned frequently.

- Thoroughly clean and dry water-damaged carpets and building materials (within 24 hours if possible) or consider removal and replacement. Water-damaged carpets and building materials can harbor mold and bacteria. It is very difficult to completely rid such materials of biological contaminants.

- Keep the house clean. House dust mites, pollens, animal dander and other allergy-causing agents can be reduced, although not eliminated, through regular cleaning. People who are allergic to these pollutants should use allergen-proof mattress encasements, wash bedding in hot (130°F) water and avoid room furnishings that accumulate dust, especially if they cannot be washed in hot water. Allergic individuals should also leave the house while it is being vacuumed because vacuuming can actually increase airborne levels of mite allergens and other biological contaminants. Using central vacuum systems that are vented to the outdoors or vacuums with high-efficiency filters may also be of help.

- Take steps to minimize biological pollutants in basements. Clean and disinfect the basement floor drain regularly. Do not finish a basement below ground level unless all water leaks are patched and outdoor ventilation and adequate heat to prevent condensation are provided. Operate a dehumidifier in the basement if needed to keep relative humidity levels between 30–50 percent.

Standards or Guidelines

There are currently no federal government standards for biologicals in school indoor air environments (as of 1999).

Chapter 4

Allergies in Children

Chapter Contents

Section 4.1

Trends in Allergic Conditions among Children

This section includes text excerpted from "Trends in Allergic
Conditions among Children: United States, 1997–2011," Centers for
Disease Control and Prevention (CDC), November 6, 2015.

Allergic conditions are among the most common medical conditions
affecting children in the United States. An allergic condition is a hypersensitivity disorder in which the immune system reacts to substances
in the environment that are normally considered harmless. Food or
digestive allergies, skin allergies (such as eczema), and respiratory
allergies (such as hay fever) are the most common allergies among children. Allergies can affect a child's physical and emotional health and
can interfere with daily activities, such as sleep, play, and attending
school. A severe allergic reaction with rapid onset, anaphylaxis, can be
life threatening. Foods represent the most common cause of anaphylaxis among children and adolescents. Early detection and appropriate
interventions can help to decrease the negative impact of allergies on
quality of life. This section presents trends in the prevalence of allergies and differences by selected sociodemographic characteristics for
children under age 18 years.

- The prevalence of food and skin allergies increased in children
  under age 18 years from 1997–2011.

- The prevalence of skin allergies decreased with age. In contrast,
  the prevalence of respiratory allergies increased with age.

- Hispanic children had a lower prevalence of food allergy, skin
  allergy, and respiratory allergy compared with children of other
  race or ethnicities. Non-Hispanic black children were more
  likely to have skin allergies and less likely to have respiratory
  allergies compared with non-Hispanic white children.

- Food and respiratory allergy prevalence increased with income
  level. Children with family income equal to or greater than 200
  percent of the poverty level had the highest prevalence rates.

The prevalence of food and skin allergies increased in children aged
0–17 years from 1997–2011. Among children aged 0–17 years, the
prevalence of food allergies increased from 3.4 percent in 1997–1999

to 5.1 percent in 2009–2011. The prevalence of skin allergies increased from 7.4 percent in 1997–1999 to 12.5 percent in 2009–2011. There was no significant trend in respiratory allergies from 1997–1999 to 2009–2011, yet respiratory allergy remained the most common type of allergy among children throughout this period (17.0% in 2009–2011). Skin allergy prevalence was also higher than food allergy prevalence for each period from 1997–2011.

Younger children were more likely to have skin allergies, while older children were more likely to have respiratory allergies.

Food allergy prevalence was similar among all age groups. Skin allergy prevalence decreased with the increase of age (14.2% among 0–4 years, 13.1% among 5–9 years, and 10.9% among 10–17 years); while respiratory allergy prevalence increased with the increase of age (10.8% among 0–4 years, 17.4% among 5–9 years, and 20.8% among 10–17 years)

Hispanic children had lower rates of all three types of allergies compared with children of other race or ethnicities. Non-Hispanic black children were more likely to have skin allergies and less likely to have respiratory allergies compared with non-Hispanic white children.

Hispanic children had a lower prevalence of food allergy (3.6%), skin allergy (10.1%), and respiratory allergy (13.0%) compared with non-Hispanic white and non-Hispanic black children. Non-Hispanic black children had a higher percentage of reported skin allergy (17.4%) compared with non-Hispanic white children (12.0%) and a lower percentage of respiratory allergy (15.6%) compared with non-Hispanic white children (19.1%).

The prevalence of both food allergy and respiratory allergy increased with the increase of income level. Among children with family income less than 100 percent of the poverty level, 4.4 percent had a food allergy and 14.9 percent had a respiratory allergy. Food allergy prevalence among children with family income between 100 percent and 200 percent of the poverty level was 5.0 percent, and respiratory allergy prevalence was 15.8 percent. Among children with family income above 200 percent of the poverty level, food allergy prevalence was 5.4 percent, and respiratory allergy prevalence was 18.3 percent. There was no significant difference in the prevalence of skin allergy by poverty status.

Section 4.2

Allergic Asthma and Children

This section includes text excerpted from the following sources: Text in this section begins with excerpts from "Asthma in Children," MedlinePlus, National Institutes of Health (NIH), May 18, 2018; Text beginning with the heading "Asthma and Allergies and Their Environmental Triggers" is excerpted from "Asthma and Allergies and Their Environmental Triggers," National Institute of Environmental Health Sciences (NIEHS), January 6, 2017.

Asthma is a chronic disease that affects your airways. Your airways are tubes that carry air in and out of your lungs. If you have asthma, the inside walls of your airways become sore and swollen. In the United States, about 20 million people have asthma. Nearly 9 million of them are children. Children have smaller airways than adults, which makes asthma especially serious for them. Children with asthma may experience wheezing, coughing, chest tightness, and trouble breathing, especially early in the morning or at night.

Many things can cause asthma, including:

- Allergens—mold, pollen, animals

- Irritants—cigarette smoke, air pollution

- Weather—cold air, changes in weather

- Exercise

- Infections—flu, common cold

When asthma symptoms become worse than usual, it is called an asthma attack. Asthma is treated with two kinds of medicines: quick-relief medicines to stop asthma symptoms and long-term control medicines to prevent symptoms.

Asthma and Allergies and Their Environmental Triggers

Asthma and allergy attacks have increased in the United States despite the fact that our outdoor air quality has improved. Some researchers think these problems have increased because kids are spending too much time indoors.

When outdoors, we are exposed to pollens and dust, and other irritants. But when indoors, we are also exposed to "allergens."

Allergens are proteins that originate from cockroaches, mold, pets, and dust mites (tiny bug-like creatures that live in dust). Allergens cause allergies.....and most people know that allergies can make you sniffle, sneeze, have runny and itchy eyes, and other cold-like symptoms. But allergens can also trigger asthma attacks, which are more serious. Asthma symptoms include wheezing (a high-pitched whistling sound heard when exhaling); coughing spells unrelated to a cold; shortness of breath, especially during exercise; and tightness in the chest. Allergic asthma affects about 3 million children (8–12% of all children) and 7 million adults in the United States each year.

What Can You Do?

Reduce the allergens from your environment! Most children with asthma are allergic to something, and so staying away from the "allergen" should help control asthma. If you have asthma or allergies, stay away from animals, remove the teddy bears, rugs, curtains and lampshades in rooms that you stay in a lot, like the bedroom. Plastic mattress and pillow covers, exterminators for pesky bugs, and the elimination of dust-traps like curtains and rugs in your bedroom may help you breathe easier. Or if it's trees and pollen that get to you, air conditioning and air filters should help. Read a fun "make-believe" story about "Dustmitezilla"—a dust mite of giant proportions!

And Research Helps Too!

Children whose parents or brothers and sisters have asthma are more likely to develop it themselves. But even though our "genes" do play some part in whether or not we'll have asthma, researchers hope to make the most progress in fighting the disease by looking at the environmental aspect of asthma. The hope is that if kids encounter fewer allergens early in life, they'll be less likely to develop allergic responses.

Section 4.3

Allergy Relief for Your Child

This section includes text excerpted from "Allergy Relief for Your Child," U.S. Food and Drug Administration (FDA), June 1, 2017.

Children are magnets for colds. But when the sniffles and sneezing won't go away for weeks, the culprit may be allergies. Long-lasting sneezing, with a stuffy or runny nose, may signal the presence of the allergic rhinitis—the collection of symptoms that affect the nose when you have an allergic reaction to something you breathe in and that lands on the lining inside the nose.

Allergies may be seasonal or can strike year-round (perennial). In most parts of the United States, plant pollens are often the cause of seasonal allergic rhinitis—more commonly called hay fever. Indoor substances, such as mold, dust mites, and pet dander, may cause the perennial kind.

Up to 40 percent of children suffer from allergic rhinitis. And children are more likely to develop allergies if one or both parents have allergies. The U.S. Food and Drug Administration (FDA) regulates over-the-counter (OTC) and prescription medicines that offer allergy relief as well as allergen extracts used to diagnose and treat allergies. Take care to read and follow the directions provided when giving any medicine to children, including these products.

Immune System Reaction

An allergy is the body's reaction to a specific substance, or allergen. Our immune system responds to the invading allergen by releasing histamine and other chemicals that typically trigger symptoms in the nose, lungs, throat, sinuses, ears, eyes, skin, or stomach lining. In some children, allergies can also trigger symptoms of asthma—a disease that causes wheezing or difficulty breathing. If a child has allergies and asthma, "not controlling the allergies can make asthma worse," says Anthony Durmowicz, M.D., a pediatric pulmonary doctor at the FDA.

Avoid Pollen, Mold, and Other Allergy Triggers

If your child has seasonal allergies, pay attention to pollen counts and try to keep your child inside when the levels are high.

- In the late summer and early fall, during ragweed pollen season, pollen levels are highest in the morning.

- In the spring and summer, during the grass pollen season, pollen levels are highest in the evening.

- Some molds, another allergy trigger, may also be seasonal. For example, leaf mold is more common in the fall.

- Sunny, windy days can be especially troublesome for pollen allergy sufferers.

It may also help to keep windows closed in your house and car and run the air conditioner.

Allergy Medicines for Children

For most children, symptoms may be controlled by avoiding the allergen, if known, and using OTC medicines. But if a child's symptoms are persistent and not relieved by OTC medicines, see a healthcare professional. Although some allergy medicines are approved for use in children as young as 6 months, the FDA cautions that simply because a product's box says that it is intended for children does not mean it is intended for children of all ages. Always read the label to make sure the product is right for your child's age.

When your child is taking more than one medication, read the label to be sure that the active ingredients aren't the same. Although the big print may say the product is to treat a certain symptom, different products may have the same medicine (active ingredient). It might seem that you are buying different products to treat different symptoms, but in fact, the same medicine could be in all the products. The result: You might accidentally be giving too much of one type of medicine to your child. Children are more sensitive than adults to many drugs. For example, some antihistamines can have adverse effects at lower doses on young patients, causing excitability or excessive drowsiness.

Allergy Shots and Children

Jay E. Slater, M.D., a pediatric allergist at the FDA, says that children who don't respond to either OTC or prescription medications, or who suffer from frequent complications of allergic rhinitis, may be candidates for allergen immunotherapy—commonly known as allergy shots. After allergy testing, typically by skin testing to detect what allergens your child may react to, a healthcare professional injects the child with "extracts"—small amounts of the allergens that trigger a reaction. The doses are gradually increased so that the body builds up immunity to these allergens. Allergen extracts are manufactured from natural substances, such as pollens, insect venoms, animal hair, and foods. More than 1,200 extracts are licensed by the FDA.

In 2014, the FDA approved three new immunotherapy products that are taken under the tongue for treatment of hay fever caused by certain pollens, two of them for use in children. All of them are intended for daily use, before and during the pollen season. They are not meant for immediate symptom relief. Although they are intended for at-home use, these are prescription medications, and first doses are taken in the presence of a healthcare provider. The products are Oralair, Grastek, and Ragwitek (which is approved for use in adults only).

In 2017, the FDA approved Odactra, the first immunotherapy product administered under the tongue for treatment of house dust mite-induced allergic rhinitis (nasal inflammation) with or without conjunctivitis (eye inflammation). Odactra is approved for use only in adults. "Allergy shots are never appropriate for food allergies," adds Slater, "but it's common to use extracts to test for food allergies so the child can avoid those foods." "In the last 20 years, there has been a remarkable transformation in allergy treatments," says Slater. "Kids used to be miserable for months out of the year, and drugs made them incredibly sleepy. But today's products offer proven approaches for relief of seasonal allergy symptoms."

Section 4.4

Food Allergy in Children

This section contains text excerpted from the following
sources: Text beginning with the heading "What Is Food Allergy?"
is excerpted from "Guidelines for the Diagnosis and Management
of Food Allergy in the United States," National Institute of Allergy
and Infectious Diseases (NIAID), May 2011. Reviewed August 2018;
Text under the heading "Food Allergy Reactions in Kids" is excerpted
from "Severe Food Allergy Reactions in Kids," National Institutes of
Health (NIH), July 9, 2012. Reviewed August 2018.

What Is Food Allergy?

A food allergy is an adverse health effect arising from a specific
immune response that occurs reproducibly on exposure to a given food.
Food allergens are the parts of food or ingredients within food (usually
proteins) that are recognized by immune cells. When an immune cell
binds to a food allergen, a reaction occurs that causes the symptoms
of food allergy.

What else you should know: Most food allergens cause reactions
even after they have been cooked or digested. Some allergens, most
often from fruits and vegetables, cause allergic reactions only when
eaten raw. Food oils, such as soy, corn, peanut, and sesame, may or
may not be allergenic (causing allergy), depending on how they are processed. "Allergy" and "allergic disease" refer to conditions that involve
changes to your immune system. These immune system changes fall
into two categories:

- **Immunoglobulin E (IgE) mediated**—the symptoms are the
  result of interaction between the allergen and a type of antibody
  known as IgE, which is thought to play a major role in allergic
  reactions

- **Non-IgE-mediated**—the symptoms are the result of interaction
  of the allergen with the immune system, but the interaction does
  not involve an IgE antibody

If you are sensitized to a food allergen, it means that your body has
made a specific IgE (sIgE) antibody to that food allergen, but you may
or may not have symptoms of food allergy.

If you can consistently tolerate a food that once caused you to have an
allergic reaction, you have outgrown the food allergy. Food intolerances

are adverse health effects caused by foods. They do not involve the immune system. For example, if you are lactose intolerant, you are missing the enzyme that breaks down lactose, a sugar found in milk.

How Common Is Food Allergy?

A survey conducted by the Centers for Disease Control and Prevention (CDC) estimated that food allergy affects 5 percent of children under the age of 5 and 4 percent of children aged 5–17 years and adults in the United States. There are eight major food allergens in the United States—milk, egg, peanut, tree nuts, soy, wheat, fish, and crustacean shellfish. Prevalence rates in the United States for some of these food allergens are provided below:

- Peanut: 0.6 percent
- Tree nuts: 0.4–0.5 percent
- Fish: 0.2 percent in children and 0.5 percent in adults
- Crustacean shellfish (crab, crayfish, lobster, shrimp): 0.5 percent in children and 2.5 percent in adults
- All seafood: 0.6 percent in children and 2.8 percent in adults
- Milk and egg: no reliable data available from U.S. studies, but based on data obtained outside the United States, this rate is likely to be 1–2 percent for young children

Can Food Allergy Be Outgrown?

Most children eventually outgrow milk, egg, soy, and wheat allergy. Fewer children outgrow peanut and tree nuts allergy. Outgrowing a childhood allergy may occur as late as the teenage years. For many children, sIgE antibodies can be detected within the first 2 years of life. A child with a high initial level of sIgE, along with clinical symptoms of food allergy, is less likely to outgrow the allergy. A decrease in sIgE antibodies is often associated with outgrowing the allergy. Food allergy also can begin in adulthood. Late-developing food allergy tends to persist.

What Other Conditions Can Occur with Food Allergy?

If someone has a food allergy, he or she is more likely to have asthma, eczema, eosinophilic esophagitis (EoE), or exercise-induced anaphylaxis (EIA).

What Are Risk Factors for Severe Allergic Reactions to Foods?

The severity of allergic reactions to foods is based on many different factors, including how much you ate and whether the food was cooked, raw, or processed. You cannot tell how severe your next allergic reaction will be based on the severity of your previous reactions. No available tests can predict how severe a future allergic reaction will be. You are more likely to have a severe allergic reaction to food if you also have asthma.

Food Allergy Reactions in Kids

Young children with allergies to milk or eggs had allergic reactions to these and other foods more often than expected, a new study reports. The researchers also found that less than a third of the children with severe allergic reactions were given epinephrine, a drug that reverses symptoms and can save lives.

Food allergies are caused by an abnormal immune system reaction to food. By some estimates, about 5 percent of children under the age of 5 are affected. In severe cases, allergic reactions can lead to a life-threatening condition called anaphylaxis. Symptoms include throat swelling, a sudden drop in blood pressure, trouble breathing, fainting, and dizziness. Epinephrine is the primary treatment for severe allergic reactions and anaphylaxis.

A research team led by Dr. David M. Fleischer of National Jewish Health in Denver and Dr. Scott H. Sicherer of the Mount Sinai School of Medicine set out to study food allergy reactions in preschool children. The scientists are part of the Consortium of Food Allergy Research (CoFAR), a research network established by National Institutes of Health's (NIH) National Institute of Allergy and Infectious Disease (NIAID).

The team followed 512 infants, ages 3–15 months old, for 3 years. The children entered the study either because they had a previous allergic reaction to milk or eggs or were thought likely to be allergic, based on a positive skin test and the presence of eczema, a chronic skin condition. At the start of the study, the caretakers were given advice and strategies for avoiding food allergens and written emergency plans with epinephrine prescriptions. Data was collected from patient questionnaires, telephone interviews, and doctor's visits.

The researchers reported in the July 2012 edition of *Pediatrics* that nearly 72 percent of the children had a food-allergic reaction over the

3-year period. Over half the children had more than 1 reaction. The overall reaction rate was nearly 1 food-allergic reaction per child per year. Most of the reactions were to milk (42%), egg (21%) and peanut (8%). Notably, in 11 percent of the cases, the foods were given to the children on purpose, despite the information that had been given to their caretakers.

Over 11 percent of the allergic reactions were severe. Of these, however, only 30 percent were treated with epinephrine. Caretakers most often either didn't recognize how severe the reaction was, didn't have epinephrine available or feared administering the drug.

"Intentional exposures to allergenic food are typically reported in teenagers, who tend to take more risks or who might be embarrassed about their food allergy," Fleischer says. "What is troubling is that in this study we found that a significant number of young children received allergenic foods from parents who were aware of the allergy."

"This study reinforces the importance of educating parents and other caregivers of children with food allergy about avoiding allergenic foods and using epinephrine to treat severe food-allergic reactions," Sicherer says. "We must work harder to thoroughly educate parents about the details of avoidance and when and how to correctly use epinephrine to manage this life-threatening condition."

Section 4.5

Exposure to Pet and Pest Allergens during Infancy

This section includes text excerpted from "Exposure to Pet and Pest Allergens during Infancy Linked to Reduced Asthma Risk," National Institute of Allergy and Infectious Diseases (NIAID), September 19, 2017.

Children exposed to high indoor levels of pet or pest allergens during infancy have a lower risk of developing asthma by 7 years of age, new research supported by the National Institutes of Health reveals. The findings, published September 19 in the *Journal of Allergy* and *Clinical Immunology*, may provide clues for the design of strategies to prevent asthma from developing.

While previous studies have established that reducing allergen exposure in the home helps control established asthma, the new findings suggest that exposure to certain allergens early in life, before asthma develops, may have a preventive effect. The observations come from the ongoing Urban Environment and Childhood Asthma (URECA) study, which is funded by the National Institutes of Health's (NIH) National Institute of Allergy and Infectious Diseases (NIAID) through its Inner-City Asthma Consortium (ICAC).

"We are learning more and more about how the early-life environment can influence the development of certain health conditions," said NIAID Director Anthony S. Fauci, M.D. "If we can develop strategies to prevent asthma before it develops, we will help alleviate the burden this disease places on millions of people, as well as on their families and communities." According to the Centers for Disease Control and Prevention (CDC), more than 8 percent of children in the United States currently have asthma, a chronic disease that intermittently inflames and narrows the airways. Asthma can result in missed time from school and work and is a major cause of emergency department visits and hospitalizations.

The URECA study investigates risk factors for asthma among children living in urban areas, where the disease is more prevalent and severe. Since 2005, URECA has enrolled 560 newborns from Baltimore, Boston, New York City and St. Louis at high risk for developing asthma because at least one parent has asthma or allergies. Study investigators have been following the children since birth, and the current research report evaluates the group through 7 years of age.

Among 442 children for whom researchers had enough data to assess asthma status at age 7 years, 130 children (29%) had asthma. Higher concentrations of cockroach, mouse and cat allergens present in dust samples collected from the children's homes during the first three years of life (at age 3 months, 2 years and 3 years) were linked to a lower risk of asthma by age 7 years. The researchers observed a similar association for dog allergen, although it was not statistically significant, meaning it could be due to chance. Additional analysis indicated that exposure to higher levels of these four allergens at age 3 months was associated with a lower risk of developing asthma.

Evidence also suggested that the microbial environment in the home during infancy may be associated with asthma risk. A previous report from URECA that assessed the microbiome of house dust collected in the first year of life suggested that exposure to certain bacteria during

47

infancy may protect 3-year-olds from recurrent wheezing, a risk factor for developing asthma. In the current report, researchers found associations between the abundance of certain types of bacteria in the house dust and an asthma diagnosis by age 7 years, suggesting that exposure to certain types of bacteria in early life might influence development of asthma. However, additional research is needed to clarify the potential roles of these microbial exposures in asthma development.

"Our observations imply that exposure to a broad variety of indoor allergens, bacteria and bacterial products early in life may reduce the risk of developing asthma," said James E. Gern, M.D., the principal investigator of URECA and a professor at the University of Wisconsin-Madison. "Additional research may help us identify specific targets for asthma prevention strategies."

In addition, the seven-year URECA results confirm previous research linking the development of childhood asthma to recognized risk factors such as prenatal exposure to tobacco smoke and maternal stress and depression. Investigators found that the presence of cotinine, which results from the breakdown of nicotine in the body, in the umbilical cord blood of newborns increased their risk of developing asthma by age 7 years. Maternal stress and depression reported during the first three years of the child's life also were associated with an increased risk of developing childhood asthma.

The URECA investigators are continuing to monitor the children. By dividing the children into groups based on characteristics of their allergies and asthma, the scientists hope to uncover additional information about which early-life factors influence the development of allergic or nonallergic asthma.

Part Two

Types of Allergic Reactions

Chapter 5

Allergic Rhinitis (Hay Fever)

Allergic rhinitis (hay fever) is a common health problem; about eight percent of adults and children in the United States have it. If you have an allergy, your immune system reacts to something that doesn't cause problems for most people. Many complementary health approaches, including both mind and body practices and natural products, have been studied for allergic rhinitis.

Hay Fever

Each spring, summer, and fall, trees, weeds, and grasses release tiny pollen grains into the air. Some of the pollen ends up in your nose and throat. This can trigger a type of allergy called hay fever.

Symptoms can include:

- Sneezing, often with a runny or clogged nose

- Coughing and postnasal drip

- Itching eyes, nose, and throat

This chapter contains text excerpted from the following sources: Text in this chapter begins with excerpts from "Seasonal Allergies (Allergic Rhinitis)," National Center for Complementary and Integrative Health (NCCIH), September 24, 2017; Text under the heading "Hay Fever" is excerpted from "Hay Fever," MedlinePlus, National Institutes of Health (NIH), June 28, 2018; Text beginning with the heading "What the Science Says" is excerpted from "Seasonal Allergies at a Glance," National Center for Complementary and Integrative Health (NCCIH), September 24, 2017.

- Red and watery eyes

- Dark circles under the eyes

Your healthcare provider may diagnose hay fever based on a physical exam and your symptoms. Sometimes skin or blood tests are used. Taking medicines and using nasal sprays can relieve symptoms. You can also rinse out your nose, but be sure to use distilled or sterilized water with saline. Allergy shots can help make you less sensitive to pollen and provide long-term relief.

What the Science Says

Many complementary health approaches have been studied for allergic rhinitis. There's some evidence that a few may be helpful.

Mind and Body Practices

- A 2015 evaluation of 13 studies of acupuncture for allergic rhinitis, involving a total of 2,365 participants, found evidence that this approach may be helpful.

- Rinsing the sinuses with a neti pot (a device that comes from the Ayurvedic tradition) or with other devices such as nebulizers or spray, pump, or squirt bottles, may be a useful addition to conventional treatment for allergic rhinitis.

Natural Products

- An evaluation of six studies of the herb butterbur for allergic rhinitis, involving a total of 720 participants, indicated that butterbur may be helpful.

- Researchers have been investigating probiotics (live microorganisms that may have health benefits) for diseases of the immune system, including allergies. Although some studies have had promising results, the overall evidence on probiotics and allergic rhinitis is inconsistent. It's possible that some types of probiotics might be helpful but that others are not.

- It's been thought that eating honey might help to relieve pollen allergies because honey contains small amounts of pollen and might help people build up a tolerance to it. Another possibility is that honey could act as an antihistamine or anti-inflammatory agent. Only a few studies have examined the effects of honey in people with seasonal allergies, and their results have been inconsistent.

- Many other natural products have been studied for allergic rhinitis, including astragalus, capsaicin, grape seed extract, omega-3 fatty acids, Pycnogenol (French maritime pine bark extract), quercetin, spirulina, stinging nettle, and an herb used in Ayurvedic medicine called tinospora or guduchi. In all instances, the evidence is either inconsistent or too limited to show whether these products are helpful.

Side Effects and Risks

- People can get infections if they use neti pots or other nasal rinsing devices improperly. The U.S. Food and Drug Administration (FDA) has information on how to rinse your sinuses safely.

  - Most important is the source of water that is used with nasal rinsing devices. According to the FDA, tap water that is not filtered, treated, or processed in specific ways is not safe for use as a nasal rinse. Sterile water is safe; over-the-counter (OTC) nasal rinsing products that contain sterile saline (salt water) are available.

  - Some tap water contains low levels of organisms, such as bacteria and protozoa, including amoebas, which may be safe to swallow because stomach acid kills them. But these organisms can stay alive in nasal passages and cause potentially serious infections. Improper use of neti pots may have caused two deaths in 2011 in Louisiana from a rare brain infection that the state health department linked to tap water contaminated with an amoeba called *Naegleria fowleri*.

- Acupuncture is generally considered safe when performed by an experienced practitioner using sterile needles. Improperly performed acupuncture can cause potentially serious side effects.

- Raw butterbur extracts contain pyrrolizidine alkaloids, which can cause liver damage and cancer. Extracts of butterbur that are almost completely free from these alkaloids are available. However, no studies have proven that the long-term use of butterbur products, including the reduced-alkaloid products, is safe.

- In healthy people, probiotics usually have only minor side effects, if any. However, in people with underlying health problems (for example, weakened immune systems), serious complications such as infections have occasionally been reported.

- Be cautious about using herbs or bee products for any purpose. Some herbs, such as chamomile and echinacea, may cause allergic reactions in people who are allergic to related plants. Also, people with pollen allergies may have allergic reactions to bee products, such as bee pollen, honey, royal jelly, and propolis (a hive sealant made by bees from plant resins). Children under one year of age should not eat honey.

- Talk to your healthcare provider about the best way to manage your seasonal allergies, especially if you're considering or using a dietary supplement. Be aware that some supplements may interact with medications or other supplements or have side effects of their own. Keep in mind that most dietary supplements have not been tested in pregnant women, nursing mothers, or children.

Chapter 6

Sinusitis

Chapter Contents

Section 6.1

What Is Sinusitis?

This section includes text excerpted from "Sinus
Infection (Sinusitis)," Centers for Disease Control
and Prevention (CDC), September 25, 2017.

A sinus infection (sinusitis) does not typically need to be treated
with antibiotics in order to get better. If you or your child is diagnosed
with a sinus infection, your healthcare professional can decide if antibiotics are needed.

Causes

Sinus infections occur when fluid is trapped or blocked in the
sinuses, allowing germs to grow. Sinus infections are usually (9 out
of 10 cases in adults; 5–7 out of 10 cases in children) caused by a virus.
They are less commonly (1 out of 10 cases in adults; 3–5 out of 10 cases
in children) caused by bacteria.

Other conditions can cause symptoms similar to a sinus infection,
including:

- Allergies

- Pollutants (airborne chemicals or irritants)

- Fungal infections

Risk Factors

Several conditions can increase your risk of getting a sinus infection:

- A previous respiratory tract infection, such as the common cold

- Structural problems within the sinuses

- A weak immune system or taking drugs that weaken the
  immune system

- Nasal polyps

- Allergies

In children, the following are also risk factors for a sinus infection:

- Going to daycare

- Using a pacifier

- Drinking a bottle while laying down
- Being exposed to secondhand smoke

Signs and Symptoms

Common signs and symptoms of a sinus infection include:

- Headache
- Stuffy or runny nose
- Loss of the sense of smell
- Facial pain or pressure
- Postnasal drip (mucus drips down the throat from the nose)
- Sore throat
- Fever
- Coughing
- Fatigue (being tired)
- Bad breath

When to Seek Medical Care

See a healthcare professional if you or your child has any of the following:

- Temperature higher than 100.4°F
- Symptoms that are getting worse or lasting more than 10 days
- Multiple sinus infections in the past year
- Symptoms that are not relieved with over-the-counter (OTC) medicines

If your child is younger than three months of age and has a fever, it's important to call your healthcare professional right away.

You may have chronic sinusitis if your sinus infection lasts more than eight weeks or if you have more than four sinus infections each year. If you are diagnosed with chronic sinusitis, or believe you may have chronic sinusitis, you should visit your healthcare professional for evaluation. Chronic sinusitis can be caused by nasal growths, allergies, or respiratory tract infections (viral, bacterial, or fungal).

Diagnosis and Treatment

Your healthcare professional will determine if you or your child has a sinus infection by asking about symptoms and doing a physical examination. Sometimes they will also swab the inside of your nose. Antibiotics may be needed if the sinus infection is likely to be caused by bacteria. Antibiotics will not help a sinus infection caused by a virus or an irritation in the air (like secondhand smoke). These infections will almost always get better on their own. Antibiotic treatment in these cases may even cause harm in both children and adults. If symptoms continue for more than 10 days, schedule a follow-up appointment with your healthcare professional for re-evaluation.

Symptom Relief

Rest, OTC medicines and other self-care methods may help you or your child feel better. For more information talk to your healthcare professional, including your pharmacist. Always use over-the-counter products as directed since many OTC products are not recommended for children of certain ages.

Prevention

There are several steps you can take to help prevent a sinus infection, including:

- Practice good hand hygiene.
- Keep you and your child up to date with recommended immunizations.
- Avoid close contact with people who have colds or other upper respiratory infections.
- Avoid smoking and exposure to secondhand smoke.
- Use a clean humidifier to moisten the air at home.

Section 6.2

Nasal Polyps

What Is a Nasal Polyp?

Nasal polyps are small, polypoidal, noncancerous growths that can occur anywhere in the mucous membranes lining the nose or the paranasal sinuses. They are overgrowths of the mucosa that frequently accompany allergic rhinitis. They are not tender and are freely movable. They may occur singly or in clusters, and they usually form where the sinuses open into the nasal cavity. While small polyps may not cause problems, larger ones can block the sinuses or the nasal airway. Nasal polyps can develop at any age, but they are most common in adults over age 40; and men are more affected than women. They are uncommon in children under ten years. When young children are diagnosed with nasal polyps, in fact, doctors should conduct further tests to rule out cystic fibrosis, a genetic disorder characterized by a buildup of mucus in the lungs. Nasal polyps occur in nearly two-thirds of cystic fibrosis patients.

Causes

It is not entirely clear why some people develop nasal polyps and others do not. Although there is no definite cause of nasal polyposis, some factors may contribute to an increased risk of developing nasal polyps. One of the most common triggers is nasal congestion arising from chronic inflammation of the sinuses, which may be caused by allergies or recurring sinus infections. A certain degree of genetic predisposition has been observed in patients with nasal polyps, and it may explain why the mucosa in some people reacts differently to inflammation. Polyps are also commonly seen in patients with late onset of asthma and aspirin sensitivity, allergic rhinitis, sinusitis, a foreign body in the nose.

Types of Nasal Polyp

It is classified as antrochoanal and ethmoidal. Antrochoanal nasal polyp (ACP) is single, unilateral. It will originate from maxillary sinus and usually found in children. Ethmoidal polyps are bilateral and usually found in adults.

Symptoms and Diagnosis

Polyposis may be asymptomatic in some people, particularly if the polyps are small. Larger polyps are usually associated with catarrh (excessive secretion of mucus), breathing difficulties, inflammation of the paranasal cavities, and loss of smell and taste. Other symptoms of nasal polyps may include postnasal drip (drainage of mucous down the back of the throat) and a dull, achy feeling in the face because of fluid buildup.

Diagnosis of nasal polyps is generally made using a procedure called nasal endoscopy. Although a routine examination with a rhinoscope (a lighted device fitted with a lens that can be inserted into the nose) can find polyps located in the nasal cavity, an endoscope (a long, flexible tool fitted with a miniature camera on its end) is required to find polyps that are deep-seated in the sinuses. The doctor may also request a computerized tomography (CT) scan to diagnose polyps and additional tests like biopsy to rule out nasal and sinus cancer and nonmalignant condition like nasal papilloma.

Pathogenesis of Nasal Polyp

The exact pathogenesis of nasal polyps is unknown. Nasal mucosa, first becomes oedematous due to collection of extracellular fluid, causing polypoidal change. Polyps which are sessile in the beginning become pedunculated due to gravity and excessive sneezing. In early stages, surfaces of nasal polyps are covered by ciliated columnar epithelium, but later on it undergoes metaplastic change to squamous type on atmospheric irritation. Submucosa shows large intercellular spaces filled with serous fluid.

The following some diseases associated with polyp formation:

- Chronic rhinosinusitis

- Cystic fibrosis (CF)

- Asthma

- Aspirin-induced asthma (AIA)

- Nasal mastocytosis

- Kartagener syndrome, etc.

Exposure to some forms of chromium can cause nasal polyps and associated disease.

Treatment Options

Although various forms of medicine can alleviate symptoms associated with nasal polyps, they may provide only temporary relief. The first line of treatment is usually nasal drops or sprays containing steroids. Steroid treatment is often beneficial if the polyps are small, and the patient is likely to experience marked improvement in breathing as the polyps shrink and free up the airways. Tapered oral steroid medications can prevent sinus inflammation associated with allergies and effectively reduce the size of inflammatory polyps, but these drugs are used sparingly because they may increase the risk of such health concerns as diabetes, high blood pressure, and osteoporosis. Steroids, both topical and oral, are also frequently used after surgery to prevent the recurrence of polyps. Doctors may also prescribe antibiotics to treat chronic sinusitis that may be associated with nasal polyps.

Endoscopic nasal surgery is the most commonly used treatment option for polyposis when the polyps are too large to respond to corticosteroids. This minimally invasive surgical procedure, known as a polypectomy, is performed with a nasal endoscope and can be done on an outpatient basis. The procedure is carried out under general anaesthesia using a suction device or a microdebrider (a minuscule, motorized shaver) to remove the polyps. The removal of nasal polyps by nasal endoscopy surgery lasts approximately 45 minutes to 1 hour. Recovery from the disease is anywhere from 1–3 weeks. If there is no bleeding, the patient is discharged after a few hours of observation. Antibiotics are usually prescribed to prevent infection at the site of surgery. Although surgery can provide symptomatic relief for a few years, the nasal polyps grow back in at least 15 percent of patients. In such cases, postoperative use of steroidal sprays and saline washes is usually prescribed to extend the period before the polyps recur.

References

1. Case-Lo, Christine. "Nasal Polyps," Healthline, October 5, 2015.

2. "Nasal Polyps—Treatment," NHS Choices, February 12, 2015.

Chapter 7

Conjunctivitis (Pink Eye)

Allergic conjunctivitis is common in people who have other signs of allergic disease, such as hay fever, asthma, and eczema. It is caused by the body's reaction to certain substances to which it is allergic, such as:

- Pollen from trees, plants, grasses, and weeds
- Dust mites
- Animal dander
- Molds
- Contact lenses and lens solution
- Cosmetics

Symptoms

Symptoms of conjunctivitis (pink eye) can include:

- Pink or red color in the white of the eye(s)
- Swelling of the conjunctiva (the thin layer that lines the white part of the eye and the inside of the eyelid) and/or eyelids
- Increased tear production
- Feeling like a foreign body is in the eye(s) or an urge to rub the eye(s)
- Itching, irritation, and/or burning

This chapter includes text excerpted from "Conjunctivitis (Pink Eye)," Centers for Disease Control and Prevention (NEI), October 2, 2017.

- Discharge (pus or mucus)
- Crusting of eyelids or lashes, especially in the morning
- Contact lenses that feel uncomfortable and/or do not stay in place on the eye
- Depending on the cause, other symptoms may occur

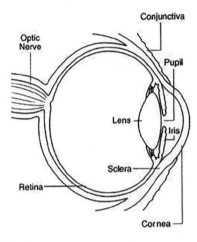

Figure 7.1. *Human Eye*

Allergic conjunctivitis

- Usually occurs in both eyes
- Can produce intense itching, tearing, and swelling in the eyes
- May occur with symptoms of allergy, such as an itchy nose, sneezing, a scratchy throat, or asthma

Viral conjunctivitis

- Can occur with symptoms of a cold, flu, or other respiratory infection
- Usually begins in one eye and may spread to the other eye within days
- Discharge from the eye is usually watery rather than thick

Bacterial conjunctivitis

- More commonly associated with discharge (pus), which can lead to eyelids sticking together
- Sometimes occurs with an ear infection

Conjunctivitis caused by irritants

• Can produce watery eyes and mucus discharge

Diagnosis

A doctor can often determine whether a virus, bacterium, or allergen is causing the conjunctivitis (pink eye) based on patient history, symptoms, and an examination of the eye. Conjunctivitis always involves eye redness or swelling, but it also has other symptoms that can vary depending on the cause. These symptoms can help a healthcare professional diagnose the cause of conjunctivitis. However, it can sometimes be difficult to make a firm diagnosis because some symptoms are the same no matter the cause.

It can also sometimes be difficult to diagnose without doing laboratory testing. Although not routinely done, your healthcare provider may collect a sample of eye discharge from the infected eye and send it to the laboratory to help them determine which form of infection you have and how best to treat it.

The cause is likely allergic if:

• Conjunctivitis occurs seasonally when pollen counts are high

• The patient's eyes itch intensely

• It occurs in someone with other signs of allergic disease, such as hay fever, asthma, or eczema

Treatment

Conjunctivitis caused by an allergen (such as pollen or animal dander) usually improves by removing the allergen from the person's environment. Allergy medications and certain eye drops (topical antihistamine and vasoconstrictors), including some prescription eye drops, can also provide relief from allergic conjunctivitis. In some cases, your doctor may recommend a combination of drugs to improve symptoms. Your doctor can help if you have conjunctivitis caused by an allergy.

Prevention

Conjunctivitis caused by allergens or irritants is not contagious unless a secondary viral or bacterial infection develops.

Chapter 8

Allergic Asthma

Chapter Contents

Section 8.1

What Is Asthma?

This section includes text excerpted from "Asthma," National
Heart, Lung, and Blood Institute (NHLBI), May 1, 2018.

Asthma is a chronic lung disease that inflames and narrows the
airways. Asthma causes recurring periods of wheezing (a whistling
sound when you breathe), chest tightness, shortness of breath, and
coughing. The coughing often occurs at night or early in the morning.
Asthma affects people of all ages, but it most often starts during childhood. In the United States, more than 25 million people are known to
have asthma. About 7 million of these people are children.

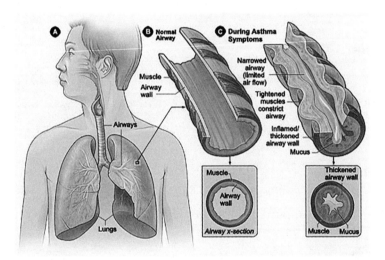

Figure 8.1. *Asthma*

*Figure A shows the location of the lungs and airways in the body. Figure B shows a
cross-section of a normal airway. Figure C shows a cross-section of an airway during
asthma symptoms.*

Outlook

Asthma has no cure. Even when you feel fine, you still have the disease and it can flare up at any time. However, with today's knowledge
and treatments, most people who have asthma are able to manage
the disease. They have few, if any, symptoms. They can live normal,
active lives and sleep through the night without interruption from

asthma. If you have asthma, you can take an active role in managing the disease. For successful, thorough, and ongoing treatment, build strong partnerships with your doctor and other healthcare providers.

Causes

The exact cause of asthma isn't known. Researchers think some genetic and environmental factors interact to cause asthma, most often early in life. These factors include:

- An inherited tendency to develop allergies, called atopy

- Parents who have asthma

- Certain respiratory infections during childhood

- Contact with some airborne allergens or exposure to some viral infections in infancy or in early childhood when the immune system is developing

If asthma or atopy runs in your family, exposure to irritants (for example, tobacco smoke) may make your airways more reactive to substances in the air.

Some factors may be more likely to cause asthma in some people than in others. Researchers continue to explore what causes asthma.

The "Hygiene Hypothesis"

One theory researchers have for what causes asthma is the "hygiene hypothesis." They believe that the Western lifestyle—with its emphasis on hygiene and sanitation—has resulted in changes in the living conditions and an overall decline in infections in early childhood. Many young children no longer have the same types of environmental exposures and infections as children did in the past. This affects the way that young children's immune systems develop during very early childhood, and it may increase their risk for atopy and asthma. This is especially true for children who have close family members with one or both of these conditions.

Risk Factors

Asthma affects people of all ages, but it most often starts during childhood. In the United States, more than 22 million people are known to have asthma. Nearly 6 million of these people are children. Young children who often wheeze and have respiratory infections—as well as certain other risk factors—are at highest risk of developing asthma that continues beyond 6 years of age. The other risk factors include having allergies, eczema (an allergic skin condition), or parents who have asthma.

Among children, more boys have asthma than girls. But among adults, more women have the disease than men. It's not clear whether or how sex and sex hormones play a role in causing asthma. Most, but not all, people who have asthma have allergies. African Americans and Puerto Ricans are at higher risk for asthma than those of other racial and ethnic groups. Some people develop asthma because of contact with certain chemical irritants or industrial dusts in the workplace. This type of asthma is called occupational asthma.

Screening and Prevention

You can't prevent asthma. However, you can take steps to control the disease and prevent its symptoms. For example:

- Learn about your asthma and ways to control it.
- Follow your written asthma action plan.
- Use medicines as your doctor prescribes.
- Identify and try to avoid things that make your asthma worse (asthma triggers). However, one trigger you should not avoid is physical activity. Physical activity is an important part of a healthy lifestyle. Talk with your doctor about medicines that can help you stay active.
- Keep track of your asthma symptoms and level of control.
- Get regular checkups for your asthma.

Signs, Symptoms, and Compilations

Common signs and symptoms of asthma include:

- **Coughing.** Coughing from asthma often is worse at night or early in the morning, making it hard to sleep.
- **Wheezing.** Wheezing is a whistling or squeaky sound that occurs when you breathe.
- **Chest tightness.** This may feel like something is squeezing or sitting on your chest.
- **Shortness of breath.** Some people who have asthma say they can't catch their breath or they feel out of breath. You may feel like you can't get air out of your lungs.

Not all people who have asthma have these symptoms. Likewise, having these symptoms doesn't always mean that you have asthma. The best way to diagnose asthma for certain is to use a lung function test, a medical history (including type and frequency of symptoms), and a physical exam.

The types of asthma symptoms you have, how often they occur, and how severe they are may vary over time. Sometimes your symptoms may just annoy you. Other times, they may be troublesome enough to limit your daily routine.

Severe symptoms can be fatal. It's important to treat symptoms when you first notice them so they don't become severe.

With proper treatment, most people who have asthma can expect to have few, if any, symptoms either during the day or at night.

What Causes Asthma Symptoms to Occur?

Many things can trigger or worsen asthma symptoms. Your doctor will help you find out which things (sometimes called triggers) may cause your asthma to flare up if you come in contact with them. Triggers may include:

- Allergens from dust, animal fur, cockroaches, mold, and pollens from trees, grasses, and flowers

- Irritants such as cigarette smoke, air pollution, chemicals, or dust in the workplace, compounds in home décor products, and sprays (such as hairspray)

- Medicines such as aspirin or other nonsteroidal anti-inflammatory drugs (NSAIDs) and nonselective beta-blockers

- Sulfites in foods and drinks

- Viral upper respiratory infections, such as colds

- Physical activity, including exercise

Other health conditions can make asthma harder to manage. Examples of these conditions include a runny nose, sinus infections, reflux disease, psychological stress, and sleep apnea. These conditions need treatment as part of an overall asthma care plan. Asthma is different for each person. Some of the triggers listed above may not affect you. Other triggers that do affect you may not be on the list. Talk with your doctor about the things that seem to make your asthma worse.

Diagnosis

Your primary care doctor will diagnose asthma based on your medical and family histories, a physical exam, and test results. Your doctor also will figure out the severity of your asthma—that is, whether it's intermittent, mild, moderate, or severe. The level of severity will determine what treatment you'll start on.

You may need to see an asthma specialist if:

- You need special tests to help diagnose asthma

- You've had a life-threatening asthma attack

- You need more than one kind of medicine or higher doses of medicine to control your asthma, or if you have overall problems getting your asthma well controlled

- You're thinking about getting allergy treatments

Medical and Family Histories

Your doctor may ask about your family history of asthma and allergies. He or she also may ask whether you have asthma symptoms and when and how often they occur. Let your doctor know whether your symptoms seem to happen only during certain times of the year or in certain places, or if they get worse at night. Your doctor also may want to know what factors seem to trigger your symptoms or worsen them. Your doctor may ask you about related health conditions that can interfere with asthma management. These conditions include a runny nose, sinus infections, reflux disease, psychological stress, and sleep apnea.

Physical Exam

Your doctor will listen to your breathing and look for signs of asthma or allergies. These signs include wheezing, a runny nose or swollen nasal passages, and allergic skin conditions, such as eczema.

Keep in mind that you can still have asthma even if you don't have these signs on the day that your doctor examines you.

Diagnostic Tests

Pulmonary Function Tests

Your doctor will use pulmonary function tests to check how your lungs are working.

- **Spirometry** measures how much air you can breathe in and out. It also measures how fast you can blow air out.

- **Bronchoprovocation tests** measure how your airways react to specific exposures. Using spirometry, this test repeatedly measures your lung function during physical activity or after you receive increasing doses of cold air or a special chemical to breathe in. Fractional concentration of exhaled nitric oxide tests measure how much nitric oxide is in the air you exhale. This test can be helpful to diagnose or guide asthma treatment in some patients.

Your doctor also may give you medicine and then test you again to see whether the results have improved.

If the starting results are lower than normal and improve with the medicine, and if your medical history shows a pattern of asthma symptoms, your diagnosis will likely be asthma.

Other Tests

Your doctor may recommend other tests if he or she needs more information to make a diagnosis. Other tests may include:

- Allergy testing to find out which allergens affect you, if any

- A test to measure how sensitive your airways are. This is called a bronchoprovocation. test. Using spirometry, this test repeatedly measures your lung function during physical activity or after you receive increasing doses of cold air or a special chemical to breathe in.

- A test to show whether you have another condition with the same symptoms as asthma, such as reflux disease, vocal cord dysfunction, or sleep apnea

- A chest X-ray or an EKG (electrocardiogram). These tests will help find out whether a foreign object or other disease may be causing your symptoms.

Diagnosing Asthma in Young Children

Sometimes it's hard to tell whether a child has asthma or another childhood condition. This is because the symptoms of asthma also occur with other conditions.

Also, many young children who wheeze when they get colds or respiratory infections don't go on to have asthma after they're six years old. A child may wheeze because he or she has small airways that become even narrower during colds or respiratory infections. The airways grow as the child grows older, so wheezing no longer occurs when the child gets colds.

A young child who has frequent wheezing with colds or respiratory infections is more likely to have asthma if:

- One or both parents have asthma

- The child has signs of allergies, including the allergic skin condition eczema

- The child has allergic reactions to pollens or other airborne allergens

- The child wheezes even when he or she doesn't have a cold or other infection

The most certain way to diagnose asthma is with a pulmonary function test (spirometry), a medical history, and a physical exam. However, it's hard to do pulmonary function tests in children younger than five years. Thus, doctors must rely on children's medical histories, signs and symptoms, and physical exams to make a diagnosis. Doctors also may use a four- to six-week trial of asthma medicines to see how well a child responds.

Treatment

Asthma is a long-term disease that has no cure. The goal of asthma treatment is to control the disease. Good asthma control will:

- Prevent chronic and troublesome symptoms, such as coughing and shortness of breath

- Reduce your need for quick-relief medicines

- Help you maintain good lung function

- Let you maintain your normal activity level and sleep through the night

- Prevent asthma attacks that could result in an emergency room visit or hospital stay

To control asthma, partner with your doctor to manage your asthma or your child's asthma. Children aged 10 or older—and younger children who are able—should take an active role in their asthma care.

Taking an active role to control your asthma involves:

- Working with your doctor to treat other conditions that can interfere with asthma management

- Avoiding things that worsen your asthma (asthma triggers). However, one trigger you should not avoid is physical activity. Physical activity is an important part of a healthy lifestyle. Talk with your doctor about medicines that can help you stay active.

- Working with your doctor and other healthcare providers to create and follow an asthma action plan. An asthma action plan gives guidance on taking your medicines properly; avoiding asthma triggers, except physical activity; tracking your level of asthma control; responding to worsening symptoms; and seeking emergency care when needed.

Asthma is treated with two types of medicines: long-term control and quick-relief medicines. Long-term control medicines help reduce airway inflammation and prevent asthma symptoms. Quick-relief, or "rescue," medicines relieve asthma symptoms that may flare up. Your initial treatment will depend on the severity of your asthma. Follow-up asthma treatment will depend on how well your asthma action plan is controlling your symptoms and preventing asthma attacks.

Your level of asthma control can vary over time and with changes in your home, school, or work environments. These changes can alter how often you're exposed to the factors that can worsen your asthma. Your doctor may need to increase your medicine if your asthma doesn't stay under control. On the other hand, if your asthma is well con-trolled for several months, your doctor may decrease your medicine. These adjustments to your medicine will help you maintain the best control possible with the least amount of medicine necessary. Asthma treatment for certain groups of people—such as children, pregnant women, or those for whom exercise brings on asthma symptoms—will be adjusted to meet their special needs.

Living With

If you have asthma, you'll need long-term care. Successful asthma treatment requires that you take an active role in your care and follow your asthma action plan.

Learn How to Manage Your Asthma

Partner with your doctor to develop an asthma action plan. This plan will help you know when and how to take your medicines. The plan also will help you identify your asthma triggers and manage your disease if asthma symptoms worsen. Children aged 10 or older—and younger children who can handle it—should be involved in creating and following their asthma action plans.

Most people who have asthma can successfully manage their symptoms by following their asthma action plans and having regular checkups. However, knowing when to seek emergency medical care is important. Learn how to use your medicines correctly. If you take inhaled medicines, you should practice using your inhaler at your doctor's office. If you take long-term control medicines, take them daily as your doctor prescribes. Record your asthma symptoms as a way to track how well your asthma is controlled. Also, your doctor may advise you to use a peak flow meter to measure and record how well your lungs are working. Your doctor may ask you to keep records of your symptoms or peak flow results daily for a couple of weeks before an office visit. You'll bring these records with you to the visit. These steps will help you keep track of how well you're controlling your asthma over time. This will help you spot problems early and prevent or relieve asthma attacks. Recording your symptoms and peak flow results to share with your doctor also will help him or her decide whether to adjust your treatment.

Ongoing Care

Have regular asthma checkups with your doctor so he or she can assess your level of asthma control and adjust your treatment as needed. Remember, the main goal of asthma treatment is to achieve the best control of your asthma using the least amount of medicine. This may require frequent adjustments to your treatments.

If you find it hard to follow your asthma action plan or the plan isn't working well, let your healthcare team know right away. They will work with you to adjust your plan to better suit your needs. Get treatment for any other conditions that can interfere with your asthma management.

Watch for Signs That Your Asthma Is Getting Worse

Your asthma might be getting worse if:

- Your symptoms start to occur more often, are more severe, or bother you at night and cause you to lose sleep

- You're limiting your normal activities and missing school or work because of your asthma

- Your peak flow number is low compared to your personal best or varies a lot from day to day

- Your asthma medicines don't seem to work well anymore

- You have to use your quick-relief inhaler more often. If you're using quick-relief medicine more than 2 days a week, your asthma isn't well controlled.

- You have to go to the emergency room or doctor because of an asthma attack

If you have any of these signs, see your doctor. He or she might need to change your medicines or take other steps to control your asthma. Partner with your healthcare team and take an active role in your care. This can help you better control your asthma so it doesn't interfere with your activities and disrupt your life.

Section 8.2

Allergy Testing for Asthma

This section includes text excerpted from "Allergy Testing for Persons with Asthma," Centers for Disease Control and Prevention (CDC), July 15, 2007. Reviewed August 2018.

What Are Allergies?

Allergy problems ("allergies") happen when a person's immune system overreacts to an allergen. An allergen is any substance that causes the immune system to overreact ("allergic reaction").

How Do Allergies Affect Asthma?

For persons with asthma and allergies, exposure to allergens can increase asthma symptoms and trigger asthma attacks. In these individuals, exposure to allergens can also cause symptoms such as sneezing, stuffy nose, or itchy eyes.

Why Is Allergy Testing for Inhalant Allergens Important in Asthma?

Inhalant allergens (e.g., pollens, molds, animal dander, and house dust mites) appear to be the most important for children and adults with asthma. Allergic individuals with asthma often experience chest, nose, or eye symptoms soon after they are exposed to inhalant allergens. Food allergens are not a common cause of asthma symptoms.

When Should Allergy Testing Be Administered in Persons with Asthma?

The recommendation is that children and adults with persistent asthma receive allergy testing, particularly for indoor inhalant allergens (animal dander, house dust mites, cockroaches, and certain molds). Also, allergy testing can be considered for persons with intermittent asthma.

What Does Allergy Testing Look For?

Allergy testing looks for a substance in the body called Immunoglobulin E (IgE). IgE is a cause of allergies. Some individuals have IgE for only one type of allergen (e.g., cat), other individuals have IgE for multiple types of allergens (e.g., cat, cockroach, and ragweed), and others have no IgE for any allergens. Allergy testing can show whether an individual has IgE for zero, one, or more than one allergen. Allergy testing for persons with asthma usually looks for IgE for inhalant allergens that are known to commonly affect asthma symptoms. Some inhalant allergen sources can be present in any season, such as animal dander, indoor mold, and cockroach. In contrast, levels of pollens and outdoor mold can vary by season, depending on the geographic region. Also, allergens tested during inhalant allergy testing can vary by geographic region, because some allergens are found only in certain parts of the United States.

How Is Allergy Testing Administered?

Allergy testing can use skin testing or blood testing to look for IgE for allergens. Each method has its benefits and its drawbacks. Compared to blood testing, allergy skin testing provides results more quickly (within one hour). However, not all healthcare providers have the resources and knowledge to conduct allergy skin testing. Also, some individuals with asthma cannot receive skin testing because of certain medical problems they have or because of certain medications they take. If allergy skin testing is not possible, blood testing for allergies can be used. Waiting for allergy blood test results usually takes longer than waiting for allergy skin test results. Persons who receive allergy blood testing usually wait at least one day (or several days or weeks) for their test results.

How Are Allergy Test Results Used?

Both allergy test results and asthma symptoms are important information for persons with asthma. Because allergies found during allergy testing do not always trigger asthma symptoms, healthcare providers can find out if an individual's asthma symptoms relate to his or her allergy test results. Sometimes, allergens found during allergy testing can affect an individual's asthma without him or her realizing it. Healthcare providers can use their expertise to assess which allergy test results are most important for each individual with asthma. If one or more allergens appear to affect an individual's asthma, the recommendation is that the individual reduce or avoid exposure to those allergens. For example, during peak pollen times and peak pollen seasons, persons with asthma who are allergic to pollens are advised to stay indoors with windows closed in an air-conditioned environment. Another recommendation is that these individuals take multiple actions to avoid exposure to allergens, because single actions alone are not as effective. For example, an integrated pest management program is recommended for persons with asthma who are allergic to cockroaches. Integrated pest management includes: blocking cockroach entry into the home by sealing cracks and holes; removing sources of cockroach food by using sealed food containers and disposing of trash frequently; and, when necessary, applying low-toxicity pesticides (out of the reach of children and pets).

Section 8.3

Asthma and Its Environmental Triggers

This section includes text excerpted from "Asthma and Its Environmental Triggers," National Institute of Environmental Health Sciences (NIEHS), February 2012. Reviewed August 2018.

Once considered a minor ailment, asthma is now the most common chronic disorder in childhood. The prevalence of asthma has progressively increased over the past 15 years. In the United States alone, nearly 40 million people—13.3 percent of adults and 13.8 percent of children—have been diagnosed with asthma.

Does Asthma Run in Families?

Asthma does run in families, which suggests that genetics play an important role in the development of the disease. If one or both parents have asthma, the child is much more likely to develop the condition—this is known as genetic susceptibility. A National Institute of Environmental Health Sciences (NIEHS) study of 615 Mexico City families showed that variations in two genes, *ORMDL3* and *GSDML*, were associated with an increased risk of childhood asthma. These results confirm a similar study conducted among European populations.

Are Allergies Related to Asthma?

Asthma can be triggered by substances in the environment called allergens. Indoor allergens from dust mites, cockroaches, dogs, cats, rodents, molds, and fungi are among the most important environmental triggers for asthma. NIEHS scientists, along with researchers from the U.S. Department of Housing and Urban Development (HUD), conducted an extensive survey known as the National Survey of Lead Hazards and Allergens in Housing (NSLAH), which showed that 46 percent of the homes had dust mite allergens high enough to produce allergic reactions, while nearly 25 percent of the homes had allergen levels high enough to trigger asthma symptoms in genetically susceptible individuals. The survey also showed that nearly two-thirds of American homes have cockroach allergens.

What Can I Do to Reduce Allergens and Asthma Attacks?

NIEHS scientists identified several strategies that reduce indoor allergens and asthma symptoms—cockroach extermination, thorough professional cleaning, and in-home visits to educate the occupants about asthma management. Using these strategies, cockroach allergens were reduced by 84 percent, well below the threshold for producing asthma symptoms. Other research showed that some simple steps—washing bedding in hot water; putting allergen-impermeable covers on pillows, box springs, and mattresses; and vacuuming and steam cleaning carpets and upholstered furniture—can significantly reduce dust mite allergen levels.

NIEHS has also collaborated with the National Institute of Allergy and Infectious Diseases (NIAID) to conduct the National Cooperative Inner-City Asthma Study (NCICAS) aimed at reducing asthma among children in the inner-city.

The program targeted six allergens that trigger asthma symptoms—dust mites, cockroaches, pet dander, rodents, secondhand smoke, and mold. Allergen-impermeable covers were placed on the mattress and box spring of the child's bed, and families were given vacuum cleaners equipped with high-efficiency particulate air (HEPA) filters. A HEPA air purifier was set up in the child's bedroom to remove tobacco smoke, dog and cat allergens, and mold. Children who received the help had 19 percent fewer clinic visits, a 13 percent reduction in the use of albuterol inhalers, and 38 more symptom-free days than those in the control group.

What about Mold?

After hurricane Katrina and the subsequent flooding in New Orleans, NIEHS partnered with the National Institute on Minority Health and Health Disparities to establish the Head-off Environmental Asthma in Louisiana (HEAL) Project. Preliminary data from the HEAL project indicates there may be an association between mold sensitivity and asthma symptoms, but more research is needed.

What about the Air Pollution Outside?

While much of the asthma research has focused on indoor allergens, scientists know that outdoor pollution also plays a major role. NIEHS-funded researchers at the Keck School of Medicine of the

University of Southern California (USC) studied air pollution in 10 Southern California cities and found that children living within 150 meters of a freeway were more likely to be diagnosed with asthma than children who lived further away. The researchers also found that children who had higher levels of nitrogen dioxide in the air around their homes were more likely to develop asthma symptoms. Nitrogen dioxide is one of many pollutants emitted from motor vehicles.

Scientists with the Columbia Center for Children's Environmental Health (CCCEH) found that New York City mothers who were exposed during pregnancy to both polycyclic aromatic hydrocarbons, air pollutants from gasoline and other fossil fuels, and secondhand tobacco smoke had children who were more likely to have asthma. Research conducted by NIEHS-funded scientists at Yale University also suggests that asthmatic children who use medication to control asthma symptoms are particularly vulnerable to the effects of ground-level ozone, a highly reactive form of oxygen that is a primary ingredient of urban smog.

Section 8.4

Occupational Asthma due to Allergen Exposure at Work

This section includes text excerpted from "Do You Have Work-Related Asthma?—A Guide for You and Your Doctor," Occupational Safety and Health Administration (OSHA), March 14, 2014. Reviewed August 2018.

What Is Work-Related Asthma?

Work-related asthma is a lung disease caused or made worse by exposures to substances in the workplace. Common exposures include chemicals, dust, mold, animals, and plants. Exposure can occur from both inhalation (breathing) and skin contact. Asthma symptoms may start at work or within several hours after leaving work and may occur with no clear pattern. People who never had asthma can develop asthma due to workplace exposures. People who have had asthma for years may find that their condition worsens due to workplace exposures. Both of these situations are considered work-related asthma. A group of chemicals called isocyanates are one of the most common chemical causes of work-related asthma. Occupational Safety and Health Administration (OSHA) is working to reduce exposures to isocyanates and has identified their use in numerous workplaces. Table 8.1. below for common products (both at home and work) and common jobs where exposure to isocyanates may occur.

Why You Should Care about Work-Related Asthma

Work-related asthma may result in long-term lung damage, loss of work days, disability, or even death. The good news is that early diagnosis and treatment of work-related asthma can lead to a better health outcome.

What to Do If You Think You Have Work-Related Asthma

If you think that you may have work-related asthma, see your doctor as soon as possible. Take this information and a copy of the safety data sheet with you.

Work-Related Asthma Quick Facts

- Work-related asthma can develop over any period of time (days to years).

- Work-related asthma may occur with changes in work exposures, jobs, or processes.

- It is possible to develop work-related asthma even if your workplace has protective equipment, such as exhaust ventilation or respirators.

- Work-related asthma can continue to cause symptoms even when the exposure stops.

- Before working with isocyanates or any other asthma-causing substances, ask your employer for training, as required under OSHA's Hazard Communication standard

Table 8.1. Products and Jobs Where Exposure to Isocyanates May Occur

Common Products	Common Jobs and Job Processes
• Polyurethane foam	• Car manufacture and repair
• Paints, lacquers, ink, varnishes, sealants, finishes	• Building construction (plaster, insulation)
• Insulation materials	• Foam blowing and cutting
• Polyurethane rubber	• Painting
• Glues and adhesives	• Truck bedliner application
	• Foundry work (casting)
	• Textile, rubber, and plastic manufacturing
	• Printing
	• Furniture manufacturing
	• Electric cable insulation

Section 8.5

Aspergillosis: People with Asthma at Highest Risk

This section includes text excerpted from "Definition of Aspergillosis," Centers for Disease Control and Prevention (CDC), November 13, 2015.

What Is Aspergillosis?

Aspergillosis is a disease caused by *Aspergillus*, a common mold (a type of fungus) that lives indoors and outdoors. Most people breathe in *Aspergillus* spores every day without getting sick. However, people with weakened immune systems or lung diseases are at a higher risk of developing health problems due to *Aspergillus*. There are different types of aspergillosis. Some types are mild, but some of them are very serious.

Types of Aspergillosis

- **Allergic bronchopulmonary aspergillosis (ABPA):** *Aspergillus* causes inflammation in the lungs and allergy symptoms such as coughing and wheezing, but doesn't cause an infection.

- **Allergic *Aspergillus* sinusitis:** *Aspergillus* causes inflammation in the sinuses and symptoms of a sinus infection (drainage, stuffiness, headache) but doesn't cause an infection.

- **Aspergilloma:** Also called a "fungus ball." As the name suggests, it is a ball of *Aspergillus* that grows in the lungs or sinuses, but usually does not spread to other parts of the body.

- **Chronic pulmonary aspergillosis (CPA):** A long-term (three months or more) condition in which *Aspergillus* can cause cavities in the lungs. One or more fungal balls (aspergillomas) may also be present in the lungs.

- **Invasive aspergillosis:** A serious infection that usually affects people who have weakened immune systems, such as people who have had an organ transplant or a stem cell transplant. Invasive aspergillosis most commonly affects the lungs, but it can also spread to other parts of the body.

- **Cutaneous (skin) aspergillosis:** *Aspergillus* enters the body through a break in the skin (for example, after surgery or a burn wound) and causes infection, usually in people who have weakened immune systems. Cutaneous aspergillosis can also occur if invasive aspergillosis spreads to the skin from somewhere else in the body, such as the lungs.

Symptoms of Aspergillosis

The different types of aspergillosis can cause different symptoms. The symptoms of allergic bronchopulmonary aspergillosis (ABPA) are similar to asthma symptoms, including:

- Wheezing
- Shortness of breath
- Cough
- Fever (in rare cases)

Symptoms of allergic Aspergillus sinusitis include:

- Stuffiness
- Runny nose
- Headache
- Reduced ability to smell

Symptoms of an aspergilloma ("fungus ball") include:

- Cough
- Coughing up blood
- Shortness of breath

Symptoms of chronic pulmonary aspergillosis include:

- Weight loss
- Cough
- Coughing up blood
- Fatigue
- Shortness of breath

Invasive aspergillosis usually occurs in people who are already sick from other medical conditions, so it can be difficult to know which symptoms are related to an Aspergillus infection. However, the symptoms of invasive aspergillosis in the lungs include:

- Fever
- Chest pain
- Cough
- Coughing up blood
- Shortness of breath

Other symptoms can develop if the infection spreads from the lungs to other parts of the body. Contact your healthcare provider if you have symptoms that you think are related to any form of aspergillosis.

Aspergillosis Risk and Prevention

Who Gets Aspergillosis?

The different types of aspergillosis affect different groups of people.

- Allergic bronchopulmonary aspergillosis (ABPA) most often occurs in people who have cystic fibrosis or asthma.

- Aspergillomas usually affect people who have other lung diseases like tuberculosis.

- Chronic pulmonary aspergillosis (CPA) typically occurs in people who have other lung diseases, including tuberculosis (TB), chronic obstructive pulmonary disease (COPD), or sarcoidosis.

- Invasive aspergillosis affects people who have weakened immune systems, such as people who have had a stem cell transplant or organ transplant, are getting chemotherapy for cancer, or are taking high doses of corticosteroids.

How Does Someone Get Aspergillosis?

People can get aspergillosis by breathing in microscopic *Aspergillus* spores from the environment. Most people breathe in *Aspergillus* spores every day without getting sick. However, people with weakened immune systems or lung diseases are at a higher risk of developing health problems due to *Aspergillus*.

Is Aspergillosis Contagious?

No. Aspergillosis can't spread between people or between people and animals from the lungs.

How Can I Prevent Aspergillosis?

It's difficult to avoid breathing in *Aspergillus* spores because the fungus is common in the environment. For people who have weakened immune systems, there may be some ways to lower the chances of developing a severe *Aspergillus* infection.

- **Protect yourself from the environment.** It's important to note that although these actions are recommended, they haven't been proven to prevent aspergillosis.

  - Try to avoid areas with a lot of dust like construction or excavation sites. If you can't avoid these areas, wear an N95 respirator (a type of face mask) while you're there.

  - Avoid activities that involve close contact to soil or dust, such as yard work or gardening. If this isn't possible:

- Wear shoes, long pants, and a long-sleeved shirt when doing outdoor activities such as gardening, yard work, or visiting wooded areas.

- Wear gloves when handling materials such as soil, moss, or manure.

- To reduce the chances of developing a skin infection, clean skin injuries well with soap and water, especially if they have been exposed to soil or dust.

- **Antifungal medication.** If you are at high risk for developing invasive aspergillosis (for example, if you've had an organ transplant or a stem cell transplant), your healthcare provider may prescribe medication to prevent aspergillosis. Scientists are still learning about which transplant patients are at highest risk and how to best prevent fungal infections.

- **Testing for early infection.** Some high-risk patients may benefit from blood tests to detect invasive aspergillosis. Talk to your doctor to determine if this type of test is right for you.

How Is Aspergillosis Diagnosed?

Healthcare providers consider your medical history, risk factors, symptoms, physical examinations, and lab tests when diagnosing aspergillosis. You may need imaging tests such as a chest X-ray or a computed tomography (CT) scan of your lungs or other parts of your body depending on the location of the suspected infection. If your healthcare provider suspects that you have an *Aspergillus* infection in your lungs, he or she might collect a sample of fluid from your respiratory system to send to a laboratory. Healthcare providers may also perform a tissue biopsy, in which a small sample of affected tissue is analyzed in a laboratory for evidence of *Aspergillus* under a microscope or in a fungal culture. A blood test can help diagnose invasive aspergillosis early in people who have severely weakened immune systems.

Treatment for Aspergillosis

Allergic Forms of Aspergillosis

For allergic forms of aspergillosis such as allergic bronchopulmonary aspergillosis (ABPA) or allergic *Aspergillus* sinusitis, the recommended treatment is itraconazole, a prescription antifungal medication. Corticosteroids may also be helpful.

Invasive Aspergillosis

Invasive aspergillosis needs to be treated with prescription anti-fungal medication, usually voriconazole. Other antifungal medications used to treat aspergillosis include lipid amphotericin formulations, posaconazole, isavuconazole, itraconazole, caspofungin, and mica-fungin. Whenever possible, immunosuppressive medications should be discontinued or decreased. People who have severe cases of asper-gillosis may need surgery.

Chapter 9

Atopic Dermatitis (Eczema)

Chapter Contents

Section 9.1

Understanding Atopic Dermatitis

This section includes text excerpted from "Atopic Dermatitis," National Institute of Arthritis and Musculoskeletal and Skin Diseases (NIAMS), July 31, 2016.

Atopic dermatitis (AD) is a skin disease. When a person has this disease the skin becomes extremely itchy. Scratching leads to redness, swelling, cracking, "weeping" clear fluid, crusting, and scaling. Often, the skin gets worse (flares), and then it improves or clears up (remissions). Atopic dermatitis is the most common kind of eczema, a term that describes many kinds of skin problems.

Who Gets It?

Atopic dermatitis is most common in babies and children. But it can happen to anyone. People who live in cities and dry climates may be more likely to get this disease.

You can't "catch" the disease or give it to other people.

What Causes It?

No one knows what causes atopic dermatitis. It is probably passed down from your parents (genetics). Your environment can also trigger symptoms. Stress can make the condition worse, but it does not cause the disease.

What Are the Symptoms?

The most common symptoms of atopic dermatitis are:

- Dry and itchy skin

- Rashes on the face, inside the elbows, behind the knees, and on the hands and feet

Scratching the skin can cause:

- Redness

- Swelling

- Cracking

- "Weeping" clear fluid

- Crusting

- Thick skin

- Scaling

Is There a Test?

At present, there is no single test to diagnose atopic dermatitis, but your doctor may:

- Ask you about your medical history, including:

  - Your family history of allergies

  - Whether you also have diseases such as hay fever or asthma

  - Exposure to irritants, such as:

    - Wool or synthetic fibers

    - Soaps and detergents

    - Some perfumes and cosmetics

    - Substances such as chlorine, mineral oil, or solvents

    - Dust or sand

    - Cigarette smoke

  - Sleep problems

  - Foods that seem to be related to skin flares

  - Previous treatments for skin-related symptoms

  - Use of steroids or other medications

- Identify factors that may trigger flares of atopic dermatitis by pricking the skin with a needle that contains something that you might be allergic to (in small amounts).

Your doctor may need to see you several times to diagnose you. In some cases, your family doctor or pediatrician may refer you to a dermatologist (doctor specializing in skin disorders) or allergist (allergy specialist) for further evaluation.

How Is It Treated?

The goals in treating atopic dermatitis are to heal the skin and prevent flares. You should watch for changes in the skin to find out what treatments help the most.

Treatments can include:

- Medications:

  - Skin creams or ointments that control swelling and lower allergic reactions

  - Corticosteroids

  - Antibiotics to treat infections caused by bacteria

  - Antihistamines that make people sleepy to help stop nighttime scratching

  - Drugs that suppress the immune system

- Light therapy

- Skin care that helps heal the skin and keep it healthy

- Avoiding things that cause an allergic reaction

Section 9.2

Atopic Dermatitis: Complications and Skin Care at Home

This section includes text excerpted from "Eczema (Atopic Dermatitis) Complications," National Institute of Allergy and Infectious Diseases (NIAID), August 28, 2015.

The skin of people with atopic dermatitis lacks infection-fighting proteins, making them susceptible to skin infections caused by bacteria and viruses. Fungal infections also are common in people with atopic dermatitis.

Bacterial Infections

A major health risk associated with atopic dermatitis is skin colonization or infection by bacteria such as *Staphylococcus aureus*. Sixty to ninety percent of people with atopic dermatitis are likely to have staph bacteria on their skin. Many eventually develop infection, which worsens the atopic dermatitis.

Viral Infections

People with atopic dermatitis are highly vulnerable to certain viral infections of the skin. For example, if infected with herpes simplex virus, they can develop a severe skin condition called atopic dermatitis with eczema herpeticum. Those with atopic dermatitis should not receive the currently licensed smallpox vaccine, even if their disease is in remission, because they are at risk of developing a severe infection called eczema vaccinatum. This infection is caused when the live vaccinia virus in the smallpox vaccine reproduces and spreads throughout the body. Furthermore, those in close contact with people who have atopic dermatitis or a history of the disease should not receive the smallpox vaccine because of the risk of transmitting the live vaccine virus to the person with atopic dermatitis.

Skin Care at Home

You and your doctor should discuss the best treatment plan and medications for your atopic dermatitis. But taking care of your skin at home may reduce the need for prescription medications. Some recommendations include:

- Avoid scratching the rash or skin.

- Relieve the itch by using a moisturizer or topical steroids. Take antihistamines to reduce severe itching.

- Keep your fingernails cut short. Consider light gloves if nighttime scratching is a problem.

- Lubricate or moisturize the skin two to three times a day using ointments such as petroleum jelly. Moisturizers should be free of alcohol, scents, dyes, fragrances, and other skin-irritating chemicals. A humidifier in the home also can help.

- Avoid anything that worsens symptoms, including:
  - Irritants such as wool and lanolin (an oily substance derived from sheep wool used in some moisturizers and cosmetics)
  - Strong soaps or detergents

- Sudden changes in body temperature and stress, which may cause sweating
- When washing or bathing:
  - Keep water contact as brief as possible and use gentle body washes and cleansers instead of regular soaps. Lukewarm baths are better than long, hot baths.
  - Do not scrub or dry the skin too hard or for too long.
  - After bathing, apply lubricating ointments to damp skin. This will help trap moisture in the skin.

Wet Wrap Therapy

Researchers at National Institute of Allergy and Infectious Diseases (NIAID) and other institutions are studying an innovative treatment for severe eczema called wet wrap therapy. It includes three lukewarm baths a day, each followed by an application of topical medicines and moisturizer that is sealed in by a wrap of wet gauze.

People with severe eczema have come to the National Institutes of Health (NIH) Clinical Center (CC) in Bethesda, Maryland, for research evaluation. Treatment may include wet wrap therapy to bring the condition under control. Patients and their caregivers also receive training on home-based skin care to properly manage flare-ups once they leave the hospital.

Chapter 10

Allergic Contact Dermatitis

Chapter Contents

97

Section 10.1

Contact Dermatitis and Latex Allergy

This section includes text excerpted from "Infection Control,"
Centers for Disease Control and Prevention (CDC),
July 10, 2013. Reviewed August 2018.

What Is Contact Dermatitis?

Occupationally related contact dermatitis can develop from frequent and repeated use of hand hygiene products, exposure to chemicals, and glove use. Contact dermatitis is classified as either irritant or allergic. Irritant contact dermatitis is common, nonallergic, and develops as dry, itchy, irritated areas on the skin around the area of contact. By comparison, allergic contact dermatitis (type IV hypersensitivity) can result from exposure to accelerators and other chemicals used in the manufacture of rubber gloves as well as from exposure to other chemicals found in the dental practice setting. Allergic contact dermatitis often manifests as a rash beginning hours after contact and, like irritant dermatitis, is usually confined to the areas of contact.

What Is Latex Allergy?

Latex allergy (type I hypersensitivity to latex proteins) can be a more serious systemic allergic reaction. It usually begins within minutes of exposure but can sometimes occur hours later. It produces varied symptoms, which commonly include runny nose, sneezing, itchy eyes, scratchy throat, hives, and itchy burning sensations. However, it can involve more severe symptoms including asthma marked by difficult breathing, coughing spells, and wheezing; cardiovascular and gastrointestinal ailments; and in rare cases, anaphylaxis and death.

What Are Some Considerations If Dental Healthcare Personnel Are Allergic to Latex?

Dental healthcare personnel who are allergic to latex will need to take precautions at work and outside the workplace since latex is used in a variety of other common products in addition to gloves. The following recommendations are based on those issued by the National Institute for Occupational Health and Safety (NIOSH).

If definitively diagnosed with allergy to natural rubber latex (NRL) protein:

- Avoid, as far as feasible, subsequent exposure to the protein and only use nonlatex (e.g., nitrile or vinyl) gloves.

- Make sure that other staff members in the dental practice wear either nonlatex or reduced protein, powder-free latex gloves.

- Use only synthetic or powder-free rubber dams.

Dental personnel can further reduce occupational exposure to NRL protein by taking the following steps:

- Using reduced protein, powder-free latex gloves

- Frequently changing ventilation filters and vacuum bags used in latex contaminated areas

- Checking ventilation systems to ensure they provide adequate fresh or recirculating air

- Frequently cleaning all work areas contaminated with latex dust

- Educating dental staff on the signs and symptoms of latex allergies

Why Are Powder-Free Gloves Recommended?

Proteins responsible for latex allergies are attached to glove powder. When powdered gloves are worn, more latex protein reaches the skin. Also, when gloves are put on or removed, particles of latex protein powder become aerosolized and can be inhaled, contacting mucous membranes. As a result, allergic dental healthcare personnel and patients can experience symptoms related to cutaneous, respiratory, and conjunctival exposure. Dental healthcare personnel can become sensitized to latex proteins after repeated exposure. Work areas where only powder-free, low-allergen (i.e., reduced-protein) gloves are used show low or undetectable amounts of allergy-causing proteins.

What Are Some Considerations for Providing Dental Treatment to Patients with Latex Allergy?

Patients with a latex allergy should not have direct contact with latex-containing materials and should be treated in a "latex safe" environment. Such patients also may be allergic to the chemicals used in manufacturing natural rubber latex gloves, as well as to metals, plastics, or other materials used to provide dental care. By obtaining thorough patient health histories and preventing patients from having contact with potential allergens, dental healthcare professionals can minimize the possibility of patients having adverse reactions. Considerations in providing safe treatment for patients with possible or documented latex allergy include (but are not limited to) the following:

- Screen all patients for latex allergy (e.g., obtain their health history, provide medical consultation when latex allergy is suspected).

- Be aware of some common predisposing conditions (e.g., spina bifida, urogenital anomalies, or allergies to avocados, kiwis, nuts, or bananas).

- Be familiar with the different types of hypersensitivity— immediate and delayed—and the risks that these pose for patients and staff.

- Consider sources of latex other than gloves. Dental patients with a history of latex allergy may be at risk from a variety of dental products including, but not limited to, prophylaxis cups, rubber dams, and orthodontic elastics.

- Provide an alternative treatment area free of materials containing latex. Ensure a latex-safe environment or one in which no personnel use latex gloves and no patient contact occurs with other latex devices, materials, and products.

- Remove all latex-containing products from the patient's vicinity. Adequately cover/isolate any latex-containing devices that cannot be removed from the treatment environment.

- Be aware that latent allergens in the ambient air can cause respiratory and or anaphylactic symptoms in people with latex hypersensitivity. Therefore, to minimize inadvertent exposure to airborne latex particles among patients with latex allergy, try to give them the first appointments of the day.

- Frequently clean all working areas contaminated with latex powder/dust.

- Frequently change ventilation filters and vacuum bags used in latex-contaminated areas.

- Have latex-free kits (e.g., dental treatment and emergency kits) available at all times.

- Be aware that allergic reactions can be provoked from indirect contact as well as direct contact (e.g., being touched by someone who has worn latex gloves). Hand hygiene, therefore, is essential.

- Communicate latex allergy procedures (e.g., verbal instructions, written protocols, posted signs) to other personnel to prevent them from bringing latex-containing materials into the treatment area.

- If latex-related complications occur during or after the procedure, manage the reaction and seek emergency assistance as indicated. Follow current medical emergency response recommendations for management of anaphylaxis.

Section 10.2

Outsmarting Poison Ivy and Other Poisonous Plants

This section includes text excerpted from "Outsmarting Poison Ivy and Other Poisonous Plants," U.S. Food and Drug Administration (FDA), November 6, 2017.

First comes the itching, then a red rash, and then blisters. These symptoms of poison ivy, poison oak, and poison sumac can emerge any time from a few hours to several days after exposure to the plant oil found in the sap of these poisonous plants. The culprit: the urushiol oil. Here are some tips to avoid it.

Recognizing Poison Ivy, Poison Oak, and Poison Sumac

- **Poison ivy:** Found throughout the United States except Alaska, Hawaii, and parts of the West Coast. Can grow as a vine or small shrub trailing along the ground or climbing on low plants, trees and poles. Each leaf has three glossy leaflets, with smooth or toothed edges. Leaves are reddish in spring, green in summer, and yellow, orange, or red in fall. May have greenish-white flowers and whitish-yellow berries.

- **Poison oak:** Grows as a low shrub in the Eastern and Southern United States, and in tall clumps or long vines on the Pacific Coast. Fuzzy green leaves in clusters of three are lobed or deeply toothed with rounded tips. May have yellow-white berries.

- **Poison sumac:** Grows as a tall shrub or small tree in bogs or swamps in the Northeast, Midwest, and parts of the Southeast. Each leaf has clusters of seven to 13 smooth-edged leaflets. Leaves are orange in spring, green in summer, and yellow, orange, or red in fall. May have yellow-greenish flowers and whitish-green fruits hang in loose clusters.

Poison Plant Rashes Aren't Contagious

Poison ivy and other poison plant rashes can't be spread from person to person. But it is possible to pick up the rash from plant oil that may have stuck to clothing, pets, garden tools, and other items that have come in contact with these plants. The plant oil lingers (sometimes for years) on virtually any surface until it's washed off with water or rubbing alcohol.

The rash will occur only where the plant oil has touched the skin, so a person with poison ivy can't spread it on the body by scratching. It may seem like the rash is spreading if it appears over time instead of all at once. But this is either because the plant oil is absorbed at different rates on different parts of the body or because of repeated exposure to contaminated objects or plant oil trapped under the fingernails. Even if blisters break, the fluid in the blisters is not plant oil and cannot further spread the rash.

Tips for Prevention

- Learn what poison ivy, oak, and sumac plants look like so you can avoid them.

- Wash your garden tools and gloves regularly. If you think you may be working around poison ivy, wear long sleeves, long pants tucked into boots, and impermeable gloves.

- Wash your pet if it may have brushed up against poison ivy, oak, or sumac. Use pet shampoo and water while wearing rubber gloves, such as dishwashing gloves. Most pets are not sensitive to poison ivy, but the oil can stick to their fur and cause a reaction in someone who pets them.

- Wash your skin in soap and cool water as soon as possible if you come in contact with a poisonous plant. The sooner you cleanse the skin, the greater the chance that you can remove the plant oil or help prevent further spread.

Tips for Treatment

Don't scratch the blisters. Bacteria from under your fingernails can get into them and cause an infection. The rash, blisters, and itch normally disappear in several weeks without any treatment.
You can relieve the itch by:

- Using wet compresses or soaking in cool water.

- Applying over-the-counter (OTC) topical corticosteroid preparations or taking prescription oral corticosteroids.

- Applying topical OTC skin protectants, such as zinc acetate, zinc carbonate, zinc oxide, and calamine dry the oozing and weeping of poison ivy, poison oak, and poison sumac. Protectants such as baking soda or colloidal oatmeal relieve minor irritation and itching. Aluminum acetate is an astringent that relieves rash.

See a doctor if:

- You have a temperature over 100 degrees Fahrenheit (°F)

- There is pus, soft yellow scabs, or tenderness on the rash

- The itching gets worse or keeps you awake at night

- The rash spreads to your eyes, mouth, genital area, or covers more than one-fourth of your skin area

- The rash is not improving within a few weeks

- The rash is widespread and severe

- You have difficulty breathing

Section 10.3

Allergic Contact Rashes

This section includes text excerpted from "Red, Itchy Rash?"
NIH News in Health, National Institutes of Health (NIH),
April 2012. Reviewed August 2018.

You've probably had a rash at some point or another, whether from poison ivy or the chickenpox or something more unusual. Why does your skin break out in red blotches like that? More important, is there anything you can do about it?

We often think of the skin as a barrier—it keeps the insides of our bodies in, and it keeps the outside world out. But our skin is also filled with special cells of the immune system. These cells protect the skin and body against viruses, bacteria and other threats. Whenever these cells detect a suspicious substance, they begin a chain reaction in the skin that leads to inflammation. The medical name for this reaction is dermatitis. But it's more commonly known as a rash.

There are many different types of dermatitis, and each has a distinct set of treatments. Sometimes the skin's immune cells react to something that directly touches the skin. Other times, the immune system flares in the skin because of a whole-body infection or illness.

The symptoms of these different types of rashes often overlap. "Itching is a common symptom for all these problems," says Dr. Stephen I. Katz, director of National Institutes of Health's (NIH) National Institute of Arthritis and Musculoskeletal and Skin Diseases (NIAMS). Many rashes are red, painful, and irritated. Some types of rash can also lead to blisters or patches of raw skin. While most rashes clear up fairly quickly, others are long lasting and need to be cared for over long periods of time.

Eczema, or atopic dermatitis, is a dry, red, itchy rash that affects up to 1 in 5 infants and young children. It often improves over time, although it can last into adulthood or start later in life. In this condition, the watertight barrier between skin cells gets weak, which lets moisture out and other things in. That's why people with atopic dermatitis have to moisturize their skin, and they're more susceptible to skin infections.

Researchers have identified specific genes that are involved in maintaining the skin barrier. People with certain versions of these genes are more likely to get atopic dermatitis.

"The skin is the outermost sentinel for fighting off bacteria and noxious agents," says Katz. "If the barrier is broken somehow, you can become more allergic to things."

A skin allergy, or allergic contact dermatitis, produces a red, itchy rash that sometimes comes with small blisters or bumps. The rash arises when the skin comes in contact with an allergen, a usually harmless substance that the immune system attacks. Allergens trigger allergic reactions. Allergens can come from certain soaps, creams and even pets.

Your immune system might not react the first time you encounter an allergen. But over time, your immune system can become sensitive to the substance. As a result, your next contact may lead to inflammation and an allergic rash.

"The most common form of dermatitis that is seen anywhere is an allergic contact dermatitis to nickel," says Katz. "Why? Because of ear piercing." Many inexpensive earrings are made of nickel, and over time, wearing nickel earrings can cause an allergic reaction to the metal.

Other common causes of allergic dermatitis are poison oak and poison ivy. The stems and leaves of these plants produce a chemical that's likely to cause allergies. If you touch one of them, wash your skin as soon as possible. The chemical can also remain in clothing for a long time, so it's important to wash any clothes or shoes—or even pets—that come into contact with these plants.

Mild cases of allergic contact dermatitis usually disappear after a few days or weeks. But if the rash persists, is extremely uncomfortable or occurs on the face, it's important to see a physician. A doctor can prescribe medications that will tone down the immune reaction in the skin. This eases swelling and itching and will protect your eyes and face.

The immune cells of the skin can also produce rashes when they react to invading germs—like bacteria, fungi and viruses. Bacterial and viral infections within your body can cause your skin to break out in spots as well. The chickenpox virus, for example, can cause itchy spots in children. Years later, in older adults, the same virus may reappear as shingles, bringing a painful rash and high fever. Vaccines can prevent several rash-causing diseases, including chickenpox, shingles and measles.

Certain drugs, including antibiotics like amoxicillin, may also cause itchy skin rashes. If you're allergic to a drug, a rash can be the first sign of a serious reaction. As with other allergies, a reaction to a drug may not occur the first time you take it. It could show up after several uses. Not all drug rashes are due to an allergy, however. If you break out in itchy spots after starting a new drug prescription, contact your doctor right away.

While most rashes get better with time, some can last a lifetime. Psoriasis, a condition where skin cells build up into thick red patches, tends to run in families. "It's a complex genetic disease, in that there's not one gene that causes psoriasis but many," says Katz. Even though none of these genes alone has a great effect on the disease, knowing which genes are involved can help researchers design potential new treatments. Other long-term diseases that can produce rashes include autoimmune diseases, such as lupus, and some forms of cancer.

If you notice an itchy or painful rash on your skin, think twice before going to the drugstore and getting some cream if you don't know the cause. "The creams that you buy can produce problems that make your original problem even worse," Katz says. Because rashes can be caused by many different things—bacteria, viruses, drugs, allergies, genetic disorders, and even light—it's important to figure out what kind of dermatitis you have.

"If you have any significant rash, you should see a dermatologist," says Katz. A dermatologist, or skin doctor, is specially trained to figure out what's causing a rash and help you get the right treatment.

Your skin is your protection. It's not just the covering that keeps your body in; it's also your first line of defense against germs and chemicals. Take care of your skin so your skin can take care of you.

Call Your Doctor If

- Your rash is so uncomfortable or painful it interferes with daily activities or sleep
- The rash is on your face
- Your rash looks worrisome or seems infected
- You break out in a rash after taking a new medication
- Your rash lasts for several days

Chapter 11

Other Allergic Skin Reactions

Chapter Contents

Section 11.1

Urticaria (Hives)

Urticaria, commonly known as hives, is a condition in which itchy, swollen red wheals or welts of different sizes appear on the skin. Although there are many possible causes of hives, they most commonly result from an allergic reaction to food or drugs. Hives can last from several minutes to several hours, or in some cases several weeks. They can be itchy, painful, and sometimes cause a burning sensation. Hives may form in one small area on the surface of the skin, or on a larger area of the body. They affect one out of every five people at some point in life. There are two distinct types of urticaria, acute and chronic. Acute urticaria typically lasts for less than six weeks. The rashes appear suddenly and disappear within a short period of time. Chronic hives, on the other hand, last for more than six weeks and sometimes for months. Although the condition is not dangerous, it can cause considerable discomfort. Angioedema is another form of hives in which the swelling occurs beneath the surface of the skin, often around the eyes and lips. Hives are generally not life threatening and do not have long-term health effects. However, when breathing difficulties, dizziness, and swelling of the throat or tongue occur along with an eruption of hives on the skin, it could signal anaphylaxis—a severe, life-threatening allergic reaction—and emergency medical care must be sought.

Causes and Treatment

Hives usually occur as a symptom of allergic reactions, when the body's immune system releases histamines and other chemicals into the bloodstream. Hives may be triggered by contact with a variety of common allergens, including foods, drugs, latex, pollen, insect bites, or dust mites. Urticaria may also occur as a result of bacterial and viral infections; immunizations; disease conditions such as vasculitis and lupus; adverse reactions to blood transfusions; or skin contact with plants such as poison ivy. In some cases, hives may also be caused by external triggers such as exercise, emotional stress, heat and cold, and sun exposure. While the cause of hives may be obvious in people with known allergies, other people may need to undergo medical testing by specialists to identify the cause. In some people with chronic hives, the underlying cause may be difficult to find. It may be helpful to keep a diary of symptoms, noting the conditions under which they occur and improve. This information can help people identify and avoid any factors that can trigger the condition.

As the first course of treatment for hives, a healthcare provider will usually prescribe antihistamine medication to negate the effects of histamines released into the bloodstream. Corticosteroids may be prescribed if the symptoms are severe. If the patient experiences hives as part of a severe allergic reaction and has symptoms of anaphylaxis, they will require an immediate shot of epinephrine. Anti-itch medications or salves may also be prescribed to provide relief from itching. Applying wet compresses or taking a cool bath with baking soda or oatmeal sprinkled in the water can also help relieve symptoms of hives.

References

1. Cole, Gary W. "Hives (Urticaria and Angioedema)," MedicineNet, n.d.

2. "Hives (Urticaria)," American College of Allergy, Asthma, and Immunology (ACAAI), 2014.

3. "Hives," Medline Plus, U.S. National Library of Medicine (NLM), September 8, 2014.

Section 11.2

Cold Urticaria

This section includes text excerpted from "Cold Urticaria," Genetic and Rare Diseases Information Center (GARD), National Center for Advancing Translational Sciences (NCATS), September 15, 2015.

Cold urticaria is a condition that affects the skin. Signs and symptoms generally include reddish, itchy welts (hives) and/or swelling when skin is exposed to the cold (i.e., cold weather or swimming in cold water). This rash is usually apparent within 2–5 minutes after exposure and can last for 1–2 hours. The exact cause of cold urticaria is poorly understood in most cases. Rarely, it may be associated with an underlying blood condition or infectious disease. Treatment generally consists of patient education, avoiding exposures that may trigger a reaction, and/or medications.

Symptoms

The signs and symptoms of cold urticaria and the severity of the condition vary. Affected people generally develop reddish, itchy welts (hives) and/or swelling when skin is exposed to the cold (i.e., cold weather or swimming in cold water). This rash is usually apparent within 2–5 minutes after exposure and lasts for 1–2 hours. Other signs and symptoms may include:

- Headache
- Anxiety
- Tiredness
- Fainting
- Heart palpitations
- Wheezing
- Joint pain
- Low blood pressure

In very severe cases, exposure to cold could lead to loss of consciousness, shock or even death.

Cause

In most cases of cold urticaria, the underlying cause is poorly understood. Although the symptoms are triggered by exposure of the skin to the cold (most often when the temperature is lower than 39 degrees Fahrenheit °F), it is unclear why this exposure leads to such a significant reaction. Rarely, cold urticaria is associated with blood conditions or infectious disease such as cryoglobulinemia, chronic lymphocytic leukaemia (CLL), lymphosarcoma, chicken pox, viral hepatitis, and mononucleosis.

Inheritance

Cold urticaria is not thought to be inherited. Most cases occur sporadically in people with no family history of the condition.

Diagnosis

A diagnosis of cold urticaria is typically suspected based on the presence of characteristic signs and symptoms. Additional testing can then be ordered to confirm the diagnosis and determine if there are other associated conditions. This generally involves a cold stimulation test in which a cold object (such as an ice cube) is applied against the skin of the forearm for 1–5 minutes. In people affected by cold urticaria, a distinct red and swollen rash will generally develop within minutes of exposure. A complete blood count and/or metabolic tests may also be performed to determine associated diseases.

Treatment

The treatment of cold urticaria generally consists of patient education, avoiding scenarios that may trigger a reaction (i.e., cold temperatures, cold water), and/or medications. Prophylactic treatment with high-dose antihistamines may be recommended when exposure to cold is expected and can not be avoided. Additionally, affected people are often told to carry an epinephrine autoinjector due to the increased risk of anaphylaxis.

Several other therapies have reportedly been used to treat cold urticaria with varying degrees of success. These include:

- Leukotriene antagonists
- Ciclosporin
- Systemic corticosteroids
- Dapsone
- Oral antibiotics
- Synthetic hormones
- Danazol

Prognosis

The long-term outlook (prognosis) for people with cold urticaria varies. In approximately 50 percent of cases, the condition either completely resolves or drastically improves within five to six years. However, some people have the disorder for many years or even lifelong.

Section 11.3

Allergic Reaction Caused by Mast Cells—Mastocytosis

This section includes text excerpted from "Mastocytosis," Genetic and Rare Diseases Information Center (GARD), National Center for Advancing Translational Sciences (NCATS), February 22, 2018.

Mastocytosis occurs when too many mast cells accumulate in the skin and/or internal organs such as the liver, spleen, bone marrow, and small intestines. Mast cells are a type of white blood cell in the immune system. Mast cells are responsible for protecting the body from infection and releasing chemicals to create inflammatory responses. The signs and symptoms of mastocytosis vary based on which parts of the body are affected. There are two main forms of mastocytosis. Cutaneous mastocytosis only affects the skin and is more common in children. Systemic mastocytosis affects more than one part of the body and is more common in adults.

Mastocytosis is usually caused by changes (known as variations or mutations) in the *KIT* gene. Most cases are caused by somatic mutations, meaning they only occur in certain parts of the body and are not inherited or passed on to the next generation. However, mastocystosis can rarely affect more than one person in a family. Mastocytosis may be suspected when a doctor sees a person has signs and symptoms of the disease. Diagnosis may be confirmed with a skin biopsy or bone marrow biopsy. Treatment of mastocytosis is based on the signs and symptoms present in each person and can include antihistamines, mast cell stabilizers, corticosteroids, and oral psoralen plus ultraviolet A (UVA) therapy.

Symptoms

The signs and symptoms of mastocytosis vary based on which parts of the body are affected. Signs and symptoms of mastocytosis are more likely to occur after a "trigger" such as a change in temperature, certain medications, emotional stress, or irritation of the skin. There are two main forms of mastocytosis:

- **Cutaneous mastocytosis:** This form only affects the skin. The most common signs and symptoms include small tan-red macules that develop on the body, especially on the upper and lower extremities and on the thorax and abdomen. Another common feature is known as Darier sign, which is the development of lesions in a new area shortly after irritation to the skin such as scratching. When cutaneous mastocytosis occurs in children, signs and symptoms tend to improve or go away completely by the time the child reaches puberty.

- **Systemic mastocytosis:** This form affects more than one part of the body such as the bone marrow, liver, and GI system. Signs and symptoms may include the skin findings associated with cutaneous mastocytosis, as well as symptoms such as low blood pressure (hypotension) abdominal pain, vomiting, diarrhea, fatigue, and frequent headaches. These symptoms may be episodic, meaning they only occur once in a while, or chronic, meaning symptoms are present during a long time. People with systemic mastocytosis may also present to the doctor with an enlarged liver and spleen (hepatosplenomegaly), anemia, or osteoporosis.

Many people affected by mastocytosis, especially systemic mastocytosis, also have symptoms of anxiety and depression. It is unknown if this is due to the stress of having these symptoms as part of daily life, or if the accumulation of mast cells may also affect the chemicals in a person's brain, causing anxiety and depression.

Cause

Most cases of mastocytosis are caused by a change (known as variation or mutation) in the *KIT* gene. This gene provides instructions to the body to make a protein that helps control many important cellular processes such as cell growth and division, survival, and movement. This protein is also important for the development of certain types of cells, including mast cells. Mast cells are cells of the immune system that protect the body against infections and produce an inflammatory response when it senses that the body is being attacked. Mutations in the *KIT* gene can lead to an overproduction of mast cells. In mastocytosis, mast cells accumulate in the skin and/or internal organs, leading to the many signs and symptoms of the disease.

Inheritance

Most cases of mastocytosis are not inherited. The change (variation or mutation) in the *KIT* gene that causes many cases of mastocytosis is typically a somatic mutation. Somatic mutations occur after the egg and sperm join (conception) and are only present in certain cells of the body. Typically, affected cells do not include the egg and sperm (germ cells). Therefore, the genetic change associated with mastocytosis typically only occurs in one person in a family, and the disease is not passed onto the next generation.

Mastocytosis can rarely affect more than one person in the same family. This is known as familial mastocytosis and occurs when a person does have the *KIT* mutation in the egg or sperm (germ cells). In these cases, the mastocytosis is inherited in an autosomal dominant manner. This means that to have mastocytosis, a person only needs a disease-causing genetic change in one copy of the *KIT* gene. A person with familial mastocytosis has a 50 percent chance with each pregnancy of passing along the changed gene to his or her child.

Diagnosis

Mastocytosis is often first suspected by a doctor when a person has signs and symptoms of the disease. A diagnosis of mastocytosis that causes skin lesions may be confirmed by a skin biopsy of the lesion. During a skin biopsy, a sample of skin tissue is taken and looked at under a microscope for the presence of dense areas of mast cells. If there are no cutaneous lesions or if the skin biopsy reveals uncertain results, a bone marrow biopsy may be performed. This procedure can also be useful in differentiating between cutaneous and systemic mastocytosis.

Blood and/or urine tests may also be used to measure the levels of specific chemicals or substances related to mast cells. High levels of certain substances support the diagnosis of mastocytosis. Some substances may be elevated in systemic mastocytosis but not in cutaneous mastocytosis. Other evaluations or tests used to confirm a diagnosis may include a bone scan, gastrointestinal workup, or genetic testing to confirm there is a mutation in the *KIT* gene. Additional tests may be ordered to rule out other diseases that may cause similar symptoms, such as anaphylaxis, pheochromocytoma, carcinoid syndrome, or Zollinger-Ellison syndrome (ZES).

Treatment

The treatment for mastocytosis depends on the particular symptoms of each person. Treatment for symptoms that affect the skin include antihistamines and oral psoralen plus UVA (PUVA) therapy. If the symptoms are not responsive to other treatment, a doctor may prescribe steroid creams, ointments, or solutions to be applied to the skin (topical corticosteroids treatment). Proton pump inhibitors can be used to treat gastrointestinal symptoms and bone pain. Different treatments work better for some people than others.

Many specialists recommended that people with mastocytosis have injectable epinephrine that they can use in case of anaphylactic shock. Other recommendations include trying to avoid known triggers of symptoms of mastocytosis.

FDA-Approved Treatments

The medication(s) listed below have been approved by the U.S. Food and Drug Administration (FDA) as orphan products for treatment of this condition.

- **Cromolyn sodium** (Brand name: Gastrocrom® (oral))—Manufactured by Azur Pharma

  FDA-approved indication: Treatment of mastocytosis.

- **Midostaurin** (Brand name: Rydapt)—Manufactured by Novartis Oncology

FDA-approved indication: Treatment of adult patients with aggressive systemic mastocytosis (ASM), systemic mastocytosis with associated hematological neoplasm (SM-AHN), or mast cell leukemia (MCL).

Statistics

Mastocytosis is described as a rare disease, but to our knowledge, the exact incidence and prevalence are not known. A disease is considered rare if it affects fewer than 200,000 people in the United States at any given time. An estimate of prevalence from a population-based study is approximately 1 case per 10,000 people.

While mastocytosis in general affects males and females in equal ratios, there appears to be a slight male predominance in childhood and a slight female predominance in adulthood. In children, 80 percent of cases appear during the first year of life, and the majority is limited to the skin. Adults who develop mastocytosis more often have systemic forms of the disease. Cutaneous forms of the disease account for less than 5 percent of adult cases.

Find a Specialist

If you need medical advice, you can look for doctors or other health-care professionals who have experience with this disease. You may find these specialists through advocacy organizations, clinical trials, or articles published in medical journals. You may also want to contact a university or tertiary medical center in your area, because these centers tend to see more complex cases and have the latest technology and treatments. If you can't find a specialist in your local area, try contacting national or international specialists. They may be able to refer you to someone they know through conferences or research efforts. Some specialists may be willing to consult with you or your local doctors over the phone or by email if you can't travel to them for care.

Section 11.4

Photosensitivity: Exposure to Light Can Cause Allergic Reactions

This section includes text excerpted from "The Sun and Your Medicine," U.S. Food and Drug Administration (FDA), September 25, 2015.

Fun in the sun can be had all year long—hiking, winter skiing, swimming, or just enjoying the warmth of the sun. However, when taking certain medicines, life in the sun can sometimes be less than fun.

Some medicines contain ingredients that may cause photosensitivity—a chemically induced change in the skin. Photosensitivity makes a person sensitive to sunlight and can cause sunburn-like symptoms, a rash or other unwanted side effects. It can be triggered by products applied to the skin or medicines taken by mouth or injected.

There are two types of photosensitivity—photoallergy and phototoxicity.

Photoallergy is an allergic reaction of the skin and may not occur until several days after sun exposure. Phototoxicity, which is more common, is an irritation of the skin and can occur within a few hours of sun exposure. Both types of photosensitivity occur after exposure to ultraviolet light—either natural sunlight or artificial light, such as a tanning booth.

There are certain types of medicines that can cause sensitivity to the sun. Some of these include:

- Antibiotics (ciprofloxacin, doxycycline, levofloxacin, ofloxacin, tetracycline, trimethoprim)

- Antifungals (flucytosine, griseofulvin, voriconazole)

- Antihistamines (cetirizine, diphenhydramine, loratadine, promethazine, cyproheptadine)

- Cholesterol lowering drugs (simvastatin, atorvastatin, lovastatin, pravastatin)

- Diuretics (thiazide diuretics: hydrochlorothiazide (HCTZ), chlorthalidone, chlorothiazide.; other diuretics: furosemide and triamterene)

- Nonsteroidal anti-inflammatory drugs (ibuprofen, naproxen, celecoxib, piroxicam, ketoprofen)

- Oral contraceptives and estrogens

- Phenothiazines (tranquilizers, antiemetics: examples, chlorpromazine, fluphenazine, promethazine, thioridazine, prochlorperazine)

- Psoralens (methoxsalen, trioxsalen)

- Retinoids (acitretin, isotretinoin)

- Sulfonamides (acetazolamide, sulfadiazine, sulfamethizole, sulfamethoxazole, sulfapyridine, sulfasalazine, sulfisoxazole)

- Sulfonylureas for type 2 diabetes (glipizide, glyburide)

- Alpha-hydroxy acids in cosmetics

Not all people who take or use the medicines mentioned will have a reaction. Also, if you experience a reaction on one occasion, it does not mean that you are guaranteed to have a reaction if you use the product again.

If you have concerns about developing a reaction, try to reduce your risk:

- When outside, seek shade, especially between 10 a.m. and 2 p.m.—some organizations recommend as late as 4 p.m.

Keep in mind that the sun's rays may be stronger when reflected off water, sand, and snow.

- Wear long-sleeved shirts, pants, sunglasses, and broad-brimmed hats to limit sun exposure.

- Use a broad sunscreen regularly and as directed. Broad-spectrum sunscreens provide protection against ultraviolet A (UVA) and ultraviolet B (UVB) radiation. A sun protection factor (SPF) 15 is the minimum number needed to provide measurable protection; however, a sunscreen with an SPF value of 30 or higher is recommended. Rarely, some sunscreen ingredients can cause photosensitivity themselves.

If you have questions about your medications and the possibility of a photosensitivity, contact your healthcare professional or pharmacists. Taking a few precautions can help limit your risk of photosensitivity and keep the sun shining on your fun.

What Is Sun Protection Factor?

When shopping for a sunscreen, consumers are faced with many choices. These choices include the sun protection factor (SPF) rating, which can vary from 8–50.

SPF is a measure of how much sunlight (ultraviolet (UV) radiation) is needed to develop sunburn after a sunscreen has been applied, compared to the amount of UV radiation required to develop sunburn on unprotected skin. The higher the SPF, the greater the protection is from UV radiation, and so the greater the sunburn protection.

It is important to know that SPF does not tell you how long you can be in the sun without getting sunburn. SPF does not mean that if you normally burn in 1 hour and you apply an SPF 8 sunscreen, it will take 8 hours for you to burn. Wrong. Instead, SPF tells you the amount of sunburn protection from UV radiation that is provided by sunscreens when they are used as directed—not burn protection time.

Several things can affect the amount of UV radiation exposure:

- Time of day

- Season

- Geographic location

- Altitude

- Weather conditions (cloudy day versus clear)

For example, a person spending 15 minutes in the sun at noon in Boston without sunscreen may not sunburn, but that same person could burn after spending 15 minutes in the sun in Miami because of the higher amount of UV radiation exposure in the geographic location.

Skin complexion, amount of sunscreen applied, and how often you reapply can also affect exposure. In order for a sunscreen to be effective, it's important that it be applied as directed, and reapplied as directed and needed based on physical activity. Participating in activities like swimming or activities that can promote heavy sweating may require more frequent reapplication.

Remember, SPF does not tell you how long you can be in the sun without getting sunburn. Instead, it's a measure of the amount of sunburn protection from UV radiation that is provided by sunscreens when they are used as directed and as needed.

Chapter 12

Anaphylaxis: Life-Threatening Allergies

Chapter Contents

Section 12.1

Anaphylaxis—Overview

This section contains text excerpted from the following
sources: Text in this section begins with excerpts from
"Anaphylaxis," MedlinePlus, National Institutes of Health (NIH),
September 21, 2016; Text beginning with the heading "Exercise-
Induced Anaphylaxis" is excerpted from "Exercise-Induced
Anaphylaxis," Genetic and Rare Diseases Information
Center (GARD), National Center for Advancing
Translational Sciences (NCATS), October 12, 2016.

Anaphylaxis is a serious allergic reaction. It can begin very quickly,
and symptoms may be life threatening. The most common causes are
reactions to foods (especially peanuts), medications, and stinging
insects. Other causes include exercise and exposure to latex. Sometimes no cause can be found.

It can affect many organs:

- Skin—itching, hives, redness, swelling

- Nose—sneezing, stuffy nose, runny nose

- Mouth—itching, swelling of the lips or tongue

- Throat—itching, tightness, trouble swallowing, swelling of the
  back of the throat

- Chest—shortness of breath, coughing, wheezing, chest pain, or
  tightness

- Heart—weak pulse, passing out, shock

- Gastrointestinal (GI) tract—vomiting, diarrhea, cramps

- Nervous system—dizziness or fainting

Exercise-Induced Anaphylaxis

Exercise-induced anaphylaxis (EIAn) is a rare disorder in which
anaphylaxis occurs in association with physical activity. Food-dependent exercise-induced anaphylaxis is a subset of this disorder in which
symptoms develop if exertion takes place within a few hours of eating
a specific food. In the case of food-dependent exercise-induced anaphylaxis, neither the food nor the exercise alone is enough to cause anaphylaxis. Vigorous forms of physical activity, such as jogging, are more

commonly associated with exercise-induced anaphylaxis, although lower levels of exertion (e.g., walking and yard work) are also capable of triggering attacks. However, the condition can be unpredictable; a given level of exercise may cause an episode on one occasion but not another. Symptoms of exercise-induced anaphylaxis may include itching, hives (urticaria), flushing, extreme fatigue, and wheezing. Affected individuals may also experience nausea, abdominal cramping, and diarrhea. Continuing the physical activity causes the symptoms to become worse. However, if the individual stops the activity when the symptoms first appear, there is usually improvement within minutes. In most cases, these conditions are sporadic, though familial cases have been reported.

Treatment

Prevention remains the best treatment for patients with exercise-induced anaphylaxis. Management should include education about safe conditions for exercise, identification and avoidance of offending foods, the importance of stopping exercise immediately if symptoms develop, the appropriate use of epinephrine, and the importance of having epinephrine available at all times. Patients may also be advised to wear a medical alert bracelet with instructions on the use of epinephrine. The following factors may increase the risk of an exercise-induced attack and are often considered cofactors: nonsteroidal anti-inflammatory drugs (NSAIDs), alcohol, certain phases of the menstrual cycle, temperature extremes, and seasonal pollen exposure. As a result, patients may be advised to minimize their exposure to these risk factors.

Prognosis

The prognosis for patients with exercise-induced anaphylaxis is generally favorable. Most patients experience fewer and less severe attacks over time. Although rare, fatalities have been reported, though many of these cases had extenuating circumstances. No cure for this disorder exists. With appropriate lifestyle changes, however, patients may be able to reduce or eliminate episodes of anaphylaxis, and prompt intervention can shorten those episodes that do occur.

Section 12.2

Abnormal Immune Cells May Cause Unprovoked Anaphylaxis

This section includes text excerpted from "Abnormal Immune Cells May Cause Unprovoked Anaphylaxis," National Institutes of Health (NIH), November 9, 2007. Reviewed August 2018.

From recurrent episodes of idiopathic anaphylaxis—a potentially life-threatening condition of unknown cause characterized by a drop in blood pressure, fainting episodes, difficulty in breathing, and wheezing. In some of these individuals, researchers have found mast cells (a type of immune cell involved in allergic reactions) that have a mutated cell surface receptor that disturbs normal processes within the cell. Scientists supported by the National Institute of Allergy and Infectious Diseases (NIAID), part of the National Institutes of Health (NIH), say the association of this mutation with unprovoked anaphylaxis is striking. The hope is that these individuals may respond to inhibitors targeting the mutated cell surface receptor.

While some people suffer anaphylaxis as part of a serious allergic reaction, in two out of three people, anaphylaxis has no known cause and thus the anaphylactic reaction is called idiopathic. Anaphylaxis occurs when mast cells release large quantities of chemicals (histamines, prostaglandins and leukotrienes) that cause blood vessels to leak, bronchial tissues to swell and blood pressure to drop. Resulting conditions such as shock and unconsciousness usually resolve in most people treated with epinephrine (adrenaline) and first aid measures. In rare cases, however, death may occur.

Abnormally low blood pressure and fainting episodes are also features of mastocytosis—a disease in which people have an excessive number of mast cells. Several years ago, Dean Metcalfe, M.D., chief of the Laboratory of Allergic Diseases at NIAID, Cem Akin, M.D., Ph.D., and their NIAID colleagues decided to find out whether idiopathic anaphylaxis might have a genetic trigger related to that seen in mastocytosis. It is known that systemic mastocytosis in adults often results from a mutation in the Kit receptor found on the surface of mast cells, a discovery first made by Dr. Metcalfe's team in 1995.

The mutation causes an abnormal growth of mast cells, as is observed in bone marrow biopsies of patients with mastocytosis. So the NIAID team asked, if the Kit mutation could make mast cells grow and cause mastocytosis, and this was associated with anaphylactic reactions, could the same mutation predispose mast cells to release chemicals responsible for idiopathic anaphylaxis?

In a two-year study conducted at the NIH Clinical Center (CC), the researchers examined 48 patients diagnosed with mastocytosis with or without associated anaphylaxis, 12 patients with idiopathic anaphylaxis, and 12 patients with neither disease. Within the group of 12 patients who had idiopathic anaphylaxis, five were found with evidence of a disorder in a line of mast cells (clonal mast cell disorder). The researchers looked for evidence of a Kit mutation in three patients by analyzing bone marrow samples, and all three samples yielded a positive result. The findings demonstrate that some patients with idiopathic anaphylaxis have an aberrant population of mast cells with mutated Kit.

"We believe the mutation may be predisposing people to idiopathic anaphylaxis," says Dr. Metcalfe. "Our findings suggest that in patients with idiopathic anaphylaxis as well as in people with severe allergies, we should look for critical genetic mutations that may change the way a mast cell reacts."

Dr. Metcalfe and his NIAID colleagues report their findings in two journals. The study that appears in an early online edition in Blood describes the presence of an abnormal mast cell population in a subset of patients with idiopathic anaphylaxis. The findings about the mechanism leading to mass cell activation by Kit and the IgE receptor responsible for allergic reactions appear online in Cellular Signalling.

According to the NIAID team, both Kit and the immunoglobulin E (IgE) receptor responsible for allergic reactions activate mast cells via a common interior protein of mast cells. They also found that the mutated Kit markedly elevates the activity of that protein, which results in increased cell signaling.

The scientists are now looking to see if artificial mast cells with mutated Kit behave or release chemicals in a manner different from normal mast cells, and also if they respond to inhibitors targeting Kit.

Section 12.3

Medical Identification Critical for People with Life-Threatening Allergies

"Medical Identification Critical for People with Life-Threatening
Allergies," © 2018 Omnigraphics. Reviewed August 2018.

In an emergency, making quick decisions with regard to medical treatment may mean the difference between life and death. It is critical for medical response personnel to be aware of any allergies or medical conditions that the patient they are treating might have. But if the patient is unconscious or unable to answer questions, they cannot provide this vital information. As a result, medical care may be delayed, or the treatment provided may be inappropriate for the patient's condition or even dangerous to their health. Wearable medical identification (ID) can play a life-saving role in such emergencies.

An individual with a serious medical condition or a life-threatening allergy can carry the information on a bracelet or necklace that is immediately identifiable. Wearable medical IDs can warn medical responders about the presence of such conditions as Alzheimer disease (AD), asthma, autism, diabetes, epilepsy, heart disease, high blood pressure, or organ transplant. They can also carry information about allergies to pharmaceutical drugs, foods, insects, or substances such as latex. They also typically display the individual's blood type, along with specific medical treatment requests such as DNR (do not resuscitate), DNI (do not intubate), or organ donation. Most medical IDs also list any medications the individual takes regularly as well as the names and phone numbers of people to contact in case of emergency. It has become common practice for emergency medical technicians (EMTs) and other first responders to look for medical IDs before proceeding with treatment.

Obtaining a Medical ID

Wearable medical IDs are available from many sources online. They come in a wide variety of attractive styles and are fully customizable for individual needs. Some wearable IDs are designed to inform emergency medical responders of the presence of a more detailed medical alert card. These cards are typically carried in a wallet, purse, or backpack and provide further information about the patient's allergies or other health issues. Patients can consult with their primary-care physicians to obtain guidance in deciding what information to include on their ID.

In addition to people with life-threatening allergies and other health conditions, parents of small children and people who serve as sole caregivers for elderly or disabled individuals should also consider wearing a medical ID bracelet or necklace. If the parent or caregiver is involved in an accident or has another type of medical emergency, the medical ID can provide contact information for alternate care providers to ensure that dependent family members will receive needed assistance and remain safe. Experts also recommend wearable medical IDs for solo travelers, athletes who run or bike alone outdoors over long distances, and people who have undergone recent surgery. At a minimum, these IDs should include contact information in case of emergency.

Reference

White, Jenna. "Top Ten Reasons People Wear Medical ID Jewelry," Lauren's Hope, February 27, 2013.

Section 12.4

Red Meat Allergy Linked to Anaphylaxis

This section includes text excerpted from "Unexplained Cases of Anaphylaxis Linked to Red Meat Allergy," National Institutes of Health (NIH), December 12, 2017.

Anaphylaxis is a life-threatening allergic reaction that can cause your airway to constrict and your blood pressure to drop dangerously low. Some people have repeated episodes of anaphylaxis for unknown reasons. Food allergies are a common cause of anaphylaxis; however, it's not always easy to identify a food to which you're allergic. Avoiding your allergy triggers is the best way to prevent anaphylaxis.

Researchers recently discovered a rare red meat allergy that starts after being bitten by a lone star tick. The allergy is to a sugar molecule called galactose-α-1,3-galactose (α-Gal), or alpha-gal, that's found in beef, pork, lamb, and other red meats.

It's difficult to identify this allergy because of its unusual time delay before symptoms appear. Allergic reactions to alpha-gal usually happen between 3–6 hours after eating red meat. In contrast, reactions to most common allergy-causing foods, like peanuts or shellfish, begin about 5–30 minutes after a person is exposed.

To investigate alpha-gal allergy as a possible cause for unexplained cases of recurrent anaphylaxis, a team led by Dr. Dean D. Metcalfe at National Institutes of Health's (NIH) National Institute of Allergy and Infectious Diseases (NIAID) analyzed 70 patients who had been diagnosed with idiopathic anaphylaxis. Idiopathic means a cause couldn't be identified. The research was supported by NIAID. Results were published in Allergy.

The researchers enrolled 46 females and 24 males between the ages of 15 and 70 years old. Six adult male participants had IgE antibodies—immune proteins associated with allergies—to alpha-gal in their blood. Each of the men had a history of tick bites and lived in states where lone star ticks reside. After implementing diets free of beef, pork, lamb, and venison, none of these participants experienced anaphylaxis for the period they were followed for the study (18 months to 3 years).

Among the six participants with the alpha-gal allergy, two also had a rare condition called indolent systemic mastocytosis, or ISM. People with ISM have an abnormally high number of mast cells, a type of immune cell that contributes to anaphylaxis and other allergic symptoms by releasing histamine and other chemicals that cause inflammation. The participants with ISM had more severe reactions than those without ISM, even though they had lower levels of antibodies to alpha-gal.

"Alpha-gal allergy appears to be yet another reason to protect oneself from tick bites," says NIAID Director Dr. Anthony S. Fauci.

"We often think of ticks as carriers of infectious diseases, such as Lyme disease, but the research strongly suggests that bites from this particular species of tick can lead to this unusual allergy," explains coauthor Dr. Melody C. Carter at NIAID. "The association is increasingly clear, but we still need to discover exactly how these two events are linked and why some people with similar exposure to tick bites seem to be more prone to developing alpha-gal allergy than others."

Part Three

Foods and Food Additives That Trigger Allergic Reactions

Chapter 13

Food Allergy: An Overview

Have you noticed food allergy warnings at restaurants? Maybe you've heard about peanut-free classrooms and flights. People who have serious reactions to certain foods must be careful about what they eat, and what others eat around them. There's no cure for food allergies. But researchers are learning more about how to prevent and treat this condition.

Allergic reactions happen when your immune system—your body's defense against germs and foreign substances—overreacts to something that's normally harmless. In the United States, most food allergies are caused by peanuts, tree nuts, fish, shellfish, eggs, milk, wheat, and soy. Allergies show up most often in children. But they can develop at any age.

Food allergy symptoms can range from mild to severe. Some people experience a life-threatening reaction called anaphylaxis. Symptoms may include trouble breathing, dizziness, and fainting. When you have a food allergy, there's no way to predict how your body will react when you're exposed. You might have a mild reaction one time and a severe reaction the next.

This chapter contains text excerpted from the following sources: Text in this chapter begins with excerpts from "Understanding Food Allergies," *NIH News in Health*, National Institutes of Health (NIH), March 2017; Text beginning with the heading "Understanding Food Allergy" is excerpted from "Understanding Food Allergy," MedlinePlus, National Institutes of Health (NIH), June 23, 2017; Text beginning with the heading "FDA's Role: Labeling" is excerpted from "Food Allergies: What You Need to Know," U.S. Food and Drug Administration (FDA), February 8, 2018.

If you think that you or your child may have a food allergy, see your healthcare provider. Your doctor will take a detailed medical history and perform a physical examination. If a diagnosis of food allergy seems likely, they may recommend a blood test or skin prick test. These results will help determine if you or your child has a food allergy.

National Institutes of Health (NIH) researchers have been working to better understand food allergies. "There has been a lot of research on peanut allergy because it is often severe, lifelong, and has a huge impact on quality of life," explains Dr. Scott Sicherer, a pediatric food allergy expert at Mount Sinai's Icahn School of Medicine. Scientists hope the progress they make on peanut allergy will help guide how to handle other food allergies.

Researchers carried out a large clinical trial called Learning Early About Peanut Allergy (LEAP). The study looked at infants' chances of developing an allergy if they ate peanut-containing foods at an early age. Six hundred and forty infants who were at high risk of developing a peanut allergy were enrolled in the trial. The infants were randomly placed in either a peanut-eating or peanut-avoiding group. They continued these diets until they were 5 years old. Infants who ate peanut-containing foods beginning early in life had an 81 percent lower chance of developing a peanut allergy.

"Based on the strength of these findings, an expert panel sponsored by NIH issued updated guidelines to help healthcare providers work with families to introduce peanut-containing foods to infants to help prevent the development of peanut allergy," Sicherer says.

The panel provided three guidelines that describe when and how to give these foods. The recommendations are based on how likely a baby is to develop peanut allergy. Talk with your doctor before you introduce any peanut-containing foods to your infant. The doctor may tell you when and how to start feeding peanut to your baby or recommend doing allergy testing first.

"It's important to understand that these guidelines are about preventing peanut allergy, not treating an existing peanut allergy," Sicherer explains.

The new guidelines may come as a surprise to some people. Almost 20 years ago, experts recommended that babies at high risk for developing peanut allergy avoid peanut-containing foods until age 3. But nearly 10 years ago, experts withdrew this recommendation. There was no proof that it worked.

"The most recent change in guidance was prompted by the very compelling results of the LEAP study," says Dr. Marshall Plaut, a food allergy expert at NIH. "The new guidelines are based on these results and the clinical knowledge of the expert panel who developed them."

Whether this strategy works for other food allergies isn't known. "More research is needed to find out if early dietary introduction of other foods may help prevent allergy to those foods," Sicherer explains.

NIH scientists are also looking at ways to treat people who already have food allergies. One promising strategy is called oral immunotherapy. It involves eating small, slowly increasing amounts of the allergy-causing food. A study tried this approach for peanut-allergic preschool children. Almost 80 percent of children given the treatment could safely eat peanut-containing foods afterward. More studies are being done to improve the safety and effectiveness of the approach. The therapy is also being studied for people with milk and egg allergies in small clinical trials.

There may be other ways to provide this type of therapy. One ongoing study is investigating using a skin patch to deliver small amounts of peanut protein to peanut-allergic patients. Early results have shown some promise among young children with peanut allergy. Researchers will continue to assess this approach.

Food allergy studies have to be done very carefully because reactions can be life threatening. "It's important to understand how much careful thought goes into ethically designing research studies, particularly those involving vulnerable populations like children," Plaut says. "Sometimes answers take longer than we would all like. But it's critical to find them in a way and at a pace that is thoughtful and safe."

For now, there are no treatments for food allergies. But avoiding allergy-causing foods can help prevent symptoms. Read food labels carefully. Wash your hands and surfaces you touch to prevent accidental contact.

Sometimes it can be difficult to avoid exposure completely. Carrying an epinephrine auto-injector can be lifesaving. This device delivers a hormone that maintains blood pressure and can open your airways.

Talk with your healthcare provider to learn more about preventing and treating food allergies.

Understanding Food Allergy

Food allergies are often misunderstood.

"This disease is common and it has a dramatic impact not only on the lives of people who have the allergy but on the lives of anyone who cares about them," says Pamela Guerrerio, M.D., Ph.D. She is chief of the Food Allergy Research Unit of the Laboratory of Allergic

Diseases (LAD) at NIH's National Institute of Allergy and Infectious Diseases (NIAID). Dr. Guerrerio spoke to NIH MedlinePlus magazine about food allergies and research to help understand and potentially prevent them.

Allergic Reactions

Allergic reactions can be scary if you've never had one before. If you have a mild allergic reaction, which could include hives, itching, sneezing, or a runny nose, you should take an antihistamine if it's available and monitor for more severe symptoms, Dr. Guerrerio said. If you have a more severe reaction, you should seek immediate medical attention at an emergency room or call 911.

Severe reactions include difficulty breathing or low blood pressure, which can cause confusion, paleness, a weak pulse, or a lack of consciousness. Dr. Guerrerio said if the reaction is severe or if it involves multiple organ systems—for example the person has hives and is also vomiting—you should administer an EpiPen if you have one and call 911.

Once the initial reaction has been treated, you should see an allergist to get tested for a food allergy and discuss a course of action.

Development and Diagnosis

Blood and skin tests can be helpful but are not enough to determine a food allergy. You must also have clinical symptoms when you eat the food. Since these tests can result in false positives, "It's important that they are interpreted within the context of the patient's entire health picture," said Dr. Guerrerio. Most allergies develop early in life, Dr. Guerrerio said, and food allergy development peaks around age one.

It is uncommon for an allergy to develop later in life, though there are exceptions. The most common food allergies in adults include shellfish and nuts.

As people with a food allergy get older, they have increased chances of developing other allergic diseases or allergies. Sometimes people grow out of an allergy. "It's really only with more research into food allergy that we're going to find better ways to diagnose, prevent, and treat the disease."

Food Allergy Studies

With so many unanswered questions surrounding food allergies, it's important that researchers continue to study them. "It's really only with more research into food allergy that we're going to find better ways to diagnose, prevent, and treat the disease," Dr. Guerrerio said.

A major, NIAID-funded study on peanut allergy prevention recently took place in the United Kingdom. This led to changes in food allergy guidelines from NIH. The study, Learning Early About Peanut Allergy (LEAP), looked at early exposure to peanuts in infants at high risk of developing a peanut allergy.

The study looked at 640 infants under the age of 1 who had either eczema, an egg allergy, or both. These conditions indicate a child is at high risk of developing a peanut allergy.

The children were split into two groups. The parents of the first group of children were told to have their child avoid peanut-containing foods completely until age 5. Parents of the second group were told to introduce peanuts into their child's diet immediately and children were to eat peanut-containing foods at least three times a week.

At age 5, the children had a peanut oral food challenge to see if they had developed a peanut allergy.

"The remarkable result was that the rate of peanut allergy was almost 80 percent lower in the group that had eaten peanut-containing products compared to the group that had avoided them," Dr. Guerrerio said.

Following the LEAP study and a follow-up study, LEAP-ON, an expert panel led by NIAID reviewed the available evidence and recommended that infants with a high risk of developing a peanut allergy be exposed to peanut-containing foods as early as 4–6 months old. The goal is to reduce the development of a peanut allergy.

Dr. Guerrerio said it's important that parents of children with a high risk for developing a peanut allergy speak to a provider before introducing peanuts into a child's diet. The provider can help determine if the child should first see an allergist for a food allergy test.

NIAID is also conducting research at the NIH Clinical Center in Bethesda, Maryland. The Institute is looking for participants for a study called "Natural History and Genetics of Food Allergy and Related Conditions."

The 10-year study aims to better understand the development of a food allergy and look at nutrition and growth in children with food allergies.

"Most of the major food allergens—such as milk, eggs, peanuts, soy, and wheat—are nutritionally dense. The concern is that children who have to avoid those foods because of their allergies will be at high risk for not getting enough nutrition. So we wanted to ask whether children with food allergy are indeed susceptible to nutritional deficiencies," Dr. Guerrerio said.

Eligible participants include anyone between the ages of 2 and 99 who has a food allergy confirmed by a doctor's testing. NIAID is also looking for healthy individuals (who do not have a food allergy) for the control group.

The FDA's Role: Labeling

To help Americans avoid the health risks posed by food allergens, U.S. Food and Drug Administration (FDA) enforces the Food Allergen Labeling and Consumer Protection Act of 2004 (FALCPA) (the Act). The Act applies to the labeling of foods regulated by the FDA which includes all foods except poultry, most meats, certain egg products, and most alcoholic beverages which are regulated by other federal agencies. The Act requires that food labels must clearly identify the food source names of any ingredients that are one of the major food allergens or contain any protein derived from a major food allergen. As a result, food labels help allergic consumers identify offending foods or ingredients so they can more easily avoid them.

What Are Major Food Allergens?

While more than 160 foods can cause allergic reactions in people with food allergies, the law identifies the eight most common allergenic foods. These foods account for 90 percent of food allergic reactions, and are the food sources from which many other ingredients are derived.

The eight foods identified by the law are:

1. Milk
2. Eggs
3. Fish (e.g., bass, flounder, cod)
4. Crustacean shellfish (e.g., crab, lobster, shrimp)
5. Tree nuts (e.g., almonds, walnuts, pecans)
6. Peanuts
7. Wheat
8. Soybeans

These eight foods, and any ingredient that contains protein derived from one or more of them, are designated as "major food allergens" by FALCPA.

How Major Food Allergens Are Listed

The law requires that food labels identify the food source names of all major food allergens used to make the food. This requirement is met if the common or usual name of an ingredient (e.g., buttermilk) that is a major food allergen already identifies that allergen's food source name (i.e., milk). Otherwise, the allergen's food source name must be declared at least once on the food label in one of two ways.

The name of the food source of a major food allergen must appear:

1. In parentheses following the name of the ingredient.
    Examples: "lecithin (soy)," "flour (wheat)," and "whey (milk)" or

2. Immediately after or next to the list of ingredients in a "contains" statement. Example: "Contains Wheat, Milk, and Soy."

Severe Food Allergies Can Be Life Threatening

Following ingestion of a food allergen(s), a person with food allergies can experience a severe, life-threatening allergic reaction called anaphylaxis.

This can lead to:

*   constricted airways in the lungs;

*   severe lowering of blood pressure and shock ("anaphylactic shock"); and

*   suffocation by swelling of the throat.

Each year in the United States, it is estimated that anaphylaxis to food results in:

*   30,000 emergency room visits

*   2,000 hospitalizations

*   150 deaths

Prompt administration of epinephrine by autoinjector (e.g., EpiPen) during early symptoms of anaphylaxis may help prevent these serious consequences.

Mild Symptoms Can Become More Severe

Initially mild symptoms that occur after ingesting a food allergen are not always a measure of mild severity. In fact, if not treated promptly, these symptoms can become more serious in a very short amount of time, and could lead to anaphylaxis.

Know the Symptoms

Symptoms of food allergies typically appear from within a few minutes to two hours after a person has eaten the food to which he or she is allergic.

Allergic reactions can include:

- Hives

- Flushed skin or rash

- Tingling or itchy sensation in the mouth

- Face, tongue, or lip swelling

- Vomiting and/or diarrhea

- Abdominal cramps

- Coughing or wheezing

- Dizziness and/or lightheadedness

- Swelling of the throat and vocal cords

- Difficulty breathing

- Loss of consciousness

About Other Allergens

Persons may still be allergic to—and have serious reactions to—foods other than the eight foods identified by the law. So, always be sure to read the food label's ingredient list carefully to avoid the food allergens in question.

What to Do If Symptoms Occur

The appearance of symptoms after eating food may be a sign of a food allergy. The food(s) that caused these symptoms should be avoided, and the affected person, should contact a doctor or healthcare provider for appropriate testing and evaluation.

- Persons found to have a food allergy should be taught to read labels and avoid the offending foods. They should also be taught, in case of accidental ingestion, to recognize the early symptoms of an allergic reaction, and be properly educated on—and armed with—appropriate treatment measures.

- Persons with a known food allergy who begin experiencing symptoms while, or after, eating a food should initiate treatment immediately, and go to a nearby emergency room if symptoms progress.

Food Allergen "Advisory" Labeling

The FALCPA's labeling requirements do not apply to the potential or unintentional presence of major food allergens in foods resulting from "cross-contact" situations during manufacturing, e.g., because of shared equipment or processing lines. In the context of food allergens, "cross-contact" occurs when a residue or trace amount of an allergenic food becomes incorporated into another food not intended to contain it. FDA guidance for the food industry states that food allergen advisory statements, e.g., "may contain (allergen)" or "produced in a facility that also uses (allergen)" should not be used as a substitute for adhering to current good manufacturing practices and must be truthful and not misleading. The FDA is considering ways to best manage the use of these types of statements by manufacturers to better inform consumers.

Reporting Adverse Effects and Labeling Concerns

If you think that you or a family member has an injury or illness that you believe is associated with having eaten a particular food, including individuals with food allergies and those with celiac disease, contact your healthcare provider immediately. Also, report the suspected foodborne illness to the FDA in either of these ways: Individuals can report a problem with a food or its labeling, such as potential misuse of "gluten-free" claims, to the FDA in either of these ways:

1. Contact MedWatch, the FDA's Safety Information and Adverse Event Reporting Program, at 800-332-1088, or file a MedWatch voluntary report at www.fda.gov/MedWatch.

2. Contact the consumer complaint coordinator in their area. The list of FDA consumer complaint coordinators is available at www.fda.gov/Safety/ReportaProblem/ ConsumerComplaintCoordinators/default.

Chapter 14

Food Allergy or Food Intolerance: How Do You Tell the Difference?

Do certain foods make you itchy or cause an upset stomach? Physical reactions to certain foods are common, but a food intolerance or a food allergy cause most such problems.

A food allergy occurs when you eat something that abnormally triggers your body's immune system. Sometimes even a tiny amount of a food can trigger such a response. The body may respond to the food allergen (something that causes an allergic reaction) with such symptoms as digestive problems, hives, or an impaired airway. In some cases, the reaction may be life threatening and cause anaphylaxis. Anaphylaxis is a severe whole body reaction to an allergen.

Foods often associated with allergic reactions:

- Fish and shellfish

- Peanuts, walnuts

- Eggs

Food intolerance is different from a food allergy. Food intolerance is a reaction to a food that does not involve the body's immune system.

This chapter includes text excerpted from "Is It Food Allergy or Food Intolerance?" U.S. Department of Veterans Affairs (VA), May 8, 2018.

While the reaction may feel as if it is a food allergy, if the immune system is not responding, it is food intolerance. Sometimes it is an additive to a food that may trigger the intolerance symptoms. Some common intolerance in adults are:

- Monosodium glutamate (MSG) is a flavor enhancer which, in large amounts, can cause such symptoms as flushing, headache, and chest discomfort. MSG is found in prepared foods such as sauces, dressing, chips, and seasonings.

- Sulfites occur in some foods, such as some wines, and used in food to increase crispness. Intolerance to sulfites can cause breathing problems for people with asthma.

Lactose intolerance defines food intolerance to a sugar, lactase, found in milk and milk products. While uncommon in young children, it is more common in adults. The enzyme needed to break down the lactase declines as people age. When lactase is not broken down by the needed enzyme, the gut may respond with symptoms such as abdominal pain, bloating, and diarrhea. Your doctor can run some laboratory tests to determine if you have lactose intolerance.

It may take a little detective work to figure out which foods trigger your allergy symptoms. But one thing that can help is to use My HealtheVet's Self-Entered Allergies (www.myhealth.va.gov/mhv-portal-web/web/myhealthevet/va-allergies-adverse-reactions) and Food Journal (www.myhealth.va.gov/mhv-portal-web/web/myhealthevet/food-journal) features. You can record what you eat and when you discover that you get allergy symptoms, look for patterns.

Chapter 15

Milk Allergy

Chapter Contents

Section 15.1

Understanding Milk Allergy

"Understanding Milk Allergy,"
© 2018 Omnigraphics. Reviewed August 2018.

Milk allergy is the most common type of food allergy, particularly among infants and children. Up to 3 percent of infants develop an allergy to milk and dairy products. While most milk allergies pertain to cow's milk, they may also include adverse reactions to milk from other mammals, like goats, sheep, or buffalo. A milk allergy is primarily caused by an abnormal response of the body's immune system to milk protein. The body produces immunoglobulin E (IgE) antibodies to neutralize the protein allergen. These antibodies trigger the release of histamines and other chemicals that produce allergic reactions.

Milk allergy, for the most part, is seen more frequently in infants than in adults. An allergy to milk can develop all of a sudden, even though the food has been well tolerated in the past. While the exact causes of milk allergy are still unclear, certain risk factors have been recognized that increase a person's likelihood of developing a milk or dairy allergy. One of the most significant factors is the existence of milk allergy or any other type of allergy in either or both parents. Besides family history, the presence of other allergic conditions, like atopic dermatitis, also raises the risk of developing milk allergy, particularly in infants.

Most milk allergies manifest within the first year of life. Although 20 percent of children outgrow their allergy by age four and 80 percent by age sixteen, some remain allergic to the food all through life. Milk allergy can manifest in both breastfed and formula-fed babies. Babies who are fed formula can develop allergy symptoms through direct ingestion of milk products. Those who are breastfed can also develop milk allergy, however, through exposure to traces of cow's milk protein that pass into the breast milk from dairy products consumed by the mother. Infants who appear to be allergic to human milk are usually reacting to foods that pass through the breast milk rather than to the breast milk itself.

Symptoms and Diagnosis

In some people, allergic reactions to milk can occur quickly, with symptoms appearing within a few minutes of ingestion of a small amount of milk. In others, the symptoms may appear gradually after a few hours, or even days. A mild allergy to milk might involve such symptoms as hives or skin rashes around the mouth. More severe reactions might include respiratory and gastrointestinal symptoms such as wheezing, flatulence, diarrhea, vomiting, blood or mucus in stools, and infantile colic.

The mechanism for non-IgE-mediated milk allergy remains largely unclear and there are no validated tests for its diagnosis. If a non-IgE-mediated allergy is suspected, the allergist may recommend an extended period of avoidance. If a milk allergy is suspected, the first step would be to consult a doctor or an allergist. After taking the patient's history, the doctor may administer a skin prick test (SPT). In this procedure, a small amount of milk or a milk protein extract is introduced under the skin with the help of a small, sterile probe. A localized allergic response in the skin, such as a red bump or flare, can indicate an allergy to milk protein. The skin prick test is usually followed up with a blood test, which gives a numerical value for IgE antibodies in the blood. These antibodies are responsible for the immediate allergic responses to milk.

An oral food challenge (OFC) is recommended when the doctor is unable to make a definitive diagnosis with SPT and serum antibody levels. In this procedure, the patient ingests measured doses of food containing milk or a milk powder to check for a possible allergic reaction. It is essential that the food challenge be carried out under medical supervision with access to emergency treatment in case the test precipitates a severe allergic reaction.

Milk allergy that is characterized by a delayed onset of mostly gastrointestinal symptoms usually involves T-cells (a type of white blood cell) rather than IgE antibodies. The mechanism for non-IgE-mediated milk allergy remains largely unclear and there are no validated tests for its diagnosis. If a non-IgE-mediated allergy is suspected, the allergist may recommend an extended period of avoidance of all milk products, followed by a phased reintroduction.

Both types of milk allergy are different from lactose intolerance, which is not an allergy. Instead, it occurs when people are unable to digest lactose, the sugar found in milk, because their body does not produce sufficient quantities of lactase, the enzyme needed to metabolize lactose. Although it is not related to milk allergy, people with lactose intolerance often experience similar symptoms after ingesting milk, such as abdominal cramps, bloating, and diarrhea.

Prevention and Treatment

As is the case for all food allergies, the only way to prevent an allergic reaction to milk is to avoid milk proteins completely. The Federal Food Allergen Labeling and Consumer Protection Act (FALCPA) of 2004 established guidelines for labeling packaged food to warn consumers about the potential presence of eight major food allergens, including milk. Therefore, people with food allergies should read product labels and ingredient statements carefully before purchasing or consuming packaged food. Milk and milk derivatives can be found in a wide range of food products, including butter, cheese, chocolate, cream, custard, pudding, and yogurt.

Mild allergic reactions to milk can be treated with antihistamines, but a severe anaphylactic reaction requires immediate medical attention. An injection of epinephrine (adrenaline) is usually given to treat anaphylaxis, and those with severe milk allergy are generally advised to carry an epinephrine auto-injector with them at all times. Following treatment with epinephrine, the patient needs to be placed in an emergency setting for further evaluation and treatment in order to prevent a recurrence of symptoms.

References

1. "Milk Allergy," Food Allergy Research and Education (FARE), 2015.

2. "Milk and Dairy Allergy," American College of Allergy, Asthma, and Immunology (ACAAI), 2014.

3. "Milk: One of the Ten Priority Food Allergens," Health Canada, December 4, 2012.

Section 15.2

Lactose Intolerance

This section includes text excerpted from "Lactose Intolerance," National Institute of Diabetes and Digestive and Kidney Diseases (NIDDK), February 2018.

Definition and Facts for Lactose Intolerance

Lactose intolerance is a condition in which you have digestive symptoms—such as bloating, diarrhea, and gas—after you consume foods or drinks that contain lactose. Lactose is a sugar that is naturally found in milk and milk products, like cheese or ice cream. In lactose intolerance, digestive symptoms are caused by lactose malabsorption. Lactose malabsorption is a condition in which your small intestine cannot digest, or break down, all the lactose you eat or drink. Not everyone with lactose malabsorption has digestive symptoms after they consume lactose. Only people who have symptoms are lactose intolerant. Most people with lactose intolerance can consume some amount of lactose without having symptoms. Different people can tolerate different amounts of lactose before having symptoms. Lactose intolerance is different from a milk allergy. A milk allergy is an immune system disorder.

How Common Is Lactose Malabsorption?

While most infants can digest lactose, many people begin to develop lactose malabsorption—a reduced ability to digest lactose—after infancy. Experts estimate that about 68 percent of the world's population has lactose malabsorption. Lactose malabsorption is more common in some parts of the world than in others. In Africa and Asia, most people have lactose malabsorption. In some regions, such as northern Europe, many people carry a gene that allows them to digest lactose after infancy, and lactose malabsorption is less common. In the United States, about 36 percent of people have lactose malabsorption.

While lactose malabsorption causes lactose intolerance, not all people with lactose malabsorption have lactose intolerance.

Who Is More Likely to Have Lactose Intolerance?

You are more likely to have lactose intolerance if you are from, or your family is from, a part of the world where lactose malabsorption is more common. In the United States, the following ethnic and racial groups are more likely to have lactose malabsorption:

- African Americans
- American Indians
- Asian Americans
- Hispanics/Latinos

Because these ethnic and racial groups are more likely to have lactose malabsorption, they are also more likely to have the symptoms of lactose intolerance.

Lactose intolerance is least common among people who are from, or whose families are from, Europe.

What Are the Complications of Lactose Intolerance?

Lactose intolerance may affect your health if it keeps you from getting enough nutrients, such as calcium and vitamin D. Milk and milk products, which contain lactose, are some of the main sources of calcium, vitamin D, and other nutrients. You need calcium throughout your life to grow and have healthy bones. If you don't get enough calcium, your bones may become weak and more likely to break. This condition is called osteoporosis. If you have lactose intolerance, you can change your diet to make sure you get enough calcium while also managing your symptoms.

Symptoms and Causes of Lactose Intolerance

What Are the Symptoms of Lactose Intolerance?

If you have lactose intolerance, you may have symptoms within a few hours after you have milk or milk products, or other foods that contain lactose. Your symptoms may include:

- Bloating
- Diarrhea
- Gas
- Nausea
- Pain in your abdomen
- Stomach "growling" or rumbling sounds
- Vomiting

Your symptoms may be mild or severe, depending on how much lactose you have.

What Causes Lactose Intolerance?

Lactose intolerance is caused by lactose malabsorption. If you have lactose malabsorption, your small intestine makes low levels of lactase—the enzyme that breaks down lactose—and can't digest all the lactose you eat or drink.

The undigested lactose passes into your colon. Bacteria in your colon break down the lactose and create fluid and gas. In some people, this extra fluid and gas cause lactose intolerance symptoms.

In some cases, your genes are the reason for lactose intolerance. Genes play a role in the following conditions, and these conditions can lead to low levels of lactase in your small intestine and lactose malabsorption:

- **Lactase nonpersistence.** In people with lactase nonpersistence, the small intestine makes less lactase after infancy. Lactase levels get lower with age. Symptoms of lactose intolerance may not begin until later childhood, the teen years, or early adulthood. Lactase nonpersistence, also called primary lactase deficiency, is the most common cause of low lactase levels.

- **Congenital lactase deficiency.** In this rare condition, the small intestine makes little or no lactase, starting at birth.

Not all causes of lactose intolerance are genetic. The following can also lead to lactose intolerance:

- Injury to the small intestine. Infections, diseases, or other conditions that injure your small intestine, like Crohn's disease or celiac disease, may cause it to make less lactase. Treatments—such as medicines, surgery, or radiation therapy—for other conditions may also injure your small intestine. Lactose intolerance caused by injury to the small intestine is called secondary lactose intolerance. If the cause of the injury is treated, you may be able to tolerate lactose again.

- Premature birth. In premature babies, or babies born too soon, the small intestine may not make enough lactase for a short time after birth. The small intestine usually makes more lactase as the baby gets older.

What Is the Difference between Lactose Intolerance and Milk Allergies?

Lactose intolerance and milk allergies are different conditions with different causes. Lactose intolerance is caused by problems digesting lactose, the natural sugar in milk. In contrast, milk allergies are caused by your immune system's response to one or more proteins in milk and milk products. A milk allergy most often appears in the first year of life, while lactose intolerance typically appears later. Lactose intolerance can cause uncomfortable symptoms, while a serious allergic reaction to milk can be life threatening.

Diagnosis of Lactose Intolerance

How Do Doctors Diagnose Lactose Intolerance?

To diagnose lactose intolerance, your doctor will ask about your symptoms, family and medical history, and eating habits. Your doctor may perform a physical exam and tests to help diagnose lactose intolerance or to check for other health problems. Other conditions, such as irritable bowel syndrome, celiac disease, inflammatory bowel disease, or small bowel bacterial overgrowth can cause symptoms similar to those of lactose intolerance.

Your doctor may ask you to stop eating and drinking milk and milk products for a period of time to see if your symptoms go away. If your symptoms don't go away, your doctor may order additional tests.

Physical Exam

During a physical exam, your doctor may:

- Check for bloating in your abdomen
- Use a stethoscope to listen to sounds within your abdomen
- Tap on your abdomen to check for tenderness or pain

What Tests Do Doctors Use to Diagnose Lactose Intolerance?

Your doctor may order a hydrogen breath test to see how well your small intestine digests lactose.

Hydrogen Breath Test

Doctors use this test to diagnose lactose malabsorption and lactose intolerance. Normally, a small amount of hydrogen, a type of gas, is found in your breath. If you have lactose malabsorption, undigested lactose causes you to have high levels of hydrogen in your breath. For this test, you will drink a liquid that contains a known amount of lactose. Every 30 minutes over a few hours, you will breathe into a balloon-type container that measures the amount of hydrogen in your breath. During this time, a healthcare professional will ask about your symptoms. If both your breath hydrogen levels rise and your symptoms get worse during the test, your doctor may diagnose lactose intolerance.

Treatment for Lactose Intolerance

How Can I Manage My Lactose Intolerance Symptoms?

In most cases, you can manage the symptoms of lactose intolerance by changing your diet to limit or avoid foods and drinks that contain lactose, such as milk and milk products. Some people may only need to limit the amount of lactose they eat or drink, while others may need to avoid lactose altogether. Using lactase products can help some people manage their symptoms.

Lactase Products

Lactase products are tablets or drops that contain lactase, the enzyme that breaks down lactose. You can take lactase tablets before you eat or drink milk products. You can also add lactase drops to milk before you drink it. The lactase breaks down the lactose in foods and drinks, lowering your chances of having lactose intolerance symptoms. Check with your doctor before using lactase products. Some people, such as young children and pregnant and breastfeeding women, may not be able to use them.

How Do Doctors Treat Lactose Intolerance?

Treatments depend on the cause of lactose intolerance. If your lactose intolerance is caused by lactase nonpersistence or congenital lactase deficiency, no treatments can increase the amount of lactase your small intestine makes. Your doctor can help you change your diet to manage your symptoms. If your lactose intolerance is caused by an injury to your small intestine, your doctor may be able to treat the cause of the injury. You may be able to tolerate lactose after treatment. While some premature babies are lactose intolerant, the condition usually improves without treatment as the baby gets older.

Eating, Diet, and Nutrition for Lactose Intolerance

How Should I Change My Diet If I Have Lactose Intolerance?

Talk with your doctor or a dietitian about changing your diet to manage lactose intolerance symptoms while making sure you get enough nutrients. If your child has lactose intolerance, help your child follow the dietary plan recommended by a doctor or dietitian.

To manage your symptoms, you may need to reduce the amount of lactose you eat or drink. Most people with lactose intolerance can have some lactose without getting symptoms.

Foods That Contain Lactose

You may not need to completely avoid foods and beverages that contain lactose—such as milk or milk products. If you avoid all milk and milk products, you may get less calcium and vitamin D than you need.

People with lactose intolerance can handle different amounts of lactose. Research suggests that many people could have 12 grams of lactose—the amount in about 1 cup of milk—without symptoms or with only mild symptoms.

You may be able to tolerate milk and milk products if you:

- Drink small amounts of milk at a time and have it with meals

- Add milk and milk products to your diet a little at a time and see how you feel

- Try eating yogurt and hard cheeses, like cheddar or Swiss, which are lower in lactose than other milk products

- Use lactase products to help digest the lactose in milk and milk products

Lactose-Free and Lactose-Reduced Milk and Milk Products

Using lactose-free and lactose-reduced milk and milk products may help you lower the amount of lactose in your diet. These products are available in many grocery stores and are just as healthy for you as regular milk and milk products.

Calcium and Vitamin D

If you are lactose intolerant, make sure you get enough calcium and vitamin D each day. Milk and milk products are the most common sources of calcium.

Many foods that do not contain lactose are also sources of calcium. Examples include:

- Fish with soft bones, such as canned salmon or sardines
- Broccoli and leafy green vegetables
- Oranges
- Almonds, Brazil nuts, and dried beans
- Tofu
- Products with labels that show they have added calcium, such as some cereals, fruit juices, and soy milk

Vitamin D helps your body absorb and use calcium. Be sure to eat foods that contain vitamin D, such as eggs and certain kinds of fish, such as salmon. Some ready-to-eat cereals and orange juice have added vitamin D. Some milk and milk products also have added vitamin D. If you can drink small amounts of milk or milk products without symptoms, choose products that have added vitamin D. Also, being outside in the sunlight helps your body make vitamin D.

Talk with your doctor or dietitian about whether you are getting the nutrients you need. For safety reasons, also talk with your doctor before using dietary supplements or any other complementary or alternative medicines or practices. Also, talk with your doctor about sun exposure and sun safety.

What Foods and Drinks Contain Lactose?

Lactose is in all milk and milk products and may be found in other foods and drinks. Milk and milk products may be added to boxed, canned, frozen, packaged, and prepared foods. If you have symptoms after consuming a small amount of lactose, you should be aware of the many products that may contain lactose, such as:

- Bread and other baked goods, such as pancakes, biscuits, cookies, and cakes

- Processed foods, including breakfast cereals, instant potatoes, soups, margarine, salad dressings, and flavored chips and other snack foods

- Processed meats, such as bacon, sausage, hot dogs, and lunch meats

- Milk-based meal replacement liquids and powders, smoothies, and protein powders and bars

- Nondairy liquid and powdered coffee creamers, and nondairy whipped toppings

You can check the ingredient list on packaged foods to see if the product contains lactose. The following words mean that the product contains lactose:

- Milk

- Lactose

- Whey

- Curds

- Milk by-products

- Dry milk solids

- Nonfat dry milk powder

A small amount of lactose may be found in some prescription and over-the-counter (OTC) medicines. Talk with your doctor about the amount of lactose in medicines you take, especially if you typically cannot tolerate even small amounts of lactose.

Section 15.3

Dark Chocolate and Milk Allergies

This section includes text excerpted from "Dark
Chocolate and Milk Allergies," U.S. Food and Drug
Administration (FDA), November 29, 2017.

If you're allergic to milk and you love dark chocolate, how do you
know whether you can indulge in a candy bar without having an allergic reaction? That's what the U.S. Food and Drug Administration
(FDA) wanted to learn, especially after receiving reports that consumers had harmful reactions after eating dark chocolate.

Milk is a permitted ingredient in dark chocolate, but it is also
one of eight major food allergens (substances that can cause reactions that are sometimes dangerous). U.S. law requires manufacturers to label food products that are major allergens, as well as
food products that contain major allergenic ingredients or proteins.
Allergens contained in a food product but not named on the label
are a leading cause of FDA requests for food recalls, and undeclared
milk is the most frequently cited allergen. Chocolates are one of
the most common sources of undeclared milk associated with consumer reactions.

The FDA tested nearly 100 dark chocolate bars for the presence of
milk. Earlier this year, the agency issued preliminary findings, and
is now releasing more information about its research. The bars tested
by the FDA were obtained from different parts of the United States,
and each bar was unique in terms of product line and/or manufacturer. Bars were divided into categories based on the statements on
the labels.

The bottom line? Unfortunately, you can't always tell if dark chocolate contains milk by reading the ingredients list. FDA researchers
found that of 94 dark chocolate bars tested, only six listed milk as an
ingredient. When testing the remaining 88 bars that did not list milk
as an ingredient, the FDA found that 51 of them actually did contain
milk. In fact, the FDA study found milk in 61 percent of all bars tested.
In part, that's because milk can get into a dark chocolate product even
when it is not added as an ingredient. Most dark chocolate is produced
on equipment that is also used to produce milk chocolate. In these
cases, it is possible that traces of milk may inadvertently wind up in
the dark chocolate.

Read 'May' as 'Likely'

To inform consumers that dark chocolate products may contain milk even if not intentionally added, many chocolate manufacturers print "advisory" messages on the label. There's quite a variety of advisory messages, such as:

- "may contain milk"
- "may contain dairy"
- "may contain traces of milk"
- "made on equipment shared with milk"
- "processed in a plant that processes dairy"
- "manufactured in a facility that uses milk"

FDA found that milk was present in three out of every four dark chocolate products with one of these advisory statements. Some products had milk levels as high as those found in products that declared the presence of milk. When the National Confectioners Association (NCA) was asked for its advice, a spokesperson said that "consumers with milk allergies should not consume dark chocolate products that come with advisory statements, since these products may indeed contain milk proteins." Another problem is that advisory messages may appear to be conflicting if they are accompanied by dairy-free or vegan statements. "Even a consumer who carefully reads the label may be confused by a statement such as "vegan" (which implies that no animal-derived products were used) along with an advisory—or "may contain" statement—referring to the presence of milk," says Stefano Luccioli, M.D., a senior medical advisor at the FDA.

Not Quite 'Dairy Free'

In addition to these advisory statements, labels for chocolate bars may make other claims. Some say "dairy-free" or "lactose free," but the FDA found milk in 15 percent of the dark chocolates with this label. And 25 percent of dark chocolate products labeled only "vegan" were found to contain milk.

No Message Doesn't Mean No Milk

You shouldn't assume that dark chocolate contains no milk if the label does not mention it at all. "Milk-allergic consumers should be aware that 33 percent of the dark chocolates with no mention of milk anywhere on the label were, in fact, found to contain milk," says Luccioli.

What Consumers Can Do

1. Consumers who are sensitive or allergic to milk should know that dark chocolate products are a high-risk food if you're highly milk-allergic.

2. Start by checking the ingredients list to see if it includes milk.

3. Read all the label statements on dark chocolate products and avoid those with an advisory statement for milk, even if these products feature also other (and conflicting) statements, such as "dairy-free" or "vegan."

4. View even products with dairy-free claims or without any mention of milk with caution, unless the manufacturer is a trusted source and/or uses dedicated equipment for making milk-free chocolate products.

"The chocolate industry will continue to make every effort to understand the needs of allergic consumers and communicate the potential presence of milk allergens in dark chocolate through advisory labeling," says Laura Shumow, director of scientific and regulatory affairs at NCA.

The FDA is evaluating the study findings and considering options for addressing the issues identified in the study. Further, allergen contamination is included in the preventive and risk-based controls mandated by the FDA Food Safety Modernization Act (FSMA). Under the proposed Preventive Controls for Human Food rule that is scheduled to become final this fall, food manufacturers would be required to implement a food safety plan that identifies safeguards in place to prevent or significantly reduce such hazards as food allergens.

The proposed rule includes provisions to prevent unintended cross-contact between foods that contain allergens and those not intended to contain them. Firms covered by the final rule would have from one to three years after the rule becomes final to comply, depending on the size of the firm.

Table 15.1. Milk Detected in Individual Dark Chocolate Products

Label/Package Statement	Total Number of Dark Chocolate Products	Number and Percent (%) of Dark Chocolate Products Testing Positive for Milk
Milk (or milk-derived component[1])	6	6 (100%)
Advisory Statements[2] (alone or combined)	59	44 (75%)
Dairy-free or lactose-free[3] statements alone	13	2 (15%)
Vegan statement alone	4	1 (25%)
No statement regarding milk	12	4 (33%)
Total	94	57 (61%)

1. Some examples of milk components include cream, milk fat, and sodium caseinate.

2. Advisory statements refers to statements regarding the possible presence of milk, such as "may contain milk (or dairy)," "made on equipment shared with milk," "processed in a plant that processes dairy," or "manufactured in a facility that uses milk." This category also includes "may contain traces" statements, as well as advisory statements combined with either a vegan or dairy-free or lactose statement.

3. Lactose-free chocolates are grouped with dairy-free products although the statement "lactose-free" does not necessarily indicate that the product is free from milk. This is because lactose is a "milk sugar," and its removal does not mean that milk proteins are removed as well.

Chapter 16

Egg Allergy

Chapter Contents

Section 16.1

Understanding Egg Allergy

Egg allergy is caused by an inappropriate response of the immune system to the protein component in egg. Egg allergy is one of the most common food allergies, second only to cow's milk allergy, and estimates suggest that it affects around 2 percent of children in the United States. In most cases, the hypersensitivity to the protein present in the albumen (egg white) or the yolk begins in infancy. Although 70 percent of egg allergies disappear by age sixteen, some people may remain allergic to eggs throughout their lives. Egg white allergy is more common than yolk allergy. While some people are allergic to semi-cooked or raw eggs but can tolerate cooked eggs well, there are those who show intolerance to the food whether it is cooked or raw, and whether it includes egg white or yolk.

The mechanism of egg allergy is much the same as in other types of food allergies. An allergic reaction occurs when immunoglobulin E (IgE), a type of antibody used by the body's immune system to fight pathogens, mistakenly recognizes a harmless food component as a harmful invader. The IgE antibodies bind to the egg protein, triggering the release of histamines and other inflammatory chemicals that can set off a series of adverse reactions. The IgE-mediated allergic reaction is rapid and occurs within half an hour of ingesting the food. Non-IgE-mediated reactions typically take longer to manifest and their exact mechanism is unclear, although studies have shown that their pathways may involve T-cells, a type of lymphocyte.

Symptoms of egg allergy can vary depending on the degree of sensitivity to the protein. Mild sensitivity may present skin reactions like rashes and hives. In some people, the hypersensitivity may cause respiratory symptoms like wheezing, nasal congestion, or sneezing, as well as gastrointestinal symptoms such as vomiting, diarrhea, and abdominal cramping. In a few cases, egg allergy can cause severe, life-threatening anaphylactic reactions, resulting in a drop in blood pressure, increased heart rate, and loss of consciousness. This type of allergic reaction requires immediate administration of the drug epinephrine and emergency care.

Testing for Egg Allergy

The first step in diagnosing an egg allergy involves reviewing the patient's history of symptoms. The allergist may also order a skin prick test (SPT), in which a measured dose of egg protein in a liquid is placed under the skin using a sterile probe. The appearance of a reddish patch or a small swelling (called a "wheal") within the first 20 minutes of administration of the protein indicates an allergic response. The allergist evaluates the degree of sensitivity to egg protein on the basis of the size of the wheal. If the diagnosis is inconclusive, the doctor may ask for a blood test to evaluate the level of allergen-specific serum IgE.

In some cases, however, egg allergy may be difficult to confirm using these initial tests. For instance, the SPT may yield a negative response even though the patient experiences allergy symptoms after ingesting egg. This problem may arise from differences in quality and stability of the allergen extracts used. Likewise, a blood test may indicate the presence of food-specific IgE despite the absence of any allergy symptoms. In such cases, allergists may resort to an oral challenge test that involves a series of trial-and-error procedures. Often recognized as the "gold standard" for food allergy diagnosis, this test involves a period of egg-free diet followed by gradual reintroduction of the suspect food in measured doses. This test has to be done under medical supervision, particularly in patients who have a history of adverse reactions to the food.

Preventing and Treating Egg Allergy

Although many children outgrow it naturally, there is no cure for egg allergy or any other type of food allergy. The only way to prevent allergic reactions to egg products is to completely avoid egg or egg derivatives. This requires a lot of diligence as egg is a versatile ingredient used in a large number of processed foods, including baked foods, desserts, soups, and pasta. People with egg allergy should be vigilant about reading labels and ingredient lists when they shop for food. They must also be careful to check whether there is a possibility that other food may have come in contact with egg during preparation. At restaurants, it may help to tell the waiter about any food sensitivities, as many restaurants offer allergy-friendly dining.

As with other food allergies, mild to moderate symptoms of egg allergy are usually treated with antihistamines, bronchodilators, or steroids. Severe, anaphylactic reactions are treated with epinephrine, which can reverse symptoms that can be fatal if left untreated.

Some vaccines contain egg protein. People with extreme sensitivity to egg protein are advised to take their shots under the supervision of an allergist or in a medical office equipped to deal with any adverse effects.

Eggs are a major source of dietary protein. A registered dietitian can suggest alternatives to egg to ensure that a person on an egg-free diet gets sufficient protein. They can also suggest egg substitutes that can be incorporated into recipes. Some commonly used substitutes in egg-free recipes include: a mix of baking powder, oil, and water; unflavored gelatin; or yeast dissolved in warm water.

References

1. "Egg Allergy," Food Allergy Research and Education (FARE), 2015.

2. "Types of Food Allergy: Egg Allergy," American College of Allergy, Asthma, and Immunology (ACAAI), 2013.

Section 16.2

Flu Vaccine and Egg Allergy

This section includes text excerpted from "Flu Vaccine and People with Egg Allergies," Centers for Disease Control and Prevention (CDC), December 28, 2017.

The Centers for Disease Control and Prevention (CDC) and its Advisory Committee on Immunization Practices (ACIP) have not changed their recommendations regarding egg allergy and receipt of influenza (flu) vaccines. The recommendations remain the same as last season (2016–2017). Based on those recommendations, people with egg allergies no longer need to be observed for an allergic reaction for 30 minutes after receiving a flu vaccine. People with a history of egg allergy of any severity should receive any licensed, recommended, and age-appropriate influenza vaccine. Those who have a history of severe allergic reaction to egg (i.e., any symptom other than hives) should be vaccinated in an inpatient or outpatient medical setting (including but not necessarily limited to hospitals, clinics, health departments, and physician offices), under the supervision of a healthcare provider who is able to recognize and manage severe allergic conditions.

Most flu shots and the nasal spray flu vaccine are manufactured using egg-based technology. Because of this, they contain a small amount of egg proteins, such as ovalbumin. However, studies that have examined the use of both the nasal spray vaccine and flu shots in egg-allergic and nonegg-allergic patients indicate that severe allergic reactions in people with egg allergies are unlikely. A CDC study found the rate of anaphylaxis after all vaccines is 1.31 per one million vaccine doses given.

Changes

Recommendations for flu vaccination of persons with egg allergy have not changed since the 2016–2017 flu season. The CDC recommends:

- Persons with a history of egg allergy who have experienced only hives after exposure to egg should receive flu vaccine. Any licensed and recommended flu vaccine (i.e., any form of IIV or RIV) that is otherwise appropriate for the recipient's age and health status may be used.

- Persons who report having had reactions to egg involving symptoms other than hives, such as angioedema, respiratory distress, lightheadedness, or recurrent emesis; or who required epinephrine or another emergency medical intervention, may similarly receive any licensed and recommended flu vaccine (i.e., any form of IIV or RIV) that is otherwise appropriate for the recipient's age and health status. The selected vaccine should be administered in an inpatient or outpatient medical setting (including, but not necessarily limited to hospitals, clinics, health departments, and physician offices). Vaccine administration should be supervised by a healthcare provider who is able to recognize and manage severe allergic conditions.

- A previous severe allergic reaction to flu vaccine, regardless of the component suspected of being responsible for the reaction, is a contraindication to future receipt of the vaccine.

163

Questions and Answers

What Is Considered an Egg Allergy? What Are the Signs and Symptoms of an Egg Allergic Reaction?

Egg allergy can be confirmed by a consistent medical history of adverse reactions to eggs and egg-containing foods, plus skin and/or blood testing for immunoglobulin E antibodies to egg proteins. Persons who are able to eat lightly cooked egg (e.g., scrambled egg) without reaction are unlikely to be allergic. Egg-allergic persons might tolerate egg in baked products (e.g., bread or cake). Therefore, tolerance to egg-containing foods does not exclude the possibility of egg allergy. Egg allergies can range in severity.

How Common Is Egg Allergy in Children and Adults?

Egg allergy affects about 1.3 percent of all children and 0.2 percent of all adults.

What Vaccine Should I Get If I Am Egg Allergic, but I Can Eat Lightly Cooked Eggs?

If you are able to eat lightly cooked egg (e.g., scrambled egg) without reaction, you are unlikely to be allergic and can get any licensed flu vaccine (i.e., any form of IIV, LAIV, or RIV) that is otherwise appropriate for your age and health status.

What Flu Vaccine Should I Get If I Get Hives after Eating Egg-Containing Foods?

If you are someone with a history of egg allergy, who has experienced only hives after exposure to egg, you can get any licensed flu vaccine (i.e., any form of IIV, LAIV, or RIV) that is otherwise appropriate for your age and health.

What Kind of Flu Vaccine Should I Get If I Have More Serious Reactions to Eating Eggs or Egg-Containing Foods Like Cardiovascular Changes or a Reaction-Requiring Epinephrine?

If you are someone who has more serious reactions to eating eggs or egg-containing foods, like angioedema, respiratory distress, lightheadedness, or recurrent emesis; or who required epinephrine or another emergency medical intervention, you can get any licensed flu vaccine (i.e., any form of IIV, LAIV, or RIV) that is otherwise appropriate for your age and health status, but the vaccine should be given by a healthcare provider who can recognize and respond to a severe allergic response.

Are There Still People with Egg Allergies Who Should Not Get the Flu Vaccine?

People with egg allergy can receive flu vaccines according to the recommendations above. A person who has previously experienced a severe allergic reaction to the flu vaccine, regardless of the component suspected of being responsible for the reaction should not get a flu vaccine again.

Why Do Flu Vaccines Contain Egg Protein?

Most flu vaccines are produced using an egg-based manufacturing process and thus contain a small amount of egg protein called ovalbumin.

How Much Egg Protein Is in the Flu Vaccine?

While not all manufacturers disclose the amount of ovalbumin in their vaccines, those that did from 2011–12 through 2014–15 reported maximum amounts of ≤1 μg/0.5 mL dose for flu shots and 0.24 μg/0.2 mL dose for the nasal spray vaccine. Cell-based flu vaccine (Flucelvax) likely has a much smaller amount of egg protein since the original vaccine virus is grown in eggs, but mass production of that vaccine does not occur in eggs. Recombinant vaccine (Flublok) is the only vaccine currently available that is completely egg free.

Can Egg Protein in the Flu Vaccine Cause Allergic Reactions in Persons with a History of Egg Allergy?

Yes, allergic reactions can happen, but they occur very rarely with the flu vaccines available in the United States. Occasional cases of anaphylaxis, a severe life-threatening reaction that involves multiple organ systems and can progress rapidly, in egg-allergic persons have been reported to the Vaccine Adverse Event Reporting System (VAERS) after administration of flu vaccine. Flu vaccines contain various components that may cause allergic reactions, including anaphylaxis. In a Vaccine Safety Datalink (VSD) study, there were 10 cases of anaphylaxis after more than 7.4 million doses of the inactivated flu vaccine, trivalent (IIV3) given without other vaccines, (rate of 1.35 per one million doses). Most of these cases of anaphylaxis were not related to the egg protein present in the vaccine. CDC and the Advisory Committee on Immunization Practices continue to review available data regarding anaphylaxis cases following flu vaccines.

How Long after the Flu Vaccination Does a Reaction Occur in Persons with a History of Egg Allergy?

Allergic reactions can begin very soon after vaccination. However, the onset of symptoms is sometimes delayed. In a Vaccine Safety Datalink study of more than 25.1 million doses of vaccines of various types given to children and adults over three years, only 33 people had anaphylaxis. Of patients with a documented time to onset of symptoms, eight cases had onset within 30 minutes of vaccination, while in another 21 cases, symptoms were delayed more than 30 minutes following vaccination, including one case with symptom onset on the following day.

Section 16.3

Beating Egg Allergy

This section includes text excerpted from "Hope for Beating Egg Allergy," National Institutes of Health (NIH), July 30, 2012. Reviewed August 2018.

Giving small daily doses of egg powder to children with egg allergy could pave the way to letting them eat the food safely, a study finds. This would make life easier on kids whose only current option is to stay away from all foods that contain eggs.

Egg allergy is one of the most common food allergies in children. There's no treatment other than completely avoiding the food. That's tough for children, parents, and caregivers; eggs can lurk in everything from marshmallows to salad dressing. And the stakes are high. Children who are allergic to eggs can have reactions ranging from hives to anaphylaxis, a life-threatening condition with symptoms that include throat swelling, a sudden drop in blood pressure, trouble breathing, and dizziness.

One possible way to help people with food allergies is oral immunotherapy. In this still-experimental approach, patients eat gradually increasing amounts of the food they're allergic to. A research team led by Dr. A. Wesley Burks at the University of North Carolina and Dr. Stacie M. Jones at the University of Arkansas for Medical Sciences (UAMS) tested oral immunotherapy for children who are allergic to eggs. The study was funded by National Institutes of Health's (NIH) National Institute of Allergy and Infectious Disease (NIAID), National Center for Research Resources (NCRR) and the National Center for Advancing Translational Sciences (NCATS).

The researchers recruited 55 children, ages 5–18, who were allergic to eggs. Forty of the participants ate daily doses of raw egg-white powder. The others received cornstarch as a placebo. Researchers increased the dose every two weeks until the children on oral immunotherapy were eating the equivalent of about one-third of an egg every day.

At 10 months, the participants went into the clinic, where they were "challenged" with increasing doses of egg-white powder and watched closely for symptoms. As reported in the July 19, 2012, issue of the *New England Journal of Medicine*, more than half of the children who had been eating egg powder daily passed the challenge, with no allergic reaction or only minor symptoms. A year later, 30 children passed a challenge with an even larger dose of egg powder. In contrast, none of the children in the placebo group passed the challenge.

Those 30 children stopped oral immunotherapy and were told to avoid all eggs for 4–6 weeks. Then they faced another challenge: a dose of egg powder and a whole cooked egg. Most kids had allergic reactions, but 11 passed the test and were allowed to eat as many eggs or egg-containing foods as they wanted in their normal diets. A year later, those children reported they still had no problems eating eggs.

The study suggests two ways that egg oral immunotherapy could help children. First, while they were eating the daily dose of egg powder, most of the children could safely eat eggs. Second, a small group of children—about one in four—were able to eat eggs even after the daily oral immunotherapy ended.

"Although these results indicate that oral immunotherapy may help resolve certain food allergies, this type of therapy is still in its early experimental stages and more research is needed," says Dr. Daniel

Rotrosen, director of National Institute of Allergy and Infectious Diseases (NIAID) Division of Allergy, Immunology, and Transplantation (DAIT). "We want to emphasize that food oral immunotherapy and oral food challenges should not be tried at home because of the risk of severe allergic reactions."

Chapter 17

Seafood Allergy

A seafood allergy is an abnormal reaction of the human body when it is exposed to proteins found in fish or shellfish. Finned fish and shellfish come from unrelated families of food, so being allergic to fish does not necessarily mean a person will also be allergic to shellfish. The fish family includes an estimated 20,000 species characterized by fins, scales, and bones, such as tuna, salmon, cod, and halibut. The shellfish family is divided into two main types of marine invertebrates: crustaceans (such as shrimp, crab, and lobster); and molluscs (including clams, mussels, oysters, and squid).

Shellfish allergies affect approximately 1 percent of people, making them twice as common as fish allergies, which affect approximately 0.5 percent of people. Unlike some other types of food allergies, seafood allergies usually develop in adulthood. An estimated 60 percent of people with shellfish allergies and 40 percent of people with fish allergies experience their first reaction as an adult. Seafood allergies tend to be lifelong, and the reactions are likely to be more severe than those associated with most other types of food allergies.

Diagnosing Seafood Allergies

If someone is allergic to fish or shellfish, the body's immune system mistakenly recognizes proteins from these species as harmful and generates antibodies to fight. When proteins from seafood enter

---

the body—whether through eating fish, touching or handling fish, or breathing in vapors of cooking fish—the body overreacts and releases histamines into the bloodstream. These chemicals produce various symptoms of allergic reactions, such as coughing, throat tightness, wheezing, watery eyes, skin rashes, stomach aches, diarrhea, or vomiting. A more serious manifestation of a seafood allergy is anaphylaxis, in which the person may experience significant difficulty breathing, a drop in blood pressure, lightheadedness, and loss of consciousness. If the person does not receive medical treatment immediately, an anaphylactic reaction can be life threatening.

Anyone who experiences an allergic reaction to seafood should seek medical advice from an allergist/immunologist—a physician specializing in diagnosing and treating allergies. The allergist will conduct a thorough history and physical examination and perform a skin-prick test or a blood test to isolate and identify the type of allergy. Once diagnosed, the patient will receive instructions on how to avoid allergens and what to do if they have an allergic reaction. The allergist may also provide a referral to a dietitian—a medical professional who specializes in dietetics and nutrition—who can offer additional guidance about which foods to avoid and which foods are safe to consume.

Avoiding Seafood

The best treatment for a seafood allergy is to avoid all forms of the allergenic food, whether it is fish or shellfish. For prepared and packaged foods, be sure to read labels thoroughly to avoid buying foods that may contain fish, even if it is not the main ingredient. The U.S. Food and Drug Administration (FDA) has made it mandatory for manufacturers to mention "fish" on the label of foods that contain fish in any form under the Food Allergen Labeling and Consumer Protection Act of 2004 (FALCPA). It is important to note that fish proteins may be present in a wide variety of foods, such as Worcestershire sauce, Caesar salad dressing, and some pasta sauces, dips, and even crackers or biscuits.

At home, make sure all surfaces that were used to prepare fish—utensils, cutting boards, countertops, etc.—are thoroughly cleaned before preparing food for an allergic family member. People with a seafood allergy should also stay away from smoke or steam from cooking fish or shellfish as they carry the protein that may cause an allergic reaction.

Avoid going to restaurants that serve seafood. Cross-contamination is a serious possibility in these establishments, so it is best to choose restaurants that do not serve seafood at all. Chinese, Vietnamese, or Thai food preparations have a risk of cross-contamination due to the predominance of fish in these cuisines. Stay away from fish markets and other places where fish is present. Even if an allergist permits a patient to eat certain types of fish or shellfish, it is important to make sure the allowable foods have not been contaminated with allergens from other types of seafood.

Some dietary supplements, like glucosamine—a supplement often prescribed for people with osteoarthritis—may be obtained from the outer coating of crustaceans. As a result, it may provoke a reaction in people allergic to shellfish. Chondroitin sulfate obtained from shark cartilage is another supplement that should be avoided by people with seafood allergies.

For people who experience severe allergic reactions to seafood, a physician may prescribe emergency allergy medication, such as an epinephrine auto-injector, to alleviate symptoms in case of an allergy attack. This medication should be carried at all times and administered at the very first sign of an allergic reaction to avoid life-threatening anaphylaxis.

References

1. "Fish/Seafood Allergy," Allergy UK, March 2012.

2. "Seafood Allergy," Asthma and Allergy Foundation of America (AAFA), 2005.

Chapter 18

Peanut and Tree Nut Allergy

Chapter Contents

Section 18.1

Understanding Peanut and Tree Nut Allergy

"Understanding Peanut and Tree Nut Allergy,"
© 2018 Omnigraphics. Reviewed August 2018.

Peanut allergy is one of the most common food allergies, and its prevalence appears to be increasing. One study indicated that the number of children with peanut allergies tripled between 1997 and 2008 in the United States. Siblings of children who are allergic to peanuts are at a higher risk of developing peanut allergies. Although most peanut allergies last a lifetime, an estimated 20 percent of children outgrow them by the age of six.

Peanuts belong to the legumes family, which also includes soybeans, peas, and lentils. They are different from nuts that grow on trees, such as almonds, walnuts, hazelnuts, cashews, Brazil nuts, and pistachios. However, an estimated 25–40 percent of people who are allergic to peanuts are also allergic to tree nuts. As a result, many experts suggest that people who are allergic to peanuts also abstain from eating foods containing tree nuts and seeds.

Peanuts and tree nuts contain structurally similar proteins. In an estimated 1.0 percent of children and 0.5 percent of adults, exposure to these proteins causes the immune system to overreact and release histamine into the bloodstream, which can trigger a severe, whole-body allergic response called anaphylaxis. The symptoms of anaphylaxis can include:

- Hives
- Swelling and rashes
- Itching
- Swelling of the lips and tongue
- Constriction of the throat
- Difficulty breathing and swallowing
- Vomiting
- Diarrhea
- Dizziness and fainting
- Drop in blood pressure

Generally, people who are allergic to nuts will develop a reaction within a few minutes of exposure. Anyone who experiences these symptoms should seek medical attention. For mild allergic reactions, the healthcare provider may prescribe antihistamines to subdue the immune response. Severe reactions require immediate treatment with epinephrine (adrenaline), typically administered in an auto-injector. Left untreated, anaphylaxis can be fatal.

Diagnosis and Treatment

Peanut and tree nut allergies can be difficult to diagnose through skin tests or blood tests. When these types of allergies are suspected, the allergist may ask the patient to avoid the food in question for two to four weeks. If the patient's symptoms improve as a result of the food-elimination diet, they are most likely allergic to that specific food. When the results are inconclusive, the allergist may request an oral food challenge. During this test, the patient consumes tiny amounts of peanuts or tree nuts in a controlled environment, with emergency medication and equipment on hand in case they have a severe allergic reaction.

The primary form of treatment for peanut and tree nut allergies is strict avoidance of these foods. Eating foods that contain peanuts or tree nuts is the most common cause of severe allergic reactions. Casual contact with the skin is less likely to trigger a severe reaction, unless the residue is transferred from the skin to the eyes, nose, or mouth. Inhaling peanut fumes does not cause an allergic reaction in most people.

People who are allergic to peanuts and tree nuts should always read food labels carefully to ensure that they do not eat products that contain even trace amounts of nuts. Under U.S. law, food manufacturers are required to note whether their products contain nuts. Many companies also voluntarily note whether products were processed in a facility or with equipment that also handles nuts.

People with peanut and tree nut allergies must also be aware of hidden or unexpected sources of nuts. Some common products that often contain peanuts or tree nuts include baked goods, candy, nougat, pralines, egg rolls, chili sauce, enchilada sauce, and mole sauce. Certain types of food establishments are considered dangerous for individuals with peanut allergies due to the risk of cross-contamination, including bakeries, ice cream shops, and African, Asian, or Mexican restaurants.

References

1. "Peanut Allergy," American College of Allergy, Asthma, and Immunology (ACAAI), 2014.

2. "Peanut Allergy," Food Allergy Research and Education (FARE), 2015.

Section 18.2

Cracking Nut-Allergy Mechanisms

This section includes text excerpted from "Cracking Nut-Allergy Mechanisms," Agricultural Research Service (ARS), U.S. Department of Agriculture (USDA), October 2013. Reviewed August 2018.

Food allergy is an immune response to eating foods that contain specific components called "allergens." An increase in food allergy of 18 percent was seen between 1997 and 2007, according to a study released by the Centers for Disease Control and Prevention (CDC). Just eight foods account for most allergic reactions. Although not all allergies are lifelong people who have allergic reactions to peanuts and tree nuts are often considered to have them throughout life.

The mechanisms underlying food allergies are not completely understood. But researchers at the Agricultural Research Service's (ARS) Food Processing and Sensory Quality Research Unit in New Orleans, Louisiana, are studying allergen-immune system interactions involved in nut allergies.

Common Peptides Are Key

People affected by nut allergy experience wide variation in the breadth and intensity of their allergic reactions. For example, among people who are allergic to a specific tree nut, one individual may be five times more allergic than another.

Tree nuts can be members of several plant families. Though thought of as nuts, peanuts are not nuts. They are members of the Leguminosae family and grow underground. Still, both nuts and legumes have commonalities: They both consist of a dry fruit contained inside a shell. Some, but not all, people who have allergies to certain nuts can still eat peanuts, and vice versa.

In New Orleans, ARS chemist Soheila Maleki has worked with university collaborators on key components of a Structural Database of Allergenic Proteins (SDAP). The computational database was developed by Catherine Schein and colleagues at the University of Texas Medical Branch, in Galveston, Texas. The team is in the process of validating SDAP's ability to help predict when an individual will react to two or more different types of nuts. This condition is called "cross-reactivity."

Foods, including peanuts and tree nuts, contain proteins, which are digested into smaller fragments called "peptides." A peptide is called an "epitope" when it is recognized by antibodies—immune system components in the bloodstream. Immunoglobulin E (IgE) is an antibody that is elevated in allergic individuals. When IgE binds to the epitopes, the food is recognized as foreign by the immune system, and an allergic reaction occurs.

The proteins between cross-reactive nuts are thought to have similar IgE antibody-recognition sites. The researchers took known IgE binding sites (epitope sequences) from peanut and nut proteins and ran those through the SDAP database in order to predict cross-reactive epitopes in other nuts.

"The database provides other sequences that are likely to be allergenic based on the known sequence," says Maleki.

The computer-generated binding sequences were then made into synthetic epitopes for testing purposes. "We needed to know if the computer predicted the novel binding sites correctly," says Maleki. "So we tested those synthesized sequences using serum from people allergic to peanut and tree nuts."

Food-allergen studies commonly involves the use of blood serum from allergic individuals because their serum's IgE recognizes allergenic epitopes. The serum, which was provided by cooperators at the University of California (UC) Davis, allowed the team to match previously unknown epitopes within the major allergenic proteins known to be common to a variety of nut and peanut allergies.

The authors found that similar immunoglobulin epitopes on allergenic proteins, as defined by SDAP, could account for some of the cross-reactivity between peanuts and tree nuts. The finding indicates that SDAP can be useful for predicting previously unidentified cross-reactive epitopes, based on their similarity to known IgE epitopes.

"The novel sequences we found and validated using the database are similar, but not identical, to the sequences we fed into the software," says Maleki. "We were able to confirm sites that the immune system sees and binds but that we could not have predicted otherwise."

The study was funded by the U.S. Environmental Protection Agency (EPA) and the National Institutes of Health (NIH) and was published in *Allergy* in 2011.

Increasing Diagnostic Reliability

Previously, Maleki had assessed the diagnostic reliability of standard peanut-allergy tests. She found that while people generally eat peanuts that have been heat treated (via roasting or boiling), the extracts that are commonly used to diagnose peanut allergies are from raw peanuts. She and colleagues hypothesized that raw peanut proteins undergo specific changes during roasting that may contribute to increases in allergenic properties.

Since then, Maleki and colleagues have published a series of studies that shed light on the molecular differences between raw and heat-treated nuts in terms of their inherent peptides that trigger human allergic reactions.

The major allergenic proteins (or allergens) of peanut are known as "Ara h 1," "Ara h 2," and "Ara h 3." For one study, Maleki looked into how the peanut-roasting process alters how well an allergic individual's immunoglobulins bind to peanut allergens. The team compared the reaction by human IgE antibody to the heated and unheated forms of Ara h 1. The study showed that roasting-induced side reactions, such as browning, increased the amount of IgE that recognizes and binds to Ara h 1—when compared to the amount that binds to Ara h 1 from raw peanuts.

"This result partly accounts for the increased allergenic properties observed in processed, roasted peanuts," says Maleki. The study was published in 2012 in *Molecular Nutrition and Food Research*.

In another study, Maleki and colleagues in Spain showed that a combination treatment of heat and high pressure (autoclaving) applied to peanuts significantly reduced allergic reaction. Autoclaving involves a higher moisture environment, similar to steaming or boiling, than roasting. As result, autoclaving does not initiate the browning effect that comes with roasting. The less allergenic reaction to the combination-treated peanuts was confirmed by skin-prick tests applied to volunteers known to have peanut allergies.

"Proteins become unfolded with autoclaving," says Maleki. "If you unfold the protein, you may reduce allergenicity." The study was published in 2012 in *Food Chemistry*.

Insights into allergen-immune system interactions will help with preventing and diagnosing serious food allergy.—By Rosalie Marion Bliss, Agricultural Research Service Information Staff.

Section 18.3

Peanut Allergy: Early Exposure Is Key to Prevention

This section includes text excerpted from "Peanut Allergy: Early Exposure Is Key to Prevention," National Institutes of Health (NIH), January 10, 2017.

With peanut allergy on the rise in the United States, you've probably heard parents strategizing about ways to keep their kids from developing this potentially dangerous condition. But is it actually possible to prevent peanut allergy, and, if so, how do you go about doing it?

A group representing 26 professional organizations, advocacy groups, and federal agencies, including the National Institutes of Health (NIH), has just issued clinical guidelines aimed at preventing peanut allergy. The guidelines suggest that parents should introduce most babies to peanut-containing foods around the time they begin eating other solid foods, typically 4–6 months of age. While early introduction is especially important for kids at particular risk for developing allergies, it is also recommended that high-risk infants—those with a history of severe eczema and/or egg allergy—undergo a blood or skin-prick test before being given foods containing peanuts. The test results can help to determine how, or even if, peanuts should be introduced in the youngsters' diets.

This recommendation is turning older guidelines on their head. In the past, pediatricians often advised parents to delay introducing peanuts and other common causes of food allergies into their kids' diets. But in 2010, the thinking began shifting when a panel of food allergy experts concluded insufficient evidence existed to show that delaying the introduction of potentially problematic foods actually protected kids. Still, there wasn't a strategy waiting to help prevent peanut or other food allergies.

As highlighted in a previous blog entry, the breakthrough came in 2015 with evidence from the NIH-funded Learning Early About Peanut Allergy (LEAP) trial. That trial, involving hundreds of babies under a year old at high risk for developing peanut allergy, established that kids could be protected by regularly eating a popular peanut butter-flavored Israeli snack called Bamba. A follow-up study later showed those kids remained allergy-free even after avoiding peanuts for a year.

Under the new recommendations, published simultaneously in six journals including the *Journal of Allergy and Clinical Immunology*, all infants who don't already test positive for a peanut allergy are encouraged to eat peanut-enriched foods soon after they've tried a few other solid foods. The guidelines are the first to offer specific recommendations for allergy prevention based on a child's risk for peanut allergy:

- Infants at high risk for peanut allergy—based on severe eczema and/or egg allergy—are suggested to begin consuming peanut-enriched foods between 4–6 months of age, but only after parents check with their healthcare providers. Infants already showing signs of peanut sensitivity in blood and/or skin-prick tests should try peanuts for the first time under the supervision of their doctor or allergist. In some cases, test results indicating a strong reaction to peanut protein might lead a specialist to recommend that a particular child avoid peanuts.

- Infants with mild to moderate eczema should incorporate peanut-containing foods into their diets by about six months of age. It's generally OK for them to have those first bites of peanut at home and without prior testing.

- Infants without eczema or any other food allergy aren't likely to develop an allergy to peanuts. To be on the safe side, it's still a good idea for them to start eating peanuts from an early age.

Once peanut-containing foods have been consumed safely, regular exposure is key to allergy prevention. The guidelines recommend that infants—and particularly those at the greatest risk of allergies—eat about 2 grams of peanut protein (the amount in 2 teaspoons of peanut butter) 3 times a week.

Of course, it's never a good idea to give infants whole peanuts, which are a choking hazard. Infants should instead get their peanuts in prepared peanut-containing foods or by stirring peanut powder into other familiar foods. They might also try peanut butter spread on bread or crackers.

The hope is that, with widespread implementation of these guidelines, many new cases of peanut allergy can be prevented.

Chapter 19

Wheat Allergy

Chapter Contents

Section 19.1

What Is Wheat Allergy?

A wheat allergy is different from gluten sensitivity and celiac disease. The majority of wheat allergies involve albumin and globulin. People with gluten sensitivity cannot tolerate gluten, which can be found in grains such as rye and barley in addition to wheat. Celiac disease is a severe form of gluten sensitivity in which the immune system reacts to gluten by producing IgG (immunoglobulin G) antibodies, which cause inflammation in the lining of the small intestine. This inflammation can cause permanent damage to the small intestine and prevent it from absorbing nutrients. For people with celiac disease, the symptoms are generally confined to the abdomen and get worse over time.

There are four proteins found in wheat: albumin, globulin, gliadin, and glutenin (also known as gluten). In an individual with a wheat allergy, the immune system develops IgE (immunoglobulin E) antibodies to one or more of these proteins. When the person consumes wheat, the antibodies attack the protein, causing abnormal clinical reactions. These reactions may range from a mild skin rash or runny nose to a severe asthma attack or life-threatening anaphylaxis. Other possible symptoms of wheat allergy include bloated stomach, nausea, vomiting, and diarrhea.

Diagnosis and Treatment

Wheat allergy is usually diagnosed by a pinprick skin test or an immunoglobulin blood test. Doctors may also ask the patient to keep a food diary, noting symptoms experienced after eating or eliminating certain foods from their diet. Wheat allergies are most commonly found in infants and toddlers. In the majority of these cases, the child outgrows the allergy within a few years and wheat can gradually be reintroduced to their diet. A family history of allergies is considered a risk factor for developing a wheat allergy.

Avoidance of wheat-based products is the best treatment for a wheat allergy. Wheat proteins are present in many food items, such as bread, pasta, breakfast cereals, crackers, pretzels, cakes, and some sauces. Wheat proteins are also found in beer, root beer, and gravy. Monosodium glutamate (MSG), used as a flavor enhancer in many foods, is another product in which wheat proteins can be found. The U.S. Food and Drug Administration (FDA) has made it mandatory for food manufacturers to mention "wheat" on the product label if wheat is present in any form. People with wheat allergies must read food labels carefully. It is also important to be aware of cross-contamination of food during preparation and clean all surfaces thoroughly.

Wheat products are a staple in many American households. Fortunately, there are a variety of alternative foods that can replace wheat, such as maize, corn, rice, potato, soy, chickpea, tapioca, oats, millets, and quinoa. Wheat-free noodles, crackers, cereals, and other products have become widely available in recent years due to rising demand by people with gluten sensitivity. A dietitian with expertise in food allergies can help people choose among the alternatives.

References

1. Nordqvist, Christian. "What Is Wheat Allergy?" Medical News Today, November 12, 2013.

2. "Wheat Allergy and Sensitivity," Sandwell and West Birmingham Hospitals NHS Trust, July 2014.

Section 19.2

Celiac Disease and Gluten Intolerance

This section includes text excerpted from "Celiac Disease," National Institute of Diabetes and Digestive and Kidney Diseases (NIDDK), June 18, 2016.

Definition and Facts for Celiac Disease

Celiac disease is a digestive disorder that damages the small intestine. The disease is triggered by eating foods containing gluten. Gluten is a protein found naturally in wheat, barley, and rye, and is common in foods such as bread, pasta, cookies, and cakes. Many prepackaged foods, lip balms and lipsticks, hair and skin products, toothpastes, vitamin and nutrient supplements, and, rarely, medicines, contain gluten.

Celiac disease can be very serious. The disease can cause long-lasting digestive problems and keep your body from getting all the nutrients it needs. Celiac disease can also affect the body outside the intestine.

Celiac disease is different from gluten sensitivity or wheat intolerance. If you have gluten sensitivity, you may have symptoms similar to those of celiac disease, such as abdominal pain and tiredness. Unlike celiac disease, gluten sensitivity does not damage the small intestine.

Celiac disease is also different from a wheat allergy. In both cases, your body's immune system reacts to wheat. However, some symptoms in wheat allergies, such as having itchy eyes or a hard time breathing, are different from celiac disease. Wheat allergies also do not cause long-term damage to the small intestine.

How Common Is Celiac Disease?

As many as one in 141 Americans has celiac disease, although most don't know it.

Who Is More Likely to Develop Celiac Disease?

Although celiac disease affects children and adults in all parts of the world, the disease is more common in Caucasians and more often diagnosed in females. You are more likely to develop celiac disease if someone in your family has the disease. Celiac disease also is more common among people with certain other diseases, such as Down syndrome, Turner syndrome, and type 1 diabetes.

What Other Health Problems Do People with Celiac Disease Have?

If you have celiac disease, you also may be at risk for:

- Addison disease
- Hashimoto disease
- Primary biliary cirrhosis
- Type 1 diabetes

What Are the Complications of Celiac Disease?

Long-term complications of celiac disease include:

- Malnutrition, a condition in which you don't get enough vitamins, minerals, and other nutrients you need to be healthy

- Accelerated osteoporosis or bone softening, known as osteomalacia

- Nervous system problems

- Problems related to reproduction

Rare complications can include:

- Intestinal cancer

- Liver diseases

- Lymphoma, a cancer of part of the immune system called the lymph system that includes the gut

In rare cases, you may continue to have trouble absorbing nutrients even though you have been following a strict gluten-free diet. If you have this condition, called refractory celiac disease, your intestines are severely damaged and can't heal. You may need to receive nutrients through an IV.

Symptoms and Causes of Celiac Disease

What Are the Symptoms of Celiac Disease?

Most people with celiac disease have one or more symptoms. However, some people with the disease may not have symptoms or feel sick. Sometimes health issues such as surgery, a pregnancy, childbirth, bacterial gastroenteritis, a viral infection, or severe mental stress can trigger celiac disease symptoms.

If you have celiac disease, you may have digestive problems or other symptoms. Digestive symptoms are more common in children and can include:

- Bloating, or a feeling of fullness or swelling in the abdomen

- Chronic diarrhea

- Constipation

- Gas

- Nausea

- Pale, foul-smelling, or fatty stools that float

- Stomach pain

- Vomiting

For children with celiac disease, being unable to absorb nutrients when they are so important to normal growth and development can lead to:

- Damage to the permanent teeth's enamel
- Delayed puberty
- Failure to thrive in infants
- Mood changes or feeling annoyed or impatient
- Slowed growth and short height
- Weight loss

Adults are less likely to have digestive symptoms and, instead, may have one or more of the following:

- Anemia
- A red, smooth, shiny tongue
- Bone or joint pain
- Depression or anxiety
- Dermatitis herpetiformis
- Headaches
- Infertility or repeated miscarriage
- Missed menstrual periods
- Mouth problems such as canker sores or dry mouth
- Seizures
- Tingling numbness in the hands and feet
- Tiredness
- Weak and brittle bones

Adults who have digestive symptoms with celiac disease may have:

- Abdominal pain and bloating
- Intestinal blockages
- Tiredness that lasts for long periods of time
- Ulcers, or sores on the stomach or lining of the intestine

Celiac disease also can produce a reaction in which your immune system, or your body's natural defense system, attacks healthy cells in your body. This reaction can spread outside your digestive tract to other areas of your body, including your:

- Bones
- Joints
- Nervous system
- Skin
- Spleen

Depending on how old you are when a doctor diagnoses your celiac disease, some symptoms, such as short height and tooth defects, will not improve.

Dermatitis Herpetiformis

Dermatitis herpetiformis is an itchy, blistering skin rash that usually appears on the elbows, knees, buttocks, back, or scalp. The rash affects about 10 percent of people with celiac disease. The rash can affect people of all ages but is most likely to appear for the first time between the ages of 30 and 40. Men who have the rash also may have oral or, rarely, genital sores. Some people with celiac disease may have the rash and no other symptoms.

Why Are Celiac Disease Symptoms so Varied?

Symptoms of celiac disease vary from person to person. Your symptoms may depend on:

- How long you were breastfed as an infant; some studies have shown that the longer you were breastfed, the later celiac disease symptoms appear
- How much gluten you eat
- How old you were when you started eating gluten
- The amount of damage to your small intestine
- Your age—symptoms can vary between young children and adults

People with celiac disease who have no symptoms can still develop complications from the disease over time if they do not get treatment.

What Causes Celiac Disease?

Research suggests that celiac disease only happens to individuals who have particular genes. These genes are common and are carried by about one-third of the population. Individuals also have to be eating food that contains gluten to get celiac disease. Researchers do not know exactly what triggers celiac disease in people at risk who eat gluten over a long period of time. Sometimes the disease runs in families. About 10–20 percent of close relatives of people with celiac disease also are affected. Your chances of developing celiac disease increase when you have changes in your genes or variants. Certain gene variants and other factors, such as things in your environment, can lead to celiac disease.

Diagnosis of Celiac Disease

How Do Doctors Diagnose Celiac Disease?

Celiac disease can be hard to diagnose because some of the symptoms are like symptoms of other diseases, such as irritable bowel syndrome (IBS) and lactose intolerance. Your doctor may diagnose celiac disease with a medical and family history, physical exam, and tests. Tests may include blood tests, genetic tests, and biopsy.

Medical and Family History

Your doctor will ask you for information about your family's health—specifically, if anyone in your family has a history of celiac disease.

Physical Exam

During a physical exam, a doctor most often:

- Checks your body for a rash or malnutrition, a condition that arises when you don't get enough vitamins, minerals, and other nutrients you need to be healthy

- Listens to sounds in your abdomen using a stethoscope

- Taps on your abdomen to check for pain and fullness or swelling

Dental Exam

For some people, a dental visit can be the first step toward discovering celiac disease. Dental enamel defects, such as white, yellow, or brown spots on the teeth, are a pretty common problem in people with celiac disease, especially children. These defects can help dentists and other healthcare professionals identify celiac disease.

What Tests Do Doctors Use to Diagnose Celiac Disease?

Blood Tests

A healthcare professional may take a blood sample from you and send the sample to a lab to test for antibodies common in celiac disease. If blood test results are negative and your doctor still suspects celiac disease, he or she may order more blood tests.

Genetic Tests

If a biopsy and other blood tests do not clearly confirm celiac disease, your doctor may order genetic blood tests to check for certain gene changes, or variants. You are very unlikely to have celiac disease if these gene variants are not present. Having these variants alone is not enough to diagnose celiac disease because they also are common in people without the disease. In fact, most people with these genes will never get celiac disease.

Intestinal Biopsy

If blood tests suggest you have celiac disease, your doctor will perform a biopsy to be sure. During a biopsy, the doctor takes a small piece of tissue from your small intestine during a procedure called an upper GI endoscopy.

Skin Biopsy

If a doctor suspects you have dermatitis herpetiformis, he or she will perform a skin biopsy. For a skin biopsy, the doctor removes tiny pieces of skin tissue to examine with a microscope. A doctor examines the skin tissue and checks the tissue for antibodies common in celiac disease. If the skin tissue has the antibodies, a doctor will perform blood tests to confirm celiac disease. If the skin biopsy and blood tests both suggest celiac disease, you may not need an intestinal biopsy.

Do Doctors Screen for Celiac Disease?

Screening is testing for diseases when you have no symptoms. Doctors in the United States do not routinely screen people for celiac disease. However, blood relatives of people with celiac disease and those with type 1 diabetes should talk with their doctor about their chances of getting the disease. Many researchers recommend routine screening of all family members, such as parents and siblings, for celiac disease. However, routine genetic screening for celiac disease is not usually helpful when diagnosing the disease.

Treatment for Celiac Disease

A Gluten-Free Diet

Doctors treat celiac disease with a gluten-free diet. Gluten is a protein found naturally in wheat, barley, and rye that triggers a reaction if you have celiac disease. Symptoms greatly improve for most people with celiac disease who stick to a gluten-free diet. In recent years, grocery stores and restaurants have added many more gluten-free foods and products, making it easier to stay gluten free. Your doctor may refer you to a dietitian who specializes in treating people with celiac disease. The dietitian will teach you how to avoid gluten while following a healthy diet. He or she will help you:

- Check food and product labels for gluten
- Design everyday meal plans
- Make healthy choices about the types of foods to eat

For most people, following a gluten-free diet will heal damage in the small intestine and prevent more damage. You may see symptoms improve within days to weeks of starting the diet. The small intestine usually heals in 3–6 months in children. Complete healing can take several years in adults. Once the intestine heals, the villi, which were damaged by the disease, regrow and will absorb nutrients from food into the bloodstream normally.

Gluten-Free Diet and Dermatitis Herpetiformis

If you have dermatitis herpetiformis—an itchy, blistering skin rash—skin symptoms generally respond to a gluten-free diet. However, skin symptoms may return if you add gluten back into your diet. Medicines such as dapsone, taken by mouth, can control the skin symptoms. People who take dapsone need to have regular blood tests to check for side effects from the medicine.

Dapsone does not treat intestinal symptoms or damage, which is why you should stay on a gluten-free diet if you have the rash. Even when you follow a gluten-free diet, the rash may take months or even years to fully heal—and often comes back over the years.

In addition to prescribing a gluten-free diet, your doctor will want you to avoid all hidden sources of gluten. If you have celiac disease, ask a pharmacist about ingredients in:

- Herbal and nutritional supplements

- Prescription and over-the-counter (OTC) medicines

- Vitamin and mineral supplements

You also could take in or transfer from your hands to your mouth other products that contain gluten without knowing it. Products that may contain gluten include:

- Children's modeling dough, such as Play-Doh

- Cosmetics

- Lipstick, lip gloss, and lip balm

- Skin and hair products

- Toothpaste and mouthwash

- Communion wafers

Medications are rare sources of gluten. Even if gluten is present in a medicine, it is likely to be in such small quantities that it would not cause any symptoms.

Reading product labels can sometimes help you avoid gluten. Some product makers label their products as being gluten-free. If a product label doesn't list the product's ingredients, ask the maker of the product for an ingredients list.

What If Changing to a Gluten-Free Diet Isn't Working?

If you don't improve after starting a gluten-free diet, you may still be eating or using small amounts of gluten. You probably will start responding to the gluten-free diet once you find and cut out all hidden sources of gluten. Hidden sources of gluten include additives made with wheat, such as:

- Modified food starch

- Malt flavoring

- Preservatives
- Stabilizers

If you still have symptoms even after changing your diet, you may have other conditions or disorders that are more common with celiac disease, such as irritable bowel syndrome (IBS), lactose intolerance, microscopic colitis, dysfunction of the pancreas, and small intestinal bacterial overgrowth.

Eating, Diet, and Nutrition for Celiac Disease

What Should I Avoid Eating If I Have Celiac Disease?

Avoiding foods with gluten, a protein found naturally in wheat, rye, and barley, is critical in treating celiac disease. Removing gluten from your diet will improve symptoms, heal damage to your small intestine, and prevent further damage over time. While you may need to avoid certain foods, the good news is that many healthy, gluten-free foods and products are available.

You should avoid all products that contain gluten, such as most cereal, grains, and pasta, and many processed foods. Be sure to always read food ingredient lists carefully to make sure the food you want to eat doesn't have gluten. In addition, discuss gluten-free food choices with a dietitian or healthcare professional who specializes in celiac disease.

What Should I Eat If I Have Celiac Disease?

Foods such as meat, fish, fruits, vegetables, rice, and potatoes without additives or seasonings do not contain gluten and are part of a well-balanced diet. You can eat gluten-free types of bread, pasta, and other foods that are now easier to find in stores, restaurants, and at special food companies. You also can eat potato, rice, soy, amaranth, quinoa, buckwheat, or bean flour instead of wheat flour.

In the past, doctors and dietitians advised against eating oats if you have celiac disease. Evidence suggests that most people with the disease can safely eat moderate amounts of oats, as long as they did not come in contact with wheat gluten during processing. You should talk with your healthcare team about whether to include oats in your diet.

When shopping and eating out, remember to:

- Read food labels—especially on canned, frozen, and processed foods—for ingredients that contain gluten

- Identify foods labeled "gluten-free;" by law, these foods must contain less than 20 parts per million, well below the threshold to cause problems in the great majority of patients with celiac disease

- Ask restaurant servers and chefs about how they prepare the food and what is in it

- Find out whether a gluten-free menu is available

- Ask a dinner or party host about gluten-free options before attending a social gathering

Foods labeled gluten-free tend to cost more than the same foods that have gluten. You may find that naturally gluten-free foods are less expensive. With practice, looking for gluten can become second nature. If you have just been diagnosed with celiac disease, you and your family members may find support groups helpful as you adjust to a new approach to eating.

Is a Gluten-Free Diet Safe If I Don't Have Celiac Disease?

In recent years, more people without celiac disease have adopted a gluten-free diet, believing that avoiding gluten is healthier or could help them lose weight. No current data suggests that the general public should maintain a gluten-free diet for weight loss or better health.

A gluten-free diet isn't always a healthy diet. For instance, a gluten-free diet may not provide enough of the nutrients, vitamins, and minerals the body needs, such as fiber, iron, and calcium. Some gluten-free products can be high in calories and sugar. If you think you might have celiac disease, don't start avoiding gluten without first speaking with your doctor. If your doctor diagnoses you with celiac disease, he or she will put you on a gluten-free diet.

Gluten-Free Food Labeling Requirements

The U.S. Food and Drug Administration (FDA) published a rule defining what "gluten-free" means on food labels. The "gluten-free" for food labeling rule requires that any food with the terms "gluten-free," "no gluten," "free of gluten," and "without gluten" on the label must meet all of the definition's requirements. While the FDA rule does not apply to foods regulated by the U.S. Department of Agriculture (USDA), including meat and egg products, it is often still observed.

Section 19.3

Going Gluten Free

This section includes text excerpted from "Going Gluten Free?" *NIH News in Health*, National Institutes of Health (NIH), May 2016.

With the growing popularity of gluten-free products at your local grocery store, you may have wondered if you should avoid eating gluten. Sidestepping gluten can be a lifestyle choice for many. But for those with a condition known as celiac disease, it's a medical necessity.

Gluten is a protein found in wheat, barley, rye, and sometimes oats—ingredients often used in breads, pastas, and desserts. Some people get gas, diarrhea, or bloating after eating gluten. These symptoms could be caused by intolerance to the protein or a wheat allergy, but celiac disease is different.

When a person with celiac disease eats or drinks anything with gluten, the body's immune system attacks the inside of the small intestine. The damage from this attack keeps the body from absorbing needed nutrients. If left untreated, celiac disease can lead to malnutrition, depression, anxiety, anemia, or weakened bones. It can also delay children's growth.

Celiac disease can be hard to spot, because its symptoms can be similar to other disorders. The condition affects about 1 percent of people worldwide; nearly 80 percent of them haven't been diagnosed, says Dr. Alessio Fasano, a celiac disease specialist at Massachusetts General Hospital. "Celiac disease is a clinical chameleon. This creates tremendous confusion and challenging situations for both healthcare professionals and people who are trying to understand what's wrong with them," Fasano says.

Your doctor can use a blood test to look for signs of celiac disease. Before the test, continue eating foods with gluten. Otherwise, the results may be negative for celiac disease even if you have it. Eating a regular diet can also help your doctor determine if you have a form of gluten sensitivity that is not celiac disease. Gluten sensitivity is something you may grow out of over time, Fasano explains, whereas celiac disease is a lifelong condition.

If your tests and symptoms suggest celiac disease, your doctor may confirm the diagnosis by removing a small piece of your intestine to inspect it for damage.

Genetic tests may be used to detect the genes that turn on the body's immune response to gluten. Such tests can help rule out celiac disease, but they can't be used for diagnoses; many people who have the genes never develop celiac disease.

Fasano's team is studying why some people with these genes don't have symptoms. The National Institutes of Health (NIH)-funded researchers will follow infants who are at increased risk because a family member has celiac disease. The team hopes its findings will help doctors predict who will get celiac disease and learn how to prevent it.

People with one autoimmune disease are at increased risk for other autoimmune diseases. Because celiac disease and type 1 diabetes share risk genes, a large international study is following newborns at risk for both conditions to identify environmental factors that may trigger or protect from these diseases.

Going on a strict 100 percent gluten-free diet for life remains the only treatment for now. "We can't take the genes out, so we remove the environmental trigger," Fasano says.

Gluten is sometimes found in unexpected sources—such as medications, vitamins, or lip balms—so check ingredient lists carefully. The U.S. Food and Drug Administration (FDA) has strict regulations for the use of "gluten-free" labels. Talking with a dietitian can also be helpful for learning about your food options.

If you suspect you may have celiac disease, talk with your doctor. Waiting too long for a diagnosis might lead to serious problems.

Chapter 20

Soy Allergy

Soy is a plant in the pea family. Soybeans, the high-protein seeds of the soy plant, contain chemical compounds called isoflavones that have a variety of uses in traditional or folk medicine. Since isoflavones are similar to the female hormone estrogen, soy products have long been used to treat such women's health concerns as menopausal symptoms, osteoporosis, and breast cancer, as well as conditions like high blood pressure, high cholesterol levels, memory loss, and prostate cancer.

Soy is available in the form of dietary supplements. In addition, soybeans can be cooked and eaten or used to make tofu, soymilk, and other foods. Soy is also commonly used as an additive in a wide variety of processed foods, including baked goods, cheese, and pasta.

Common Soy Containing Foods in the United States

Edamame (green soybeans), miso (soybean pastes), soy nuts, soy milk, soy protein, soy apricot, tamari, and tempeh (fermented soybean products) are some soy-containing food products. As per the U.S. Food and Drug Administration (FDA) regulations under Food Allergen Labeling and Consumer Protection Act (FALCPA), the major eight food allergens which includes soy, should be mentioned in the label in plain language.

"Soy Allergy," © 2018 Omnigraphics. Reviewed August 2018.

Symptoms and Diagnosis

Despite its potential health benefits, soy is a fairly common food allergy. Soy allergy occurs when the human immune system overreacts to the protein in soy, causing the body to produce immunoglobulin E (IgE) antibodies. The IgE antibodies gets attached to mast cells when some allergens i.e., soy proteins is taken, it cross links the IgE molecules causing the release of Histamine and other chemicals that are typically involved in an allergic response. Soy allergy affects approximately 0.4 percent of children in the United States. A majority of children outgrow soy allergy by the age of three or four years., So it is relatively less common in adults.

Reactions to soy or its derivatives may involve a range of allergic symptoms like tingling in the mouth, hives, itching or eczema, swelling of the hips, face, tongue, and throat or other parts of the body wheezing and abdominal cramps. Anaphylaxis—a severe, life-threatening whole-body allergic response—may occur in some people with soy allergy, but it is rather rare. The most common symptoms of a soy allergy are pruritus (itching) around the lips, mouth, face, or other parts of the body; allergic rhinitis (nasal congestion, sneezing, and watery eyes); and nausea, vomiting, and diarrhea.

How the Allergy Is Diagnosed

A soy allergy is initially diagnosed with a skin prick test (SPT), wherein a measured dose of a liquid containing soy protein extract is introduced into the top layer of the skin with a sterile probe. The appearance of a red bump or flare on the skin indicates a sensitivity to soy and helps the allergist make a diagnosis. A blood test may also be done to measure the amount of IgE antibody in the blood.

Avoiding Soy Products

There is no cure for soy allergy. The only way to prevent symptoms from occurring is to exclude soy products from the diet and avoid foods containing soy in any form. Soy is one of the eight common allergens covered under the federal Food Allergen Labeling and Consumer Protection Act. As a result, food manufacturers are required to state on the label whether a product contains soy or has been manufactured in a facility or with equipment that also produces soy-containing products. People with soy allergy should read food labels carefully and avoid ingesting products that contain even traces of soy. If the information on the label is insufficient, they should contact the manufacturer for clarification.

Soy is widely used as an ingredient in commercial foods. In fact, it is estimated that soy plays a role in the production of 20,000–30,000 food products, either directly as an ingredient or indirectly as animal feed. Soy fat and oils are used in foods like margarine and mayonnaise. Soy isolates find use in meat products, soups, sauces, and imitation dairy products. Tofu, which is clotted soymilk, is a popular ingredient in many savory and sweet dishes. Soy meals and soy flour are part of many types of cereals, breads, and pasta. Lecithin, a derivative of soy, is a common additive in a variety of baked food, chocolates, and confections. Most individuals who are allergic to soy can safely tolerate refined soybean oil and lecithin, but they should check with their allergist before consuming these ingredients. Child nutrition staff should always carefully read labels to make sure whether the food is free from soy.

Research on a Hypoallergenic Strain of Soy

To address growing concerns about food allergies all over the world, scientists have worked to produce a genetically modified (GM) variety of soybean that eliminates P34, the protein in soybeans that is responsible for causing food allergy. They hope to create a "hypoallergenic soy" that will not trigger allergic reactions. Animal studies using the hypoallergenic variety are underway and will serve as a springboard for human trials. Commercial use of this new form of soy is a long way off, however, pending regulatory approvals in countries that are wary of using GM food technology.

References

1. Agricultural Research Service (ARS). "Allergic to Certain Foods?" U.S. Department of Agriculture (USDA), February 13, 2009.

2. National Food Service Management Institute (NFSMI). "Food Allergy Fact Sheet: Soy Allergies," University of Mississippi, 2012.

Chapter 21

Ingredients and Food Additives That Trigger Reactions

Chapter Contents

Section 21.1

Seed Allergy

Food allergies are on the increase in the United States, particularly among children. The mechanism involved in hypersensitivity to seeds is more or less similar to that involved in allergic reactions to peanuts tree nuts and other major food allergens. Seeds represent the embryonic stage of plants and are usually encased in a hard, protective covering, the seed coats. They contain reserve macronutrients for the growing seedling in the form of carbohydrates, lipids, and proteins. Some storage proteins, in particular, are a source of allergenicity in a wide range of tree nuts and seeds. Named 2S albumins, this major protein group has been isolated in the seeds of several mono- and di-cotyledonous plants, including sesame, mustard, pumpkin, and poppy. While these globular proteins play a protective role in plants as a defense against pathogenic bacteria and fungi, they can induce an immune system-mediated adverse reaction in the body similar to that expressed in response to the fungal attack.

Seed allergies are being commonly reported as edible seeds and their oils are being increasingly used in processed foods. Studies have also shown that the allergenic potency of seed proteins can be attributed to its high resistance to both thermal processing and proteases (enzyme group that catalyze the breakdown of proteins). While allergic reactions to seeds other than sesame seeds are reported with less frequency, seed allergy in general is becoming a subject of increasing interest to clinical and nutritional studies.

Symptoms of Seed Allergies

Hypersensitivity reactions to seed protein allergens range from mild symptoms, such as urticaria and laryngeal irritation, to immediate and severe systemic reactions, such as angioedema and anaphylaxis.

A life-threatening reaction, anaphylaxis is usually associated with one or more of the following symptoms:

- shortness of breath, or wheezing
- diarrhea and stomach cramps
- swelling of face, tongue, or throat

- low blood pressure
- dizziness
- loss of consciousness

Some Common Seeds with Potential for Allergenicity

Sesame Allergy

Allergy to sesame seed ranks ninth among food allergies in the United States and affects approximately 0.1 percent of the country's population. Sesame seeds are traditionally used as toppings in bread, cookies, crackers, and ready-to-eat breakfast cereals and are being increasingly reported for their allergenicity in recent years. Sesame allergy is most prevalent in Middle Eastern and Mediterranean countries, where the seed is incorporated in a variety of dishes, including convenience food, snacks, oil, and tahini, a widely used condiment prepared from toasted, hulled, and ground sesame seeds. Severity of symptoms may range from mild (rashes, itchy throat, and oral allergy) to severe and potentially fatal anaphylaxis requiring immediate medical assistance. Sesame seed allergy is compounded by the lack of consistency, or clarity, in food label listing. Often, terms such as "gingelly," "tahini," or simply "condiment" on food labels may be misleading, putting sesame-allergic people at risk of a severe systemic reaction.

Sunflower Seed Allergy

Sunflower kernels are harvested for their seeds and oil, which are used for human consumption and also for cattle fodder and bird food. Their leaves and hulls are used to produce fertilizer. People may report allergic reactions after eating whole-grain bread, or ready-to-eat breakfast cereals because sunflower allergens have high heat resistance and remain stable even when exposed to high baking temperatures in the order of 200°C. Oils extracted from sunflower kernels are less likely to trigger hypersensitivity as they do not contain proteins, the primary causal factor for seed allergy. Symptoms associated with sunflower seed allergy usually include urticaria, conjunctivitis, allergic rhinitis, and bronchial asthma, while severe reactions such as angioedema and anaphylactic shock are experienced to a lesser extent.

Occupational allergies associated with sunflower seeds have also been reported among bird breeders and workers in the sunflower-processing industry, and some studies attribute these to cross-reactivity of sunflower pollen with sunflower seeds. Cross-reactivity occurs when the body's immune response to a specific allergen induces a similar adaptive immune response in homologous (structurally related) food. In the case of sunflower seeds, the antibodies produced in response to allergenic proteins present in them can produce similar reactions in response to other plant derivatives such as pollen.

Mustard Allergy

Mustard is a common condiment in many cuisines around the world and is incorporated as seeds or powder in a variety of dishes, including salad dressings, marinades, curries, bread, soups, deli meat, and sauces.
Mustard seeds are of three major types:

- white, also called yellow mustard

- brown, or oriental mustard

- black

Yellow mustard is often a hidden ingredient in salad dressings or dips, and allergic reactions to the seed are reported from time to time, although with less frequency than sesame. The Brassicaceae family to which mustard belongs also includes other edibles such as cabbage, cauliflower, broccoli, canola, turnip, and Brussel sprouts. The seeds or sprouts of these edibles contain proteins similar to the proteins in mustard and are likely to trigger hypersensitivity arising from cross reactivity. As in most seed-induced allergies, the storage protein, 2S albumin, has been identified as the causal factor in mustard allergy. Mild symptoms of hypersensitivity may occur within two hours of ingesting mustard and may include conjunctivitis, rhinitis, sneezing, and skin manifestations such as pruritus, urticaria, erythema, or eczema. Gastrointestinal and respiratory reactions associated with mustard allergy, such as wheezing or diarrhea, are considered moderately severe in their manifestations, particularly in individuals with a history of asthma. The mustard allergens are also known to induce IgE-mediated anaphylaxis, which is accompanied by a dramatic drop in blood pressure. This response could prove fatal and requires immediate treatment with epinephrine (adrenaline) and a subsequent visit to the emergency room.

Diagnosis of Seed Allergies

A seed allergy is usually established with a skin prick test (SPT). This test is performed by placing a small quantity of a seed protein extract on a small prick made on the skin (usually forearm) and examining the size of the wheal (swelling) after 10–15 minutes. A blood test is another important diagnostic tool that can also be to confirm a diagnosis of seed allergy. The serum IgE test involves measurement of serum concentrations of immunoglobulin E (IgE) specific to a food allergen. Serum IgE tests are particularly significant when symptoms such as severe eczema preclude skin prick testing, or when certain antihistamine medications used to treat food allergies are likely to interfere with the reliability of skin prick tests.

Management of Seed Allergies

Seed allergy management primarily focuses on allergen avoidance. The mainstay of successful avoidance is access to proper information on possible contamination of the food by allergens. Despite increasing incidence of sesame allergy, the seed, or its products, is not recognized as a priority allergen by the current regulatory framework in the United States, and the Food Allergen Labeling and Consumer Protection Act of 2004 (FALCPA) has not included it in precautionary allergen labeling, as it has with the eight major allergens. This means that educating the patient on how to avoid the allergen is extremely important, particularly in the cases of highly sensitive individuals. Despite careful allergen avoidance, accidental exposures are known to occur. This is particularly seen in older children who are generally under less direct supervision. An accidental exposure may trigger a severe anaphylactic reaction requiring prompt epinephrine administration. Individuals with severe presentations of seed allergy must keep a preloaded adrenaline injection device available at all times. Adults and older children should be able to recognize the signs and symptoms of anaphylaxis and self-administer the medication.

References

1. "Sesame Allergy: Current Perspectives," National Center for Biotechnology Information (NCBI), April 27, 2017.

2. "Anaphylaxis," Mayo Clinic, January 5, 2018.

3. "Murphy Leads Group in Calling on FDA to Label and Regulate All Sesame Products," United States Senate, March 26, 2018.

Section 21.2

Food Additives and Intolerance

This section includes text excerpted from "Food Ingredients of
Public Health Concern," Food Safety and Inspection Service (FSIS),
U.S. Department of Agriculture (USDA), July 3, 2017.

Some individuals may be intolerant of certain food additives and
color additives. Food intolerances are often confused with allergic
reactions, but the adverse effects of food intolerances do not involve
the same immunological mechanisms as an allergic reaction. Food
intolerances generally do not result in life-threatening reactions
like food allergies; however, they are still of public health signif-
icance, and Food Safety and Inspection Service (FSIS) is equally
concerned about all food ingredients that may cause adverse health
effects.

Some people experience gastrointestinal disturbance when they
drink milk. Often, the gastrointestinal disturbance is not an allergic
reaction to milk proteins but intolerance to lactose, a sugar molecule
in milk and milk products. People intolerant to lactose are generally
deficient in lactase, the enzyme that breaks down lactose in the intestinal tract. As people get older, their lactase levels tend to decline. In
individuals with insufficient levels of lactase, bacteria in the intestine
break down lactose, which produces gas, bloating, cramping, and sometimes diarrhea. It is not just whole milk that is the problem for these
individuals, as a variety of food products may contain milk derivatives
that contain lactose.

Sulfites, including sulfur dioxide, sodium sulfite, sodium bisulfite,
potassium bisulfite, sodium metabisulfite, and potassium metabisulfite, have been used as food preservatives. One of the main uses of
sulfiting agents is to prevent browning of processed fruits, vegetables,
and shellfish. Sulfites are not used directly on meat or poultry products, but other ingredients added to meat or poultry products may
contain sulfites.

People who have an intolerance to sulfites can experience symptoms including chest tightness, hives, stomach cramps, diarrhea, and
breathing problems. The underlying mechanisms for sulfite intolerance are not completely understood. For some individuals, though, the
sensitivity to sulfites may be an allergic type of response. People with
asthma appear to be at an increased risk of having asthma symptoms
following exposure to sulfites.

The presence of sulfiting agents must be declared on the label if their concentration in the finished meat or poultry food product is 10 ppm or higher. However, some finished meat and poultry food products may be comprised of multiple separate components, e.g., potatoes or apple cobbler in a frozen dinner. For these products, if a separate component contains 10 ppm or more sulfiting agents, the sulfiting agents must be declared even though the total product contains less than 10 ppm of sulfiting agents. When sulfiting agents are required to be declared on a label, they must be:

1. declared by their specific name or as "sulfiting agents," and

2. listed in the ingredients statement in order of predominance or at the end of the ingredients statement with the statement, "This Product Contains Sulfiting Agents" (or the specific name of the sulfite compound).

FD&C Yellow No. 5, or tartrazine, has been used as a color additive in a variety of food products. Some consumers appear to have an intolerance to tartrazine. In these consumers, tartrazine may cause symptoms similar to an allergic reaction, i.e., hives and swelling, but the reaction is not considered a true allergy. Tartrazine was also thought to be associated with the onset of asthma attacks, but more recent scientific evidence indicated tartrazine was an unlikely cause of asthma symptoms. To help protect people who may be intolerant to tartrazine, the U.S. Food and Drug Administration (FDA) requires that any food for human use that contains Yellow No. 5 must specifically declare it as an ingredient.

Monosodium Glutamate (MSG) is included as a flavor enhancer in a number of meat and poultry products. Some individuals have reported headaches, chest tightness, nausea, diarrhea, and sweating following consumption of products containing MSG. There is scientific debate over whether MSG causes adverse health effects in individuals. Nonetheless, given the significant consumer concern about this ingredient, FSIS urges companies to ensure that its use is properly declared in labeling.

Gluten is the protein found in cereal grains, including wheat, barley, rye, and oats. It is what helps give dough its elasticity. Some individuals have a condition known as celiac disease, which is basically intolerance to gluten. Although it is not an allergic reaction, it does involve immunological mechanisms that result in inflammation and damage to the lining of the small intestine. Persons with celiac disease experience fatigue, bloating, cramping, chronic diarrhea, and nutrient malabsorption. FSIS permits statements highlighting the presence of certain gluten-containing ingredients. If an establishment wishes to make a special claim that a meat or poultry product is gluten-free, then it must be able to support that special claim.

Nitrate and nitrites are different compounds, both of which are composed of nitrogen and oxygen. They are used as curing agents in many meat and poultry products, including hot dogs, bologna, salami and other processed meats. These compounds contribute to the characteristic cured flavor and reddish-pink color of cured products. They are also important in inhibiting the growth of *Clostridium spp.* These compounds may cause headaches and hives in some people. In excessive amounts, nitrate or nitrite can be toxic. In addition to labeling requirements, the amount of nitrite or nitrate added to a product is restricted by regulation.

Some products that traditionally include nitrite or nitrate can be manufactured without the use of added nitrite or nitrate. Such products are formulated to only include naturally occurring sources of nitrite or nitrate, such as celery juice powder, parsley, cherry powder, beet powder, spinach, or sea salt. Such products must be labeled appropriately. For example, an "uncured" bacon product should include a declaration such as "Uncured Bacon, No Nitrates or Nitrites added except those naturally occurring in___" on the product label. In addition, such products generally must bear the statement "Not Preserved, Keep Refrigerated Below 40°F At All Times," as the naturally occurring sources of nitrite or nitrate do not inhibit the outgrowth of Clostridium spp. to the same extent as the highly purified chemical forms. Exceptions to this refrigeration handling statement would be finished products that have been dried according to other requirements or that contain a sufficient amount of salt to achieve an internal brine concentration of 10 percent or more.

Section 21.3

Sulfite Sensitivity

The U.S. Food and Drug Administration (FDA) has identified sulfites as one of the top-ten food allergens that affect one out of every 100 people living in the United States. Sulfites are used in food as preservatives to prevent discoloration or browning and to help deter spoilage. They are also used in the preparation, storage, and distribution of a wide variety of beverages. The wine industry, for example, has used sulfite as an ingredient for centuries, relying on its antioxidant and antibacterial properties to help keep wine fresh longer. During the 1970s and 1980s, the use of sulfites in food and beverages increased significantly, and in August 1986, the FDA banned the use of sulfites in fresh fruits and vegetables due to a growing number of cases of serious physical reactions to sulfites among many individuals.

In addition to their use as a food and beverage additive, sulfites are also commonly found in pharmaceutical products. These chemicals are often added to a number of medications, including those prescribed to treat asthma and allergic reactions, as a means of stabilizing and preserving the drugs for longer shelf life.

The exact causes of sulfite sensitivity are unclear; however, many experts believe there could be genetic or environmental factors involved. It also appears that individuals affected with asthma are particularly at risk for developing sulfite sensitivity. People often confuse sulfite sensitivity with an allergy; however, food allergies are usually caused by proteins in food, while the chemical sulfite does not contain proteins but is a salt of sulfurous acid.

Symptoms

The symptoms of sulfite sensitivity, which can range from mild to severe, take a minimum of 15–30 minutes to surface. They can include headache, hives, sneezing, sinus congestion, tightness of the throat, asthma attacks, runny nose, wheezing, shortness of breath, abdominal pain, nausea, coughing, skin inflammation, and skin rash.

Other health conditions that seem to have a link to sulfites include fibromyalgia, diabetes, depression, candida and other fungal infections, joint pain, immune deficiencies, skin conditions, irritable bowel syndrome (IBS), muscle weakness, nosebleeds, bloating, yeast infections, indigestion, heart palpitations, chronic fatigue syndrome (CFS), tooth pain, ear infections, and lethargy. In many cases, people can relieve some of these symptoms by maintaining a sulfite-free diet.

Asthma symptoms have been very closely linked to the intake of sulfites. Although these can vary from person to person, symptoms can range from mild wheezing to life-threatening asthma reactions. Consumption of food or beverages containing sulfite can trigger asthma attacks, but the inhalation of sulfur dioxide from foods containing sulfites may also cause asthmatic symptoms. In rare cases, sulfites have also been known to cause anaphylaxis, a severe, life-threatening allergic reaction.

Diagnosis

In order to diagnose sulfite sensitivity, a healthcare provider will ask for a complete medical history, including a detailed description of symptoms. The healthcare provider may also ask about the patient's location when the symptoms occurred, as well as the type of food and beverages consumed. A doctor will conduct a thorough physical examination and will likely order lab work that might include blood tests and allergy skin tests.

For asthma attacks linked to sulfites, the healthcare provider may recommend a challenge procedure. This involves capsules or solutions of sulfites in increasing dosages over a period of two or more hours. Initially, a small dose of sulfite is administered to the sulfite-sensitive person. Mild doses are given to make sure only slight wheezing occurs and more severe reactions are avoided. But certain individuals who are sulfite-sensitive may not react to small doses, and in these cases, a heavier dose may be required. If an asthmatic reaction takes place, then the lung function is measured, and the reaction is quickly reversed with the help of an inhaled bronchodilator medication.

Treatment

Avoidance is the best cure for sulfite sensitivity. Once a diagnosis is confirmed, a healthcare provider will determine a course of treatment. Many symptoms can be reduced or eliminated by avoiding foods, beverages, and medications that contain sulfites.

The following are some steps commonly recommended to address sulfite sensitivity:

- Knowing the names of sulfites and recognizing them on food labels

- Avoiding foods that contain sulfite ingredients
- Reading drug labels carefully, and consulting with a pharmacist for sulfite-free medications
- If allergy seems to be severe, carrying a dose of epinephrine to treat severe reactions

Certain medications might be prescribed by a healthcare provider to treat allergic reactions and other symptoms:

- Epinephrine for life-threatening allergic reactions
- For asthma, an inhaler to help relieve airway inflammation
- Antihistamines for swelling and itching
- Corticosteroids for several swelling and itching

Foods That May Contain Sulfites

Individuals with sulfite sensitivity need to educate themselves about foods that contain sulfites. Ingredients to look for on a food labels include sulfur dioxide, potassium bisulfite, sodium bisulfite, sodium metabisulfite, sodium sulfite, and potassium metabisulfite.

Some food items that may contain sulfite include maraschino cherries, all cheeses, wine vinegar, olives, pickles, and horseradish. Foods that contain gelatin, maple syrup, jams, jellies, and corn syrup can also have sulfites added to them, as can pizza, pie crust, tortillas, pasta, noodles, and crackers.

Alcoholic beverages, such as beer, wine, and mixed drinks, may contain sulfites to control or prevent fermentation, and beer and wine can also have natural sulfites in them. Sulfites might also be present in some nonalcoholic beverages, including fruit and vegetable juices and different kinds of tea.

Fish, meat, and other perishable food products require preservation until they are consumed, so many of them contain sulfites. For example, sulfites are used to help shellfish keep their color, preventing black spots on shrimp and lobster. They are added to meat to increase color so that the product looks fresher. Canned seafood, dried codfish, and seafood soups can contain sulfite, as can dried fruits and many other preserved products.

References

1. "Sulfite Sensitivity," Cleveland Clinic, December 30, 2016.

2. "Sulfite Allergies," Sulfites.org, n.d

3. "Health Library: Sulfite Sensitivity," Winchester Hospital, n.d.

4. "List of Foods for Sulfite Sensitivity," SFGate.com, n.d.

Section 21.4

Histamine Intolerance

This section includes text excerpted from "Bad Bug Book,"
U.S. Food and Drug Administration (FDA), October 24, 2017.

Scombrotoxin

Toxin

Scombrotoxin is a combination of substances, histamine prominent among them. Histamine is produced during decomposition of fish, when decarboxylase enzymes made by bacteria that inhabit (but do not sicken) the fish interact with the fish's naturally occurring histidine, resulting in histamine formation. Other vasoactive biogenic amines resulting from decomposition of the fish, such as putrescine and cadaverine, also are thought to be components of scombrotoxin. Time/temperature abuse of scombrotoxin-forming fish (e.g., tuna and mahi-mahi) create conditions that promote the formation of the toxin. Scombrotoxin poisoning is closely linked to the accumulation of histamine in these fish.

The U.S. Food and Drug Administration (FDA) has established regulatory guidelines that consider fish containing histamine at 50 ppm or greater to be in a state of decomposition and fish containing histamine at 500 ppm or greater to be a public health hazard. The European Union issued Council Directive (91/493/EEC) in 1991, which states that when 9 samples taken from a lot of fish are analyzed for histamine, the mean value must not exceed 100 ppm; two samples may have a value of more than 100 ppm, but less than 200 ppm; and no sample may have a value exceeding 200 ppm.

Disease

The disease caused by scombrotoxin is called scombrotoxin poisoning or histamine poisoning. Treatment with antihistamine drugs is warranted when scombrotoxin poisoning is suspected.

- **Mortality:** No deaths have been confirmed to have resulted from scombrotoxin poisoning.

- **Dose:** In most cases, histamine levels in illness-causing (scombrotoxic) fish have exceeded 200 ppm, often above 500 ppm. However, there is some evidence that other biogenic amines also may play a role in the illness.

- **Onset:** The onset of intoxication symptoms is rapid, ranging from minutes to a few hours after consumption.

- **Disease/complications:** Severe reactions (e.g., cardiac and respiratory complications) occur rarely, but people with preexisting conditions may be susceptible. People on certain medications, including the antituberculosis drug isoniazid, are at increased risk for severe reactions.

- **Symptoms:** Symptoms of scombrotoxin poisoning include tingling or burning in or around the mouth or throat, rash or hives, drop in blood pressure, headache, dizziness, itching of the skin, nausea, vomiting, diarrhea, asthmatic-like constriction of air passage, heart palpitation, and respiratory distress.

- **Duration:** The duration of the illness is relatively short, with symptoms commonly lasting several hours, but, in some cases, adverse effects may persist for several days.

- **Route of entry:** Oral.

- **Pathway:** In humans, histamine exerts its effects on the cardiovascular system by causing blood-vessel dilation, which results in flushing, headache, and hypotension. It increases heart rate and contraction strength, leading to heart palpitations, and induces intestinal smooth-muscle contraction, causing abdominal cramps, vomiting, and diarrhea. Histamine also stimulates motor and sensory neurons, which may account for burning sensations and itching associated with scombrotoxin poisoning. Other biogenic amines, such as putrescine and cadaverine, may potentiate scombrotoxin poisoning by interfering with the enzymes necessary to metabolize histamine in the human body.

Frequency

Scombrotoxin poisoning is one of the most common forms of fish poisoning in the United States. From 1990–2007, outbreaks of scombrotoxin poisoning numbered 379 and involved 1,726 people, per reports to the Centers for Disease Control and Prevention (CDC). However, the actual number of outbreaks is believed to be far greater than that reported.

Sources

Fishery products that have been implicated in scombrotoxin poisoning include tuna, mahi-mahi, bluefish, sardines, mackerel, amberjack, anchovies, and others. Scombrotoxin-forming fish are commonly distributed as fresh, frozen, or processed products and may be consumed in a myriad of product forms. Distribution of the toxin within an individual fish or between cans in a case lot can be uneven, with some sections of a product capable of causing illnesses and others not. Cooking, canning, and freezing do not reduce the toxic effects. Common sensory examination by the consumer cannot ensure the absence or presence of the toxin. Chemical analysis is a reliable test for evaluating a suspect fishery product. Histamine also may be produced in other foods, such as cheese and sauerkraut, which also has resulted in toxic effects in humans.

Diagnosis

Diagnosis of the illness is usually based on the patient's symptoms, time of onset, and the effect of treatment with antihistamine medication. The suspected food should be collected; rapidly chilled or, preferably, frozen; and transported to the appropriate laboratory for histamine analyses. Elevated levels of histamine in food suspected of causing scombrotoxin poisoning aid in confirming a diagnosis.

Target Populations

All humans are susceptible to scombrotoxin poisoning; however, as noted, the commonly mild symptoms can be more severe for individuals taking some medications, such as the antituberculosis drug isoniazid. Because of the worldwide network for harvesting, processing, and distributing fishery products, the impact of the problem is not limited to specific geographic areas or consumption patterns.

Food Analysis

The official method (AOAC 977.13) for histamine analysis in seafood employs a simple alcoholic extraction and quantitation by fluorescence spectroscopy. Putrescine and cadaverine can be analyzed by Association of Official Agricultural Chemists (AOAC) Official Method 996.07. Several other analytical procedures to quantify biogenic amines have been published in the literature.

Chapter 22

Other Health Problems Related to Food Allergic Reactions

Chapter Contents

Section 22.1

Eosinophilic Esophagitis

This section includes text excerpted from "Eosinophilic Esophagitis,"
MedlinePlus, National Institutes of Health (NIH), May 7, 2018.

What Is Eosinophilic Esophagitis?

Eosinophilic esophagitis (EoE) is a chronic disease of the esophagus.
Your esophagus is the muscular tube that carries food and liquids
from your mouth to the stomach. If you have EoE, white blood cells
called eosinophils build up in your esophagus. This causes damage and
inflammation, which can cause pain and may lead to trouble swallowing and food getting stuck in your throat. EoE is rare. But because it
is a newly recognized disease, more people are now getting diagnosed
with it. Some people who think that they have reflux (GERD) may
actually have EoE.

What Causes Eosinophilic Esophagitis?

Researchers are not certain about the exact cause of EoE. They
think that it is an immune system/allergic reaction to foods or to substances in your environment, such as dust mites, animal dander, pollen, and molds. Certain genes may also play a role in EoE.

Who Gets Eosinophilic Esophagitis?

EoE can affect anyone, but it is more common in people who

- are male;
- are Caucasian;
- have other allergic diseases, such as hay fever, eczema, asthma
  and food allergies; and
- have family members with EoE.

What Are the Symptoms of Eosinophilic Esophagitis?

The most common symptoms of EoE can depend on your age.
In infants and toddlers:

- Feeding problems

- Vomiting

- Poor weight gain and growth

- Reflux that does not get better with medicines

In older children:

- Vomiting

- Abdominal pain

- Trouble swallowing, especially with solid foods

- Reflux that does not get better with medicines

- Poor appetite

In adults:

- Trouble swallowing, especially with solid foods

- Food getting stuck in the esophagus

- Reflux that does not get better with medicines

- Heartburn

- Chest pain

How Is Eosinophilic Esophagitis Diagnosed?

To diagnose EoE, your doctor will:

- **Ask about your symptoms and medical history.** Since other conditions can have the same symptoms of EoE, it is important for your doctor to take a thorough history.

- **Do an upper gastrointestinal (GI) endoscopy.** An endoscope is a long, flexible tube with a light and camera at the end of it. Your doctor will run the endoscope down your esophagus and look at it. Some signs that you might have EoE include white spots, rings, narrowing, and inflammation in the esophagus. However, not everyone with EoE has those signs, and sometimes they can be signs of a different esophagus disorder.

- **Do a biopsy.** During the endoscopy, the doctor will take small tissue samples from your esophagus. The samples will be checked for a high number of eosinophils. This is the only way to make a diagnosis of EoE.

- **Do other tests as needed.** You may have blood tests to check for other conditions. If you do have EoE, you may have blood or other types of tests to check for specific allergies.

What Are the Treatments for Eosinophilic Esophagitis?

There is no cure for EoE. Treatments can manage your symptoms and prevent further damage. The two main types of treatments are medicines and diet.

Medicines used to treat EoE are:

- Steroids, which can help control inflammation. These are usually topical steroids, which you swallow either from an inhaler or as a liquid. Sometimes doctors prescribe oral steroids (pills) to treat people who have serious swallowing problems or weight-loss.

- Acid suppressors such as proton pump inhibitors (PPIs), which may help with reflux symptoms and decrease inflammation.

Dietary changes for EoE include:

- Elimination diet. If you are on an elimination diet, you stop eating and drinking certain foods and beverages for several weeks. If you are feeling better, you add the foods back to your diet one at a time. You have repeat endoscopies to see whether or not you are tolerating those foods. There are different types of elimination diets:

  - With one type, you first have an allergy test. Then you stop eating and drinking the foods you are allergic to.

  - For another type, you eliminate foods and drinks that commonly cause allergies, such as dairy products, egg, wheat, soy, peanuts, tree nuts and fish/shellfish.

- Elemental diet. With this diet, you stop eating and drinking all proteins. Instead, you drink an amino acid formula. Some people who do not like the taste of the formula use a feeding tube instead. If your symptoms and inflammation go away completely, you may be able to try adding foods back one at a time, to see whether you can tolerate them.

Which treatment your healthcare provider suggests depends on different factors, including your age. Some people may use more than one kind of treatment. Researchers are still trying to understand EoE and how best to treat it.

If your treatment is not working well enough and you have a narrowing of the esophagus, you may need dilation. This is a procedure to stretch the esophagus. This makes it easier for you to swallow.

Section 22.2

Food Protein-Induced Enterocolitis Syndrome

This section includes text excerpted from "ICD-9-CM Coordination and Maintenance—Diagnosis Agenda," Centers for Disease Control and Prevention (CDC), September 19, 2012. Reviewed August 2018.

Food protein-induced enterocolitis syndrome (FPIES) is a gastrointestinal food allergy, which causes symptoms of vomiting usually within 1–3 hours after eating the causative food. There often may also be diarrhea within 5–8 hours, which may be bloody. Vomiting and diarrhea may be so severe as to cause dehydration, and even shock; lethargy and pallor may also occur. It usually occurs in infants, with onset most often before 3 months, but up to 1 year, and usually it resolves by about 3 years of age. It most often is due to milk or soy proteins, but may also be due to rice, or other food proteins. FPIES has also been described in adults, particularly due to shellfish. The symptoms of vomiting and diarrhea with FPIES generally resolve quickly with the elimination of the causative food from the diet. In chronic cases, there may be weight loss and failure to thrive. Definitive diagnosis of FPIES may require physician-supervised oral food challenges to be done in an inpatient setting, to demonstrate the response.

Food protein-induced proctocolitis is another distinct gastrointestinal food allergy, which causes blood-streaked stools, and usually presents in the first months of life. It can cause anemia. It has been called by different terms, including allergic proctocolitis, food-induced eosinophilic proctocolitis, milk protein-induced proctocolitis, and eosinophilic colitis. The last term is the title for ICD-10-CM code K52.82.

While many allergies are Immunoglobulin E (IgE) mediated (e.g., anaphylactic shock), FPIES and food protein-induced proctocolitis are not IgE mediated. They are thought to be cell mediated. In some cases of FPIES, IgE may also be present, but would not be considered to be related.

Another non-IgE mediated food allergy is food protein-induced enteropathy. It also occurs in young infants, and causes chronic diarrhea, weight loss, and failure to thrive. It is also treated by strict dietary elimination of the allergen, and is usually outgrown by age 2 or 3 years.

Oral allergy syndrome involves symptoms of itching, swelling, or tingling of the lips, mouth, or throat, in response to a food, often to raw fruits or vegetables. This is considered a gastrointestinal allergy, which is IgE mediated, and may also be considered an adverse food reaction.

A request to consider the creation of specific ICD-10-CM diagnosis codes for FPIES and food protein-induced proctocolitis (FPIP) was received from the International Association for FPE.

Section 22.3

Oral Allergy Syndrome and Other Conditions

This section includes text excerpted from "Characterizing Food Allergy and Addressing Related Disorders," National Institute of Allergy and Infectious Diseases (NIAID), April 26, 2016.

In addition to studying common food allergies, such as peanut, milk and egg allergies, National Institute of Allergy and Infectious Diseases (NIAID) funds research on disorders that are related to, or occur alongside, food allergy. Research related to these increasingly diagnosed conditions may offer insight on treatment and prevention.

Oral Allergy Syndrome

Oral allergy syndrome is an allergic reaction to certain raw fruits and vegetables, such as apples, cherries, kiwis, celery, tomatoes, melons, and bananas. Oral allergy syndrome occurs in people with hay fever, or cold-like symptoms caused by allergies. The syndrome is most likely to occur in those allergic to birch, grass and ragweed pollens because some of the protein allergens in these types of pollen are similar in structure to the proteins of certain fruits.

Those with oral allergy syndrome generally do not experience life-threatening reactions, but they can experience a rash, itching, swelling and sneezing if they eat or even just hold these raw fruits and vegetables. Similar to the experimental baked food approach to treating other food allergies, symptoms typically do not occur after consuming cooked or baked fruits and vegetables, as cooking or processing fruits and vegetables easily breaks down the proteins that cause oral allergy syndrome.

Conditions Often Mistaken for Food Allergy

People can feel ill after eating specific foods for reasons other than food allergy. Though these disorders may have some symptoms in common, these illnesses should not be confused with food allergy.

A problem often confused with food allergy is food intolerance, which is also an abnormal response to a food product, but differs from an allergy. A common example is an intolerance to lactose, a sugar found in many milk products that can cause an uncomfortable buildup of gas in the gastrointestinal tract. Gluten intolerance, or celiac disease, occurs when the immune system responds abnormally to gluten, a component of barley, wheat, and rye. However, unlike food allergies, these disorders do not involve IgE antibodies. The National Institute of Diabetes and Digestive and Kidney Disorders (NIDDK) conducts research on lactose and gluten intolerance.

Foodborne illness, or food poisoning, can also be confused with food allergy because of similar symptoms, such as abdominal cramping. Foodborne illness, however, is caused by microbes, microbial products, and other toxins that can contaminate foods that were improperly preserved or processed.

Chapter 23

Advice for Consumers about Food Labels

Chapter Contents

Section 23.1

Questions and Answers about Food Labels

This section includes text excerpted from "Food Allergen Labeling and Consumer Protection Act of 2004 Questions and Answers," U.S. Food and Drug Administration (FDA), July 18, 2006. Reviewed August 2018.

The Food Allergen Labeling and Consumer Protection Act (FALCPA) will improve food labeling information for the millions of consumers who suffer from food allergies. The Act will be especially helpful to children who must learn to recognize the allergens they must avoid.

The following questions and answers will be useful in answering questions about FALCPA, food allergen labeling, gluten, and advice for consumers.

Food Allergen Labeling and Consumer Protection Act

What Is the Food Allergen Labeling and Consumer Protection Act of 2004?

FALCPA is an amendment to the Federal Food, Drug, and Cosmetic Act (FFDCA) and requires that the label of a food that contains an ingredient that is or contains protein from a "major food allergen " declare the presence of the allergen in the manner described by the law.

Why Did Congress Pass This Act?

Congress passed this Act to make it easier for food allergic consumers and their caregivers to identify and avoid foods that contain major food allergens. In fact, in a review of the foods of randomly selected manufacturers of baked goods, ice cream, and candy in Minnesota and Wisconsin in 1999, U.S. Food and Drug Administration (FDA) found that 25 percent of sampled foods failed to list peanuts or eggs as ingredients on the food labels although the foods contained these allergens.

When Does the Food Allergen Labeling and Consumer Protection Act Become Effective?

FALCPA applies to food products that are labeled on or after January 1, 2006.

What Is a Major Food Allergen?

FALCPA identifies eight foods or food groups as the major food allergens. They are milk, eggs, fish (e.g., bass, flounder, cod), Crustacean shellfish (e.g., crab, lobster, shrimp), tree nuts (e.g., almonds, walnuts, pecans), peanuts, wheat, and soybeans.

The Food Allergen Labeling and Consumer Protection Act Identifies Only Eight Allergens. Aren't There More Foods Consumers Are Allergic To?

Yes. More than 160 foods have been identified to cause food allergies in sensitive individuals. However, the eight major food allergens identified by FALCPA account for over 90 percent of all documented food allergies in the United States and represent the foods most likely to result in severe or life-threatening reactions.

How Serious Are Food Allergies?

It is estimated that 2 percent of adults and about 5 percent of infants and young children in the United States suffer from food allergies. Approximately 30,000 consumers require emergency room treatment and 150 Americans die each year because of allergic reactions to food.

Does the Food Allergen Labeling and Consumer Protection Act Apply to Imported Foods as Well?

FALCPA applies to both domestically manufactured and imported packaged foods that are subject to FDA regulation.

The FDA Held Public Meetings on Allergens and Gluten; What Were the Outcomes of Those Meetings?

The FDA held two meetings. The first meeting, a Food Advisory Committee Meeting held in June 2005, evaluated the FDA's draft report, "Approaches to Establish Thresholds for Major Food Allergens and for Gluten in Food."

The FDA held a second public meeting in August 2005 to obtain expert comment and consultation from stakeholders to help the FDA develop a regulation to define and permit the voluntary use on food labeling of the term "gluten-free" (Public Meeting On: Gluten-Free Food Labeling). The meeting focused on food manufacturing, analytical methods, and consumer issues related to reduced levels of gluten in food. Information presented during and following the meeting provided the

FDA important and relevant data regarding current industry practices in the production of foods marketed as "gluten-free," challenges faced by manufacturers of "gluten-free" foods, and consumer perceptions and expectations of what "gluten-free" means to them. The FDA is using this information to develop its proposal on the use of the term "gluten-free."

Will the FDA Establish a Threshold Level for Any Allergen?

The FDA may consider a threshold level for one or more food allergens.

Labeling

How Will Food Labels Change as a Result of the Food Allergen Labeling and Consumer Protection Act?

FALCPA requires food manufacturers to label food products that contain an ingredient that is or contains protein from a major food allergen in one of two ways.

The first option for food manufacturers is to include the name of the food source in parenthesis following the common or usual name of the major food allergen in the list of ingredients in instances when the name of the food source of the major allergen does not appear elsewhere in the ingredient statement.

For example:

Ingredients: Enriched flour (wheat flour, malted barley, niacin, reduced iron, thiamin mononitrate, riboflavin, folic acid), sugar, partially hydrogenated soybean oil, and/or cottonseed oil, high fructose corn syrup, whey (milk), eggs, vanilla, natural and artificial flavoring) salt, leavening (sodium acid pyrophosphate, monocalcium phosphate), lecithin (soy), mono-and diglycerides (emulsifier).

The second option is to place the word "Contains" followed by the name of the food source from which the major food allergen is derived, immediately after or adjacent to the list of ingredients, in the type size that is no smaller than the type size used for the list of ingredients. For example: Contains wheat, milk, egg, and soy.

Will the Ingredient List Be Specific about What Type of Tree Nut, Fish, or Shellfish Is in the Product?

FALCPA requires the type of tree nut (e.g., almonds, pecans, walnuts); the type of fish (e.g., bass, flounder, cod); and the type of Crustacean shellfish (e.g., crab, lobster, shrimp) to be declared.

After January 1, 2006, Will I Still Find Products on the Supermarket or Grocery Shelf without the Improved Labeling?

Yes. FALCPA does not require food manufacturers or retailers to remove or relabel products from supermarket shelves that do not reflect the additional allergen labeling so long as the products were labeled before January 1, 2006. Therefore, the FDA advises consumers with allergies to always read a product's ingredient statement in conjunction with any "contains" statement.

Does the Food Allergen Labeling and Consumer Protection Act Require the Use of a "May Contain" Statement in Any Circumstance?

No. Advisory statements are not required by FALCPA.

Are Flavors, Colors, and Food Additives Subject to the Allergen Labeling Requirements?

Yes. FALCPA requires that food manufacturers label food products that contain ingredients, including a flavoring, coloring, or incidental additive that are, or contain, a major food allergen using plain English to identify the allergens.

Are There Any Foods Exempt from the New Labeling Requirements?

Yes. Under FALCPA, raw agricultural commodities (generally fresh fruits and vegetables) are exempt as are highly refined oils derived from one of the eight major food allergens and any ingredient derived from such highly refined oil.

Can Food Manufacturers Ask to Have a Product Exempted from the New Labeling Requirements?

Yes. FALCPA provides mechanisms by which a manufacturer may request that a food ingredient covered by FALCPA may be exempt from FALCPA's labeling requirements. An ingredient may be exempt if it does not cause an allergic response that poses a risk to human health or if it does not contain allergenic protein.

What Does the FDA Require in Order for a Product to Be Exempt?

FALCPA states that any person can petition the Secretary of Health and Human Services for an exemption either through a petition process or a notification process.

The petition process requires scientific evidence (including the analytical method used to produce the evidence) that demonstrates that such food ingredient, as derived by the method specified in the petition, does not cause an allergic response that poses a risk to human health.

The notification process must include scientific evidence (including the analytical method used) that demonstrates that the food ingredient (as derived by the production method specified in the notification) does not contain allergenic protein.

If either the petition or the notification is granted by the Secretary, the result is that the ingredient in question is not considered a "major food allergen" and is not subject to the labeling requirements.

How Will the FDA Make Sure Food Manufacturers Adhere to the New Labeling Regulations?

As a part of its routine regulatory functions, the FDA inspects a variety of packaged foods to ensure that they are properly labeled.

What Is Cross-Contact?

Cross-contact is the inadvertent introduction of an allergen into a product. It is generally the result of environmental exposure during processing or handling, which may occur when multiple foods are produced in the same facility. It may occur due to use of the same processing line, through the misuse of rework, as the result of ineffective cleaning, or from the generation of dust or aerosols containing an allergen.

Are Mislabeled Food Products Removed from the Market?

Yes. A food product that contains an undeclared allergen may be subject to recall. In addition, a food product that is not properly labeled may be misbranded and subject to seizure and removed from the marketplace.

The number of recalls due to undeclared allergens (8 of the most common allergens only) remained steady between 1999 and 2001.

In 2002, recall actions nearly doubled, rising from 68–116. This rise may be attributed to the increased awareness of food allergies among consumers and manufacturers and increased attention from FDA inspectors to issues related to food allergy in manufacturing plants.

Gluten

Why Is There a Concern about Gluten?

Gluten describes a group of proteins found in certain grains (wheat, barley, and rye.) It is of concern because people with celiac disease cannot tolerate it. Celiac disease (also known as celiac sprue) is a chronic digestive disease that damages the small intestine and interferes with absorption of nutrients from food. Findings estimate that 2 million people in the United States have celiac disease or about 1 in 133 people.

What Does the Food Allergen Labeling and Consumer Protection Act Require with Regard to Gluten?

FALCPA requires the FDA to issue a proposed rule that will define and permit the voluntary use of the term "gluten free" on the labeling of foods by August 2006 and a final rule no later than August 2008.

What Has the FDA Done in Response to the Food Allergen Labeling and Consumer Protection Act Mandate?

The FDA held a public meeting in August 2005 to obtain expert comment and consultation from stakeholders to help the FDA develop a regulation to define and permit the voluntary use on food labeling of the term "gluten-free" (Public Meeting On: Gluten-Free Food Labeling). The meeting focused on food manufacturing, analytical methods, and consumer issues related to reduced levels of gluten in food.

Advice for Consumers

How Can I Avoid Foods to Which I'm Allergic?

The FDA advises consumers to work with healthcare providers to find out what food(s) can cause an allergic reaction. In addition, consumers who are allergic to major food allergens should read the ingredient statement on food products to determine if products contain

233

a major allergen. A "Contains _____ " statement, if present on a label, can also be used to determine if the food contains a major food allergen.

But I Don't Understand What Some of the Terms Mean. How Will I Know What They Are?

FALCPA was designed to improve food labeling information so that consumers who suffer from food allergies—especially children and their caregivers—will be able to recognize the presence of an ingredient that they must avoid. For example, if a product contains the milk-derived protein casein, the product's label would have to use the term "milk" in addition to the term "casein" so that those with milk allergies would clearly understand the presence of an allergen they need to avoid.

What about Food Prepared in Restaurants? How Will I Know That the Food I Ordered Does Not Contain an Ingredient to Which I Am Allergic?

FALCPA only applies to packaged FDA-regulated foods. However, the FDA advises consumers who are allergic to particular foods to ask questions about ingredients and preparation when eating at restaurants or any place outside the consumer's home.

How Will the Food Allergen Labeling and Consumer Protection Act Apply to Foods Purchased at Bakeries, Food Kiosks at the Mall, and Carry out Restaurants?

FALCPA's labeling requirements extend to retail and food-service establishments that package, label, and offer products for human consumption. However, FALCPA's labeling requirements do not apply to foods that are placed in a wrapper or container in response to a consumer's order—such as the paper or box used to provide a sandwich ordered by a consumer.

When Will Consumers See the Food Labels Change?

FALCPA applies to food products that are labeled on or after January 1, 2006, so the FDA anticipates that consumers will begin to see new labels on or after that date. However, the FDA cautions consumers that there will be a transition period of undetermined length after January 1, 2006, during which it is likely that consumers will see packaged food on store shelves and in consumers' homes without the revised allergen labeling.

Where Can I Find More Information on Food Allergens?

See the following websites for additional information on food allergens:

- U.S. Food and Drug Administration (FDA): Information about Food Allergens (www.fda.gov/Food/ IngredientsPackagingLabeling/FoodAllergens/default.htm)

- U.S. Department of Agriculture (USDA): Food Safety and Inspection Service (www.fsis.usda.gov/wps/portal/fsis/home)

- The National Institute of Health (NIH): National Institute of Allergies and Infectious Diseases (NIAID) (www.niaid.nih.gov)

- The National Library of Medicine (NLM): MedlinePlus Food Allergy (medlineplus.gov/foodallergy.html)

Section 23.2

How to Read a Label for Your Food Allergy

> This section contains text excerpted from the following sources: Text in this section begins with excerpts from "Have Food Allergies? Read the Label," U.S. Food and Drug Administration (FDA), May 11, 2011. Reviewed August 2018; Text beginning with the heading "Finding Food Allergens Where They Shouldn't Be" is excerpted from "Finding Food Allergens Where They Shouldn't Be," U.S. Food and Drug Administration (FDA), October 23, 2014. Reviewed August 2018.

Since 2006, it has been much easier for people allergic to certain foods to avoid packaged products that contain them, says Rhonda Kane, a registered dietitian and consumer safety officer at the U.S. Food and Drug Administration (FDA).

This is because a federal law requires that the labels of most packaged foods marketed in the United States disclose—in simple-to-understand terms—when they are made with a "major food allergen."

Eight foods, and ingredients containing their proteins, are defined as major food allergens. These foods account for 90 percent of all food allergies:

- Milk
- Egg
- Fish, such as bass, flounder, or cod
- Crustacean shellfish, such as crab, lobster, or shrimp
- Tree nuts, such as almonds, pecans, or walnuts
- Wheat
- Peanuts
- Soybeans

The law allows manufacturers a choice in how they identify the specific "food source names," such as "milk," "cod," "shrimp," or "walnuts," of the major food allergens on the label. They must be declared either in:

- the ingredient list, such as "casein (milk)" or "nonfat dry milk," or
- a separate "Contains" statement, such as "Contains milk," placed immediately after or next to the ingredient list.

"So first look for the 'Contains' statement and if your allergen is listed, put the product back on the shelf," says Kane. "If there is no 'Contains' statement, it's very important to read the entire ingredient list to see if your allergen is present. If you see its name even once, it's back to the shelf for that food too."

There are many different ingredients that contain the same major food allergen, but sometimes the ingredients' names do not indicate their specific food sources. For example, casein, sodium caseinate, and whey are all milk proteins. Although the same allergen can be present in multiple ingredients, its "food source name" (for example, milk) must appear in the ingredient list just once to comply with labeling requirements.

"Contains" and "May Contain" Have Different Meanings

If a "Contains" statement appears on a food label, it must include the food source names of all major food allergens used as ingredients.

For example, if "whey," "egg yolks," and a "natural flavor" that contained peanut proteins are listed as ingredients, the "Contains" statement must identify the words "milk," "egg," and "peanuts."

Some manufacturers voluntarily include a "may contain" statement on their labels when there is a chance that a food allergen could be present. A manufacturer might use the same equipment to make different products. Even after cleaning this equipment, a small amount of an allergen (such as peanuts) that was used to make one product (such as cookies) may become part of another product (such as crackers). In this case, the cracker label might state "may contain peanuts."

Be aware that the "may contain" statement is voluntary, says Kane. "You still need to read the ingredient list to see if the product contains your allergen."

When in Doubt, Leave It Out

Manufacturers can change their products' ingredients at any time, so Kane says it's a good idea to check the ingredient list every time you buy the product—even if you have eaten it before and didn't have an allergic reaction.

"If you're unsure about whether a food contains any ingredient to which you are sensitive, don't buy the product, or check with the manufacturer first to ask what it contains," says Kane. "We all want convenience, but it's not worth playing Russian roulette with your life or that of someone under your care."

Finding Food Allergens Where They Shouldn't Be

If you're allergic to a food ingredient, you probably look for it on the food product's label. But some labels may not be as reliable as they should be. In fact, allergens not listed on the label, referred to as "undeclared allergens," are the leading cause of food recalls requested by the FDA.

The FDA is working on three fronts to reduce the number of such recalls: by researching the causes of these errors; working with industry on best practices; and developing new ways to test for the presence of allergens.

Federal law requires that labels of FDA-regulated foods marketed in the United States identify major food allergens. In some people, these allergens—milk, eggs, fish, crustacean shellfish, tree nuts, wheat, peanuts, and soybeans—can cause potentially life-threatening reactions. A food product with a label that omits required allergen information is misbranded and can be seized by FDA. However, firms generally recall such food products from the marketplace voluntarily.

Help Report Food-Allergic Reactions

The first step is learning more about the problem. Steven Gendel, Ph.D., FDA food allergen coordinator, emphasizes that consumers can help by reporting food-allergic reactions to the FDA consumer complaint coordinator in their district. "We look at every complaint to determine the appropriate course of action," he says.

"What we're trying to learn," Gendel explains, "is what foods are most affected, what allergens are most involved, and how labeling errors might have happened. Those answers will help us to reduce the number of recalls for undeclared allergens."

Recalled Foods and the Allergens Involved

Looking for these answers, Gendel has sifted through FDA-collected recall data and found some clear trends.

For example, from September 2009 to September 2012, about one-third of foods reported to the FDA as serious health risks involved undeclared allergens. The five food types most often involved in food allergen recalls were bakery products; snack foods; candy; dairy products and dressings (such as salad dressings, sauces, and gravies).

The allergens most often involved in recalls were milk, wheat, and soy. Consumers can find out what products have been recalled at the FDA's (www.fda.gov/safety/recalls/default.htm#additional-info) website and at the Food Allergy Research and Education (FARE) (www.foodallergy.org/common-allergens/allergy-alerts) website, as well as from the companies that make the products.

Within the candy category, there were many reports of undeclared milk in products containing dark chocolate. For example, undeclared milk led to several recalls for chocolate-coated snack bars with labels that the products were "dairy-free" or "vegan." "This represented a significant risk for milk-allergic consumers," says Gendel.

The Source of the Problem

Recall data show that such labeling errors occur most commonly because of the use of the wrong label. This may happen when similar products made with different ingredients, including allergens, are sold in look-alike packages.

Gendel also found mistakes associated with the use of new technologies, such as computerization and the ability to print labels directly on packaging. This can save costs but also create new opportunities for errors.

The data suggest that food allergen recalls can be reduced through improved industry awareness and simple changes in the way packages, labels and ingredients are handled and tracked within production facilities.

To encourage improvements, the FDA shares its findings with industry at conferences and cooperates with the Food Safety Preventive Controls Alliance (FSPCA). FSPCA's mission is to enhance safe food production by developing training and outreach programs that support preventive controls described in the FDA Food Safety Modernization Act (FSMA).

FDA Exploring New Ways to Test for Allergens

Of course, keeping unwanted allergens out of food requires good methods for detecting them.

The most common test used worldwide is the enzyme-linked immunosorbent assay (ELISA), which uses antibodies (parts of the immune system that help neutralize viruses and bacteria) and spectroscopic detection to test for allergens.

Mark Ross, Ph.D., an FDA chemist, says ELISA is the standard test because it is easy to use, relatively low-cost, and has been improved by scientists over time. But ELISA, like similar tests used in medicine, can produce false positive results, so backup methods are needed. In addition, some allergens are so similar that scientists need another test besides ELISA to tell them apart.

Ross is working with other FDA researchers to develop methods for analyzing allergens based on mass spectrometry, a technology that more effectively determines the allergen protein content of a complex mixture of proteins, fats, sugars, and chemicals in a food.

"If someone wants us to analyze a food for peanut allergen, with mass spectrometry we can detect and differentiate among the 11 different allergenic proteins in a peanut," he says. FDA researchers are also developing deoxyribonucleic acid (DNA)-based methods, in particular to detect fish and shellfish allergens.

Chapter 24

Tips on Avoiding Food Allergy Reactions

Chapter Contents

Section 24.1

A Food Diary Can Reduce Risk of Reactions

Food allergies have emerged as a growing health crisis. They affect 15 million people in the United States, including 4 percent of adults and 8 percent of children, and account for 200,000 emergency room visits per year. When someone develops a food allergy, the body's immune system overreacts to the allergenic food by releasing histamines and other chemicals into the bloodstream. This process can cause a number of different symptoms to occur, such as hives, rashes, nasal congestion, breathing difficulties, diarrhea, nausea, and vomiting. Although some people experience only minor symptoms, food allergies can also trigger anaphylaxis, a severe, whole-body allergic reaction that is potentially fatal.

It is not always easy to identify which food can trigger an allergic reaction. For some people, the symptoms could be obviously related to a particular food, and for others the symptoms could appear mysteriously, making the allergen difficult to pinpoint. Not even diagnostic tests conducted by experts can precisely recognize food allergens in all cases. To help people identify the cause and manage their food allergy on an everyday basis, one of the best methods is to keep a written record of everything they eat.

Keeping a Food Diary

A food journal should be maintained on an everyday basis and record the details of every meal, beverage, snack, and dietary supplement. In addition, each entry should include any noticeable symptoms after a meal, even just a general feeling of indigestion or fatigue. The details that should be noted in the food diary include the symptoms experienced, whether they were mild or severe, and their duration. Other information that could be included in the journal include any medications taken; any exposure to environmental allergens such as pollen, dust mites, mold, perfumes, latex, or pet dander; any other illnesses or conditions experienced, such as the common cold, hepatitis, and insect bites; and any symptoms that were a result of physical stimuli, such as heat, cold, pressure, exercise, and extreme sun exposure.

It is important to note that a food item may contain a number of ingredients. Any kind of ingredient may cause an allergic reaction, which could range from mild to severe. If the symptoms occur while eating in a place other than home—for instance, at a restaurant—it would be helpful to talk to the chef and ask for a list of all the ingredients used in the food consumed.

If the allergic reaction is due to processed or prepackaged food, the label should be saved and the quantity consumed should be noted. All the information noted in the food diary can help an allergist make an informed diagnosis of the cause of allergy symptoms and determine the best course of treatment. A number of helpful food journal applications are available for mobile phone and tablet users to keep track of their allergies. Identifying and avoiding food culprits can help people maintain their health wisely and enjoy a better quality of life.

Reference

"Identifying Your Food Intolerances," Allergy UK, October 2012.

Section 24.2

Working with a Dietitian If Your Child Has Food Allergies

"Working with a Dietitian If Your Child Has Food Allergies," © 2018 Omnigraphics. Reviewed August 2018.

Learning that a child has food allergies can be frightening for parents. Once an allergist has diagnosed food allergies, many parents feel overwhelmed by the challenge of eliminating allergenic foods while also providing their child with healthy, nutritious meals. Without proper meal planning and supplementation, the dietary restrictions caused by food allergies can affect nutrient intake and potentially harm a child's growth, development, and future health.

Up to 90 percent of food-related allergic reactions in the United States can be traced to eight foods: cow's milk, eggs, wheat, soy, peanuts, tree nuts, fish, and shellfish. Yet these foods are high in vitamins, minerals, and other important nutrients. Nuts, for instance, are rich in vitamin E, niacin, manganese, magnesium, and chromium. As a result, at least 25 percent of children with food allergies experience vitamin and mineral deficiencies.

When certain foods must be eliminated from a child's diet, parents need to find ways to replace the nutrients that they provide. Many parents find it helpful to work with a registered dietitian in order to create meal plans that are appetizing and nutritious while also eliminating allergens. Dietitians can help ease parental anxiety by providing individualized education about how to avoid certain foods and substitute safe alternatives. They can also help families ensure that the child with food allergies receives adequate nutrition to promote growth and development. Finally, a registered dietitian can devise an action plan to help families cope with situations in which the child might encounter allergens.

Choosing a Qualified Dietitian

Training for dietitians in the United States includes four years of college to obtain a bachelor's degree in nutrition and dietetics, followed by a stipulated period of internship or professional practice. Dietitians are also required to pass a registration examination conducted by the Commission on Dietetic Registration (CDR) before they can become a Registered Dietitian (RD). Many dietitians specialize in certain areas by working under other professional dietitians. They also keep abreast with the latest developments in the field by attending seminars and workshops regularly.

Parents of children with food allergies who are interested in working with a dietitian should first assess the person's qualifications and experience. Experts advise asking prospective dietitians about their education, training, and professional memberships. It may also be helpful to know how long they have treated patients with food allergies and what specialized training they have undertaken to gain proficiency in treating food allergies. The American Dietetic Association (ADA) maintains a searchable list of registered dietitians on its website (www.eatright.org).

How the Dietitian Can Help

During the initial consultation with parents of a child with food allergies, a dietitian is likely to ask what the child eats on a regular basis, what foods have been identified as allergens, and what symptoms the child has experienced. This information will help the dietitian develop a meal plan for the child that includes safe alternative foods and provides all the nutrients the child needs to grow and thrive. The dietitian's goal is to provide suggestions for healthy, nutritious meals that offer a variety of food choices that the child will enjoy.

The dietitian can also provide parents with expert advice on how to avoid allergenic foods, from reading product labels to recognizing places where cross-contamination or accidental exposure could occur—such as school classrooms, restaurants, movie theaters, or airplanes. The dietitian can also give parents an extensive list of safe alternatives that they can substitute for allergy-inducing foods in meals or recipes.

Many dietitians ask families to keep a diary of the child's daily meals—noting any allergy symptoms observed—in order to facilitate meal planning. The dietitian will also monitor the child's growth and development through regular follow-up sessions and suggest dietary changes over time to meet their nutritional needs. Since children often outgrow allergies to certain foods, the dietitian can watch for these changes and help parents reintroduce the foods in a gradual and safe manner.

References

1. Bowers, Elizabeth Shimer. "Can a Dietitian Help with Children's Food Allergies?" Everyday Health, May 27, 2015.

2. Feuling, Mary Beth. "The Balancing Act: Nutrition and Food Allergy," Children's Hospital of Wisconsin, October 2015.

Section 24.3

Protecting Yourself from Food Allergies

This section contains text excerpted from the following
sources: Text in this section begins with excerpts from "Protecting
Yourself from Food Allergies," Foodsafety.gov, U.S. Department of
Health and Human Services (HHS), May 10, 2010. Reviewed
August 2018; Text beginning with the heading "How Can You Help?"
is excerpted from "Children and Adolescents with Food Allergies—
How Can You Help?" Centers for Disease Control and
Prevention (CDC), November 5, 2015.

The Director of the U.S. Food and Drug Administration's (FDA)
Food Labeling and Standards Staff has the responsibility to ensure
that consumers have accurate, complete, and informative labels on
the food that they buy. One of the areas that is a top concern for us
from a food safety perspective is food allergies. If you or a member
of your family suffer from food allergies, you must protect yourself
at all times. While some allergies are just irritating, approximately
30,000 Americans go to the emergency room each year to get treated
for severe food allergies.

What is a food allergy? It is a specific type of adverse food reaction
involving the immune system. The body produces an allergic antibody
to a food. Once a specific food is eaten and binds with the antibody, an
allergic response occurs.

A food allergy is not the same as a food intolerance or other nonallergic food reactions. A food intolerance is an abnormal response to a
food or additive, but it does not involve the immune system. Compared
to food intolerances, food allergies pose a much greater health risk.

In fact, it is estimated that 150–200 Americans die each year
because of allergic reactions to food.

What are the symptoms of a food allergy?

The most common symptoms are:

- Hives, itching, or skin rash

- Swelling of the lips, face, tongue and throat, or other parts of the
body

- Wheezing, nasal congestion, or trouble breathing

- Abdominal pain, diarrhea, nausea, or vomiting

- Dizziness, lightheadedness, or fainting

In a severe allergic reaction to food, you may have more extreme versions of the above reactions. Or you may experience life-threatening symptoms such as:

- Swelling of the throat and air passages that makes it difficult to breathe

- Shock, with a severe drop in blood pressure

- Rapid, irregular pulse

- Loss of consciousness

To reduce the risks, the FDA is working to ensure that major allergenic ingredients in food are accurately labeled. Since 2006, food labels must state clearly whether the food contains a major food allergen. The following are considered to be major food allergens:

- Milk

- Eggs

- Peanuts

- Tree nuts such as almonds, walnuts, and pecans

- Soybeans

- Wheat

- Fish

- Shellfish such as crab, lobster, and shrimp

These foods account for 90 percent of all food allergies in the United States. So, remember to take all measures to protect yourself and your family members who suffer from food allergies. In addition to avoiding food items that cause a reaction, it's recommended that you:

- Wear a medical alert bracelet or necklace stating that you have a food allergy

- Carry an auto-injector device containing epinephrine (adrenaline)

- Seek medical help immediately if you experience a food allergic reaction

How Can You Help?

Food allergies are a growing concern for many people and affect about 1 of 25 school-aged children. Among those with food allergies,

1 of 5 will have an allergic reaction while at school. Anaphylaxis is a severe allergic reaction that has rapid onset and may cause death, and 1 of 4 students who have a severe and potentially life-threatening reaction at school have no previous known food allergy. Schools should have a food allergy management and prevention plan to help support the needs of students with allergies. They should also teach staff members, as well as students and family members, about food allergies. This can create and maintain a healthy, safe, and inclusive educational environment.

Knowing the answers to the following questions can help you support your child's school to address food allergies. If you don't know the answers to these questions, check out the school handbook or school website, attend a school wellness meeting or Parent-Teacher Association (PTA) meeting, or simply ask your child's teacher.

1. Is there a full-time registered nurse in the school building at all times or a school-based health center to help children with chronic medical conditions or emergencies?

2. How does the school identify and share information about students with food allergies?

3. Is the school aware of the Centers for Disease Control and Prevention (CDC) Voluntary Guidelines for Managing Food Allergies in Schools and Early Care and Education Programs?

4. Is it required that each student with food allergies have an individualized health plan or emergency care plan on file? Has the child been evaluated for a Section 504 Plan, if appropriate?

5. Are students allowed to carry their medication (such as emergency epinephrine) at school?

6. Does the school or district have stock epinephrine that can be used for any student having a life-threatening allergic reaction, and are nurses, teachers, and other staff appropriately trained to administer it?

7. What are school or district protocols for students suspected of having an allergic reaction at school, on the school bus, on a field trip, or in cases of emergency or lockdown?

8. Are other school staff, such as teachers, bus drivers, and food services staff, trained to recognize and respond to a student who may be having an allergic reaction?

9. What practices are used to safely prepare and serve foods to students with food allergies within the cafeteria, classroom, school parties, and other school events?

10. Is food sharing among students allowed? Is the student with food allergies protected during classroom parties and activities involving food without having to be isolated from the activity?

11. Is there a bullying prevention policy in the school or district that discourages bullying or encourages awareness or anti-stigma of students with medical conditions?

Ideas for Parent

You can be involved in your child's school by attending meetings, workshops, or training events offered by the school; communicating with school staff and other parents; volunteering for school events or in your child's classroom; reinforcing healthy messages and practices your child learns at school; helping make decisions about health in the school; and being part of community activities supported by the school. Here are some specific ideas for how you can support your child's school in addressing food allergies.

• Have an ongoing conversation with your child to discuss their food allergies, their feelings about having food allergies, and if they feel safe and supported at school.

• Work with your child's healthcare provider to establish a current emergency care plan and for timely completion of required school forms. Encourage communication between school health services and your child's healthcare provider.

• Provide emergency medication to the school nurse or other school health official.

• Ensure that there is a current individualized healthcare plan, and assist with setting goals.

• Communicate with your child's teachers, counselors, and school health services staff about your child's food allergies and how they are coping while at school.

• Work with teachers and other staff to identify nonfood rewards for your child, thereby reducing exposure to allergens.

• Talk with school nutrition services about your child's allergies and advanced menu viewing.

- Volunteer with your child, or get involved in school health events to educate staff and other families about food allergies. Inquire about the student health education curriculum.

- Join a group, such as the PTA, school wellness committee, or school health advisory council, that addresses the needs of a supportive and healthy school environment.

- Share research-based websites or written materials about food allergies with teachers, nurses, and administrators, when possible.

Part Four

Airborne, Chemical, and Other Environmental Allergy Triggers

Chapter 25

Overview of Airborne Allergens

Watery red eyes, runny nose, sneezing, coughing—these familiar symptoms mean spring is in the air. Millions of people suffer from seasonal allergies triggered by airborne pollen—not just in spring but in summer and fall, too—and now evidence suggests their numbers will rise in a changing climate. The evidence so far is preliminary, but it points to a confluence of factors that favor longer growing seasons for the noxious weeds and other plants that trigger seasonal allergies and asthma attacks. Carbon dioxide (CO_2), in addition to being the principal global warming gas, can also be thought of as plant food—it's the source of carbon needed to make sugars during photosynthesis. When exposed to warmer temperatures and higher levels of CO_2, plants grow more vigorously and produce more pollen than they otherwise would.

Physicians who treat allergic airway diseases are already reporting an uptick in symptoms that they attribute to climate change. In a statement published last year, the World Allergy Organization (WAO), comprising 97 medical societies from around the world, opined that climate change will affect the start, duration, and intensity of the pollen season and exacerbate the synergistic effects of pollutants and respiratory infections on asthma.

This chapter includes text excerpted from "Pollen Overload: Seasonal Allergies in a Changing Climate," National Institute of Environmental Health Sciences (NIEHS), April 1, 2016.

"We're seeing increases in both the number of people with allergies and what they're allergic to," says Leonard Bielory, a professor, and allergy specialist at the Rutgers University Center for Environmental Prediction (CEP) and attending physician at Robert Wood Johnson University Hospital (RWJUH). "Should warming continue," he says, "then more people will be exposed to seasonal allergens with subsequent effects on public health."

Allergies on the Rise

Seasonal allergies and asthma impose significant health burdens, with an estimated 10–30 percent of the global population afflicted by allergic rhinitis (or hay fever) and 300 million people worldwide affected by asthma. Trend data suggest that the prevalence of asthma, including forms of the disease triggered by pollen, mold, and other allergenic substances, is on the rise. Childhood asthma rates in the United States, for instance, doubled from 1980–1995 before slowing to a more gradual (albeit ongoing) increase. Kate Weinberger, a postdoctoral associate at Brown University, says trends in seasonal allergy prevalence are more difficult to track because symptoms in most cases don't trigger emergency room visits or other types of medical care.

There is evidence suggesting that hay fever prevalence is rising in many parts of the world, particularly in urban areas, although some published studies date back to the late 1990s. A newer report from France's Rhône-Alpes Center of Epidemiology and Health Prevention shows that hay fever prevalence rose from 8 percent of the local population in 2004 to 12 percent in 2015. Michel Thiboudon, director of the French National Aerobiological Monitoring Network (RNSA), attributes the rising prevalence to increased exposures to highly allergenic ragweed. Climate change has been projected to accelerate ragweed's spread throughout the European continent.

Bielory says it's likely that other environmental factors, such as changing diets and better hygiene, contribute to the prevalence of asthma and hay fever by limiting early exposure to allergens and altering the immune system's normal development. However, much remains unknown about the relationship between aeroallergens and exacerbation of asthma, especially less severe attacks that aren't reflected in hospital visit data.

Seasonal allergies in North America generally begin in spring, when trees begin to flower and disperse their allergenic pollen into the air— they include, among others, oak and birch in the South and Northeast, and mountain cedar in the West. Late spring and early summer bring the emergence of various allergenic grasses and weeds, such as mugwort and nettle, which introduces another round of symptoms. The ragweed season comes last, starting in late summer and persisting until the plants die with the first frost. A resurgence in grass pollen also occurs in early fall, Bielory says.

Pollen grains contain the male gametes (sperm cells) of the flowering plant; they are covered in proteins that female gametes of the same species will recognize. It's those same coating proteins that trigger allergic reactions in sensitized people, with the degree of sensitization varying among individuals. According to Lewis Ziska, a research plant physiologist with the U.S. Department of Agriculture (USDA), the intensity of an allergic reaction depends on three interrelated factors: how much pollen a given species emits into the air, the duration of exposure, and the allergenicity of the pollen. In ragweed, these factors coalesce in a perfect storm of allergic misery. "What's unique about ragweed is that it produces so much pollen—roughly a billion grains per plant," Ziska says. "And the Amb a 1 protein [contained in the ragweed pollen coat] is also highly reactive with the immune system."

Regional Differences

Ziska conducted studies in the 1990s to explore potential links between pollen production, rising CO_2 levels, and warming temperatures. He grew ragweed in chambers containing up to 600 ppm ambient CO_2. That's the atmospheric concentration that the Intergovernmental Panel on Climate Change predicts by the year 2050, assuming no changes in current emissions. (At present, the atmospheric concentration level is just over 400 ppm.) Ziska found that the size of the experimental ragweed plants and their pollen output increased in tandem with rising CO_2.

Ziska then modeled future climate conditions using a novel surrogate: He and his colleagues compared how ragweed grew in urban and rural locations. Their rationale was that cities are heat sinks (because they're paved in dark surfaces that absorb and later re-radiate solar heat) as well as sources of CO_2 (from traffic and industrial emissions). Ziska's team planted ragweed in urban Baltimore, where measured CO_2 levels were 30 percent higher and temperatures 3.5°F hotter on average than they were outside the city. Their findings showed that urban ragweed plants grew faster, flowered earlier, and produced more pollen than those grown outside the city.

Climate change–related warming is anticipated to increase as one moves up in latitude. To assess the effect of warming temperatures on the length of ragweed's flowering season, Ziska's team, including Bielory, studied measures of airborne pollen collected from 10 sampling stations extending from east Texas to Saskatoon, 2,200 kilometers to the north. The results, though not unexpected, were remarkable: Between 1995 and 2009, they found the pollen seasons lengthened by 13–27 days, with greater increases the farther north they looked.

During a study published in 2014, Bielory and colleagues reached a similar conclusion. This team studied pollen measures taken from 50 sampling stations across the contiguous United States between 1994 and 2010. They reported that pollen seasons for allergenic species were lengthening more in the north than in the south, and that total counts of daily airborne pollen were getting larger. As Ziska's research also showed, the lengths of the southern pollen seasons were either unchanged or had actually shortened with time.

That finding goes to the heart of the geographic complexities underlying climate change and its influence on biological systems. Ziska explains that CO_2 and atmospheric water vapor exert competing influences on warming trends—water vapor suppresses warming in wetter, rainier southern latitudes, in part by boosting cloud cover, while CO_2 accelerates warming in dryer regions farther from the equator.

The implications of these phenomena are consistent with the health data. Jonathan Silverberg, an assistant professor at Northwestern University Feinberg School of Medicine, and his colleagues studied rates of childhood hay fever, pollen counts and weather conditions throughout the United States, and found they were lowest in wetter areas with higher humidity levels.

Meanwhile, in Europe ragweed has dramatically expanded its range since it was first introduced to the continent in the 1800s, and scientists anticipate its spread will accelerate further with climate change. Modeling by the French Climate and Environment Sciences Laboratory predicts a four-fold jump in levels of airborne ragweed pollen by 2050, with the biggest increases occurring in northern and eastern parts of Europe. Apart from ongoing seed dispersal, the models estimate higher CO_2 levels and warmer temperatures will help lengthen ragweed's pollen season.

A study published in 2014 showed that pollen seasons have already become longer in western Poland. The authors focused on allergenic species other than ragweed—namely, nettle, sorrel, broad-leaf dock, and various grasses. According to their sampling results, species-specific pollen seasons lengthened by two to nearly four days between 1996 and 2011, a trend the authors attributed mainly to warmer summer temperatures and later pollen season end dates.

Accessing Pollen Data

European pollen databases are more accessible and widespread than those in the United States, says Richard Flagan, a professor of environmental science and engineering at the California Institute of Technology. He says that's chiefly because European national weather agencies take responsibility for sampling and organizing the information in ways that scientists can use for research.

By contrast, pollen sampling in the United States is performed by a constellation of agencies and allergy clinics. At present, 84 of these sampling stations submit their data to a volunteer organization called the National Allergy Bureau™ (NAB), which is organized by the American Academy of Allergy, Asthma & Immunology (AAAAI). Bielory says the AAAAI provides quality control in the form of training and certification for contributors on how to sample airborne pollen.

The NAB provides daily pollen counts to local media outlets, but it won't release any data for research without the consent of the sampling stations that collected it. To access those data, scientists have to submit formal requests describing their research plans. The NAB passes approved requests to the appropriate member stations, which have 30 days to respond.

Flagan describes his efforts to access NAB data as "an exercise in frustration" that was frequently met with unanswered phone calls and e-mails. "Moreover, the way these stations collect data isn't compatible with science," he says. "We have at best a semi-qualitative historical record supplied by people who do not focus on the statistics of the measurement—that record has some scientific value, but you have to look at it with a big grain of salt. In reality, the pollen database in the United States is abysmal."

The USDA's Ziska says the NAB has become more cooperative and responsive to the needs of outside researchers. But he adds that since NAB sampling stations use different tools and methodologies to collect pollen, rather than one uniform system, their data can be difficult to aggregate and compare.

Bielory, who contributes to the NAB, agrees on the need for a national monitoring system that collects, stores, analyzes, and shares pollen data for the purpose of advancing science and health policy issues. The Council of State and Territorial Epidemiologists, a professional association for public health epidemiologists, proposed such a system in a draft white paper that it planned to finalize at its June 2016 annual conference.

Lab Results Hint at Possibilities

Even as researchers grapple with limited field data, they continue to produce compelling results in climate-controlled chambers that predict future effects on allergenic species. In her research at the University of Massachusetts Amherst, Kristina Stinson, an assistant professor of environmental conservation, grows ragweed in greenhouses containing CO_2 at levels ranging from 360 ppm—just under the current ambient concentration—to 720 ppm. Stinson says higher CO_2 levels could force evolutionary changes in ragweed. A study she published in 2011 showed that genotypes that, at current CO_2 levels devoted more resources to reproduction as CO_2 levels rose. In other words, she says, more genotypes overall were flowering. Stinson says that while she didn't measure pollen output directly, "we do note that more vigorous flowering and higher pollen production are usually correlated."

Her colleague Jennifer Albertine, a postdoctoral researcher at the University of Massachusetts Amherst, generated comparable results with timothy grass, a widespread perennial in North America and Europe and a major cause of early summer allergies. Albertine studied the effects of CO_2 at both 400 and 800 ppm. She found that timothy grass exposed to 800 ppm CO_2 produced roughly twice as much pollen as the lower-exposed grass.

Albertine also tested the effects of boosting ground-level ozone, which ordinarily slows plant growth by inducing oxidative damage. Coupled climate/tropospheric chemistry modeling indicates ozone levels could rise significantly by the end of the century as emissions of precursor pollutants also continue rising. Albertine's study didn't reveal any growth-limiting effect of ozone on grasses raised in elevated CO_2. But she did find that the grasses responded to higher ozone levels by making less of their allergenic protein (Phl p 5). However, any reduction in the plant's allergenic protein content, Albertine predicted, would be offset by a corresponding increase in pollen production, for a net boost in allergenic threat. (Similarly, Ziska's research showed that when raised in greenhouses containing up to 600 ppm CO_2, ragweed plants produced 60–80 percent more of their allergenic protein, Amb a 1.27.)

Stinson acknowledges that, although greenhouses allow for a controlled assessment of how atmospheric conditions affect allergenic plants, they don't replicate the real world, where other pollutants, humidity, rainfall, and additional soil nutrients—especially nitrogen—also influence plant growth and pollination patterns. With funding from the U.S. Environmental Protection Agency (EPA), she's now collaborating with David Foster, director of the 3,750-acre Harvard Forest, on a project to map ragweed hotspots in New England. Their field studies so far, which have been submitted for publication, show that ragweed plants from urban and rural areas differ in the extent and timing of flower production and in their responses to CO_2.

Among other research questions, Stinson hopes to explore spatial patterns in how people experience the effects of climate change on pollen production. "We may find that urban populations from a particular demographic might be disproportionately affected by how climate change affects allergenicity," she says.

Connecting the Dots on Health

Stinson says that connecting climate-induced trends in allergenicity with public health impacts could be challenging. It will require that scientists have better access to pollen data than they currently do in addition to health outcomes data that might be correlated with rising pollen exposure levels.

Weinberger, of Brown University, has studied the relationship between daily spring pollen counts and health outcomes in New York City (NYC). Results published last year showed that mid-spring peaks in tree pollen were associated with over-the-counter (OTC) allergy medication sales and emergency room visits for asthma attacks, especially among children. By contrast, unpublished research she's conducted showed no similar relationship between allergy drug sales and peak exposures to ragweed pollen in the fall. Weinberger says that's possibly because allergy medication purchased in the spring might last for months; in the absence of sales data, researchers wouldn't be able to detect a relationship to symptoms.

Despite the data gaps that remain, many healthcare professionals believe the trend is real, as evidenced by surveys of physicians who treat seasonal allergies. One survey involved members of the American Thoracic Society (ATS), including pulmonologists, critical care clinicians, pediatricians, and other specialists. Over half the participants queried in the survey reported increases in allergic symptoms among their own patients that the doctors believed were related to climate change. A survey of AAAAI members, currently in press, reached a similar conclusion: In this case, specialists were asked "(How) do you think your patients are being affected by climate change or might be affected in the next 10–20 years?" Nearly two-thirds reported seeing "increased care for allergic sensitization and symptoms of exposure to plants or mold."

Mona Sarfaty, director of the Program on Climate and Health at George Mason University, led both those surveys. She says that to her surprise, neither study detected regional difference in physician responses. "Instead, greater allergy symptoms seemed to be showing up across the country," she says, with only the symptoms themselves varying by location. "So a doctor in Michigan who ordinarily sees relief from mold allergies with the arrival of cold weather might see them persisting later into the year," she explains, "while a doctor in Southern California might be reporting grass allergies all year round." Sarfaty says that doctors who claimed not to believe in climate change were less likely to report these trends.

Kim Knowlton, a senior scientist with the Natural Resources Defense Council (NRDC), who also holds a faculty post at the Columbia University Mailman School of Public Health, acknowledges the need for more research. "What we have to do is tease out the chain of events starting with higher temperatures and CO_2 levels, to effects on allergenicity, to human health symptoms," she says. "The studies so far are compelling, but we need more comprehensive studies at larger scales." For the tens of millions who have allergies and asthma, this is more than an inconvenience, she says—"Those illnesses can keep you out of school and work, and for some they are absolutely life-threatening. So these are really substantial health concerns."

Chapter 26

Pollen Allergy

Chapter Contents

Section 26.1

Pollen Allergy: Overview

This section includes text excerpted from "Pollen," National Institute of Environmental Health Sciences (NIEHS), July 24, 2018.

Ragweed Pollen

Ragweed and other weeds such as curly dock, lambs quarters, pigweed, plantain, sheep sorrel, and sagebrush are some of the most prolific producers of pollen allergens. Although the ragweed pollen season runs from August to November, ragweed pollen levels usually peak in mid-September in many areas in the country. In addition, pollen counts are highest between 5:00 a.m. to 10:00 a.m. and on dry, hot, and windy days.

Preventive Strategies

- Avoid the outdoors between 5:00 a.m. to 10:00 a.m. Save outside activities for late afternoon or after a heavy rain, when pollen levels are lower.

- Keep windows in your home and car closed to lower exposure to pollen. To keep cool, use air conditioners, and avoid using window and attic fans.

- Be aware that pollen can also be transported indoors on people and pets.

- Dry your clothes in an automatic dryer rather than hanging them outside. Otherwise, pollen can collect on clothing and be carried indoors.

Grass Pollen

As with tree pollen, grass pollen is regional as well as seasonal. In addition, grass pollen levels can be affected by temperature, time of day and rain. Of the 1,200 species of grass that grow in North America, only a small percentage of these cause allergies. The most common grasses that can cause allergies are:

- Bermuda grass
- Johnson grass

- Kentucky bluegrass
- Orchard grass
- Sweet vernal grass
- Timothy grass

Preventive Strategies

- If you have a grass lawn, have someone else do the mowing. If you must mow the lawn yourself, wear a mask.
- Keep grass cut short.
- Choose ground covers that don't produce much pollen, such as Irish moss, bunch, and dichondra.
- Avoid the outdoors between 5:00 a.m. to 10:00 a.m. Save outside activities for late afternoon or after a heavy rain, when pollen levels are lower.
- Keep windows in your home and car closed to lower exposure to pollen. To keep cool, use air conditioners, and avoid using window and attic fans.
- Be aware that pollen can also be transported indoors on people and pets.
- Dry your clothes in an automatic dryer rather than hanging them outside. Otherwise, pollen can collect on clothing and be carried indoors.

Tree Pollen

Trees can aggravate your allergy whether or not they are on your property, since trees release large amounts of pollen that can be distributed miles away from the original source. Trees are the earliest pollen producers, releasing their pollen as early as January in the Southern states and as late as May or June in the Northern states.

Most allergies are specific to one type of tree such as:

- Catalpa
- Elm
- Hickory
- Olive

- Pecan
- Sycamore
- Walnut

or to the male cultivar of certain trees. The female of these species are totally pollen-free:

- Ash
- Box elder
- Cottonwood
- Date palm
- Maple (red)
- Maple (silver)
- Phoenix palm
- Poplar
- Willow

Some people, though, do show cross-reactivity among trees in the alder, beech, birch and oak family, and the juniper and cedar family.

Preventive Strategies

- If you buy trees for your yard, look for species that do not aggravate allergies such as crape myrtle, dogwood, fig, fir, palm, pear, plum, redbud, and redwood trees or the female cultivars of ash, box elder, cottonwood, maple, palm, poplar, or willow trees.

- Avoid the outdoors between 5:00 a.m. to 10:00 a.m. Save outside activities for late afternoon or after a heavy rain, when pollen levels are lower.

- Keep windows in your home and car closed to lower exposure to pollen. To keep cool, use air conditioners, and avoid using window and attic fans.

- Be aware that pollen can also be transported indoors on people and pets.

- Dry your clothes in an automatic dryer rather than hanging them outside. Otherwise, pollen can collect on clothing and be carried indoors.

Section 26.2

Ragweed Therapy Offers Allergy Sufferers Longer Relief

This section includes text excerpted from "Experimental
Ragweed Therapy Offers Allergy Sufferers Longer Relief with
Fewer Shots," National Institutes of Health (NIH), October 4, 2006.
Reviewed August 2018.

Americans accustomed to the seasonal misery of sneezing, runny noses, and itchy, watery eyes caused by ragweed pollen might one day benefit from an experimental allergy treatment that not only requires fewer injections than standard immunotherapy, but leads to a marked reduction in symptoms that persists for at least a year after therapy has stopped, according to a study in The *New England Journal of Medicine (NEJM)*. The research was sponsored by the Immune Tolerance Network (ITN), which is funded by the National Institute of Allergy and Infectious Diseases (NIAID) and the National Institute of Diabetes and Digestive and Kidney Diseases (NIDDK), both components of the National Institutes of Health (NIH), and the Juvenile Diabetes Research Foundation (JDRF) International.

"As many as 40 million Americans suffer from seasonal allergies caused by airborne pollens produced by grasses, trees, and weeds," says NIH Director Elias A. Zerhouni, M.D. "Finding new therapies for allergy sufferers is certainly an important research goal."

"This innovative research holds great promise for helping people with allergies," says NIAID Director Anthony S. Fauci, M.D. "A short course of immunotherapy that reduces allergic symptoms over an extended period of time will significantly improve the quality of life for many people."

Ragweed is one of the most common pollens in the United States and is prevalent in the Northeast, Midwest and the South. In Baltimore, where the *NEJM* study was conducted, the ragweed pollen season lasts from mid-August to October.

Physicians treat people suffering from mild and moderate ragweed allergies with antihistamines or nasal corticosteroids. However, when people with allergies do not respond to these treatments or experience severe symptoms, the next therapeutic option is a course of subcutaneous injections of the allergen, which is called allergen immunotherapy. Although this standard immunotherapy is often effective, it has two major drawbacks. First, it can cause systemic allergic reactions, such as anaphylaxis, a hypersensitivity reaction that can lead to severe and sometimes life-threatening physical symptoms. Second, to provide longlasting relief, standard immunotherapy may require frequent injections over a three- to five-year period. The large number of injections over such an extended period of time often results in many people not completing the treatment.

In the study detailed in *NEJM*, lead investigator Peter Creticos, M.D., medical director of the Johns Hopkins Asthma and Allergy Center in Baltimore, and his research team found that an investigational therapy based on the major ragweed allergen, Amb a 1, coupled to a unique short, synthetic sequence of deoxyribonucleic acid (DNA) that stimulates the immune system, reduced allergy symptoms in adults for at least one year when given just once a week over a six-week period. The therapeutic agent was provided by Dynavax Technologies Corporation (DVAX), based in Berkeley, California (CA).

"For almost 100 years, we've been using the tedious process of giving allergy sufferers one to two shots a week for up to 4–5 years to ensure its success," Dr. Creticos says. "This study is an important immunotherapy advance in that we've shown you can induce long-lasting relief from allergic rhinitis with just a few weeks of injections."

The study initially involved 25 adult volunteers, ages 23–60, with a history of seasonal allergic rhinitis, positive skin test reactions to ragweed pollen, and an immediate reaction when nasally challenged with ragweed. Prior to the start of the 2001 fall ragweed season, the study participants received six injections, each a week apart, of either the investigational therapy in increasingly higher doses or a placebo. They received no other injections throughout the course of the study. Fourteen volunteers received the study drug; 11 were given the placebo. The therapy was well-tolerated and caused only limited local reactions, which required neither medication nor change in treatment dose. No clinically significant, therapy-related adverse events occurred.

Throughout the 2001 and 2002 ragweed seasons, the volunteers were monitored for allergy-related symptoms, including the number of sneezes and the degree of postnasal drip, allergy medication use, and quality-of-life (QOL) scores. Compared with the placebo recipients, the group that received the therapy experienced dramatically better outcomes that continued throughout the 2002 ragweed season even though therapy ended one year earlier.

Clearly, the regimen of only six injections showed therapeutic promise when compared with the current therapy, the study authors note. However, because the results are based on a small number of volunteers and the long-term safety of the therapy is unknown, they say additional clinical trials with longer-term follow-up to adequately assess the therapy's safety and effectiveness are necessary.

How the experimental therapy relieves ragweed allergy symptoms is not fully understood at this time. When exposed to ragweed pollen, people who are allergic to ragweed experience an increase in IgE (immunoglobulin) antibodies; immunotherapy blocks this increase in IgE. Researchers believe the experimental therapy tempers the release of immune regulatory proteins called cytokines, which blocks increases in the level of IgE antibodies.

"Using ragweed as a model allergen system with a predictable seasonal pattern of symptoms and pollen counts, it is possible to correlate pollen levels with symptoms and measure treatment effects on symptoms. This enables us to better understand immune response to allergens and serves as an approach to similar therapies to manage other allergic reactions for which there are currently no treatments, such as food allergies," says Marshall Plaut, M.D., chief of the Allergic Mechanisms Section of NIAID's Division of Allergy, Immunology, and Transplantation (DAIT).

Chapter 27

Household Allergens: Animal Dander, Cockroach, Dust Mite, Hair Dye, and Mold Allergy

Chapter Contents

Section 27.1

Dust Mite Allergy

This section contains text excerpted from the following sources: Text in this section begins with excerpts from "Dust Mites," National Institute of Environmental Health Sciences (NIEHS), April 20, 2017; Text under the heading "U.S. Food and Drug Administration Approves Odactra for House Dust Mite Allergies" is excerpted from "FDA Approves Odactra for House Dust Mite Allergies," U.S. Food and Drug Administration (FDA), March 1, 2017.

Dust mites are tiny microscopic relatives of the spider and live on mattresses, bedding, upholstered furniture, carpets, and curtains. These tiny creatures feed on the flakes of skin that people and pets shed daily and they thrive in warm and humid environments. No matter how clean a home is, dust mites cannot be totally eliminated. However, the number of mites can be reduced by following the suggestions below.

Preventive Strategies

- Use a dehumidifier or air conditioner to maintain relative humidity at about 50 percent or below.

- Encase your mattress and pillows in dust-proof or allergen impermeable covers (available from specialty supply mail order companies, bedding, and some department stores).

- Wash all bedding and blankets once a week in hot water (at least 130–140°F) to kill dust mites. Nonwashable bedding can be frozen overnight to kill dust mites.

- Replace wool or feathered bedding with synthetic materials and traditional stuffed animals with washable ones.

- If possible, replace wall-to-wall carpets in bedrooms with bare floors (linoleum, tile or wood) and remove fabric curtains and upholstered furniture.

- Use a damp mop or rag to remove dust. Never use a dry cloth since this just stirs up mite allergens.

- Use a vacuum cleaner with either a double-layered microfilter bag or a high-efficiency particulate air (HEPA) filter to trap allergens that pass through a vacuum's exhaust.

- Wear a mask while vacuuming to avoid inhaling allergens, and stay out of the vacuumed area for 20 minutes to allow any dust and allergens to settle after vacuuming.

U.S. Food and Drug Administration Approves Odactra for House Dust Mite Allergies

The U.S. Food and Drug Administration (FDA) approved Odactra, the first allergen extract to be administered under the tongue (sublingually) to treat house dust mite (HDM)-induced nasal inflammation (allergic rhinitis), with or without eye inflammation (conjunctivitis), in people 18 through 65 years of age.

"House dust mite allergic disease can negatively impact a person's quality of life," said Peter Marks, M.D., Ph.D., director of the FDA's Center for Biologics Evaluation and Research (CBER). "The approval of Odactra provides patients an alternative treatment to allergy shots to help address their symptoms."

House dust mite allergies are a reaction to tiny bugs that are commonly found in house dust. Dust mites, close relatives of ticks and spiders, are too small to be seen without a microscope. They are found in bedding, upholstered furniture, and carpeting. Individuals with house dust mite allergies may experience a cough, runny nose, nasal itching, nasal congestion, sneezing, and itchy and watery eyes.

Odactra exposes patients to house dust mite allergens, gradually training the immune system in order to reduce the frequency and severity of nasal and eye allergy symptoms. It is a once-daily tablet, taken year round, that rapidly dissolves after it is placed under the tongue. The first dose is taken under the supervision of a healthcare professional with experience in the diagnosis and treatment of allergic diseases. The patient is to be observed for at least 30 minutes for potential adverse reactions. Provided the first dose is well tolerated, patients can then take Odactra at home. It can take about eight to 14 weeks of daily dosing after initiation of Odactra for the patient to begin to experience a noticeable benefit.

The safety and efficacy of Odactra was evaluated in studies conducted in the United States, Canada, and Europe, involving approximately 2,500 people. Some participants received Odactra, while others received a placebo pill. Participants reported their symptoms and the need to use symptom-relieving allergy medications. During treatment, participants taking Odactra experienced a 16–18 percent reduction in symptoms and the need for additional medications compared to those who received a placebo.

The most commonly reported adverse reactions were nausea, itching in the ears and mouth, and swelling of the lips and tongue. The prescribing information includes a boxed warning that severe allergic reactions, some of which can be life-threatening, can occur. As with other FDA-approved allergen extracts administered sublingually, patients receiving Odactra should be prescribed auto-injectable epinephrine. Odactra also has a Medication Guide for distribution to the patient.

Odactra is manufactured for Merck, Sharp & Dohme Corp., (a subsidiary of Merck and Co., Inc., Whitehouse Station, N.J.) by Catalent Pharma Solutions Limited, United Kingdom.

The FDA, an agency within the U.S. Department of Health and Human Services (HHS), protects the public health by assuring the safety, effectiveness, and security of human and veterinary drugs, vaccines and other biological products for human use, and medical devices. The agency also is responsible for the safety and security of our nation's food supply, cosmetics, dietary supplements, products that give off electronic radiation, and for regulating tobacco products.

Section 27.2

Cockroach Allergy

This section contains text excerpted from the following
sources: Text in this section begins with excerpts from "Cockroaches,"
National Institute of Environmental Health Sciences (NIEHS),
April 30, 2018; Text beginning with the heading "Health Concerns"
is excerpted from "Cockroaches and Schools," U.S. Environmental
Protection Agency (EPA), May 29, 2018.

Cockroaches are one of the most common and allergenic of indoor pests. Studies have found a strong association between the presence of cockroaches and increases in the severity of asthma symptoms in individuals who are sensitive to cockroach allergens. These pests are common even in the cleanest of crowded urban areas and older dwellings. They are found in all types of neighborhoods. The proteins found in cockroach saliva are particularly allergenic but the body and droppings of cockroaches also contain allergenic proteins.

Preventive Strategies

- Keep food and garbage in closed, tight-lidded containers. Never leave food out in the kitchen.

- Do not leave out pet food or dirty food bowls.

- Eliminate water sources that attract these pests, such as leaky faucets and drain pipes.

- Mop the kitchen floor and wash countertops at least once a week.

- Plug up crevices around the house through which cockroaches can enter.

- Limit the spread of food around the house and especially keep food out of bedrooms.

- Use bait stations and other environmentally safe pesticides to reduce cockroach infestation.

Health Concerns

Cockroaches and their droppings may trigger an asthma attack. Their feces, saliva, eggs, and outer covering, or cuticles left behind on surfaces contain substances that are allergic to humans, especially those with asthma or other respiratory conditions. Within and on the surface of their bodies, cockroaches carry bacteria that can cause salmonella, *staphylococcus*, and *streptococcus* if deposited in food. Additionally, cockroach feces, skin sheddings, and saliva can cause asthma and allergies, especially in children.

Cockroach Management Tips

To keep students and staff healthy, Integrated pest management (IPM) helps schools stay free of cockroach infestations:

- Don't allow dirty dishes to accumulate in the sink and remain there overnight.

- Keep food scraps in the refrigerator or in containers with tight-fitting lids.

- If small animals are in the classroom, keep the food in tightly sealed containers, and do not allow food to remain in the bowls overnight.

  - Feed only what the animal will eat at the time of feeding.

- Remove garbage from the classroom and kitchen areas on a routine basis.

  - Keep outside containers covered, especially at night.

- Periodically check and clean the evaporation pan under the refrigerator or freezer.

- Check the critical area between the stove and cabinet where grease and food scraps often accumulate.

  - Pull the stove out periodically and clean thoroughly.

Section 27.3

Mold Allergy

This section includes text excerpted from "Mold—General Information—Basic Facts," Centers for Disease Control and Prevention (CDC), December 20, 2017.

What Are Molds?

Molds are fungi that can be found both indoors and outdoors. No one knows how many species of fungi exist but estimates range from tens of thousands to perhaps three hundred thousand or more. Molds grow best in warm, damp, and humid conditions, and spread and reproduce by making spores. Mold spores can survive harsh environmental conditions, such as dry conditions, that do not support normal mold growth.

What Are Some of the Common Indoor Molds?

- Cladosporium
- Penicillium
- Alternaria
- Aspergillus

How Do Molds Affect People?

Some people are sensitive to molds. For these people, exposure to molds can lead to symptoms such as stuffy nose, wheezing, and red or itchy eyes, or skin. Some people, such as those with allergies to molds or with asthma, may have more intense reactions. Severe reactions may occur among workers exposed to large amounts of molds in occupational settings, such as farmers working around moldy hay. Severe reactions may include fever and shortness of breath.

People with a weakened immune system, such as people receiving treatment for cancer, people who have had an organ or stem cell transplant, and people taking medicines that suppress the immune system, are more likely to get mold infections. Exposure to mold or dampness may also lead to development of asthma in some individuals. Interventions that improve housing conditions can reduce morbidity from asthma and respiratory allergies.

Where Are Molds Found?

Molds are found in virtually every environment and can be detected, both indoors and outdoors, year round. Mold growth is encouraged by warm and humid conditions. Outdoors they can be found in shady, damp areas or places where leaves or other vegetation is decomposing. Indoors they can be found where humidity levels are high, such as basements or showers.

How Can People Decrease Mold Exposure?

Sensitive individuals should avoid areas that are likely to have mold, such as compost piles, cut grass, and wooded areas. Inside homes, mold growth can be slowed by controlling humidity levels and ventilating showers and cooking areas. If there is mold growth in your home, you should clean up the mold and fix the water problem. Mold growth can be removed from hard surfaces with commercial products, soap and water, or a bleach solution of no more than 1 cup of household laundry bleach in 1 gallon of water. Follow the manufacturers' instructions for use.

If you choose to use bleach to clean up mold:

- Never mix bleach with ammonia or other household cleaners. Mixing bleach with ammonia or other cleaning products will produce dangerous, toxic fumes.

- Open windows and doors to provide fresh air.

- Wear rubber boots, rubber gloves, and goggles during cleanup of affected area.

- If the area to be cleaned is more than 10 square feet, consult the U.S. Environmental Protection Agency (EPA) guide titled Mold Remediation in Schools and Commercial Buildings. Although focused on schools and commercial buildings, this document also applies to other building types. You can get it by going to the EPA website.

- Always follow the manufacturer's instructions when using bleach or any other cleaning product.

Specific Recommendations

- Keep humidity levels as low as you can—no higher than 50 percent–all day long. An air conditioner or dehumidifier will help you keep the level low. Bear in mind that humidity levels change over the course of a day with changes in the moisture in the air and the air temperature, so you will need to check the humidity levels more than once a day.

- Use an air conditioner or a dehumidifier during humid months.

- Be sure the home has adequate ventilation, including exhaust fans.

- Add mold inhibitors to paints before application.

- Clean bathrooms with mold killing products.

- Do not carpet bathrooms and basements.

- Remove or replace previously soaked carpets and upholstery.

What Areas Have High Mold Exposures?

- Antique shops
- Greenhouses
- Saunas
- Farms
- Mills
- Construction areas
- Flower shops
- Summer cottages

I Found Mold Growing in My Home, How Do I Test the Mold?

Generally, it is not necessary to identify the species of mold growing in a residence, and Centers for Disease Control and Prevention (CDC) does not recommend routine sampling for molds. Current evidence indicates that allergies are the type of diseases most often associated with molds. Since the susceptibility of individuals can vary greatly either because of the amount or type of mold, sampling and culturing are not reliable in determining your health risk. If you are susceptible to mold and mold is seen or smelled, there is a potential health risk; therefore, no matter what type of mold is present, you should arrange for its removal. Furthermore, reliable sampling for mold can be expensive, and standards for judging what is and what is not an acceptable or tolerable quantity of mold have not been established.

Section 27.4

Animal Dander Allergy

This section includes text excerpted from "Pets and Animals," National Institute of Environmental Health Sciences (NIEHS), April 20, 2017.

Many people think animal allergies are caused by the fur or feathers of their pet. In fact, allergies are actually aggravated by:

- Proteins secreted by oil glands and shed as dander

- Proteins in saliva (which stick to fur when animals lick themselves)

- Aerosolized urine from rodents and guinea pigs

Keep in mind that you can sneeze with and without your pet being present. Although an animal may be out of sight, their allergens are not. This is because pet allergens are carried on very small particles. As a result pet allergens can remain circulating in the air and remain on carpets and furniture for weeks and months after a pet is gone.

Allergens may also be present in public buildings, schools, etc., where there are no pets.

Preventive Strategies

- Remove pets from your home if possible.

- If pet removal is not possible, keep them out of bedrooms and confined to areas without carpets or upholstered furniture.

- If possible, bathe pets weekly to reduce the amount of allergens.

- Wear a dust mask and gloves when near rodents.

- After playing with your pet, wash your hands and clean your clothes to remove pet allergens.

- Avoid contact with soiled litter cages.

- Dust often with a damp cloth.

Section 27.5

Hair Dye Allergy

This section includes text excerpted from "Hair Dyes,"
U.S. Food and Drug Administration (FDA), November 3, 2017.

The U.S. Food and Drug Administration (FDA) often receives questions about the safety and regulation of hair dyes. Most of these products belong to a category called "coal-tar" hair dyes. Color additives, with the exception of coal-tar hair dyes, need FDA approval before they're permitted for use in cosmetics. FDA's ability to take action against coal-tar hair dyes associated with safety concerns is limited by law. It's important to follow the directions on the label. It is also important to be an informed consumer and understand the risks.

What Are Coal-Tar Hair Dyes?

The term "coal-tar colors" dates back to the time when these coloring materials were by-products of the coal industry. Most are made from petroleum, nowadays, but the original name is still used. Coal-tar hair dyes—those coal-tar colors used for dyeing hair—include permanent, semi-permanent, and temporary hair dyes. Coal-tar colors are also called "synthetic-organic" colors. That's because, to a chemist, a "synthetic" compound is one formed from simpler compounds and an "organic" compound is one that contains carbon atoms.

What the Law Says about Coal-Tar Hair Dyes

Under the Federal Food, Drug, and Cosmetic Act (FD&C Act), a law passed by Congress, color additives must be approved by FDA for their intended use before they are used in FDA-regulated products, including cosmetics. Other cosmetic ingredients do not need FDA approval. FDA can take action against a cosmetic on the market if it is harmful to consumers when used in the customary or expected way and used according to labeled directions.

How the law treats coal-tar hair dyes:

- The FDA cannot take action against a coal-tar hair dye, as long as the label includes a special caution statement and the product comes with adequate directions for consumers to do a skin test before they dye their hair. This is the caution statement:

Caution—This product contains ingredients which may cause skin irritation on certain individuals and a preliminary test according to accompanying directions should first be made. This product must not be used for dyeing the eyelashes or eyebrows; to do so may cause blindness. (FD&C Act, 601(a))

- Coal-tar hair dyes, unlike color additives in general, do not need FDA approval. (FD&C Act, 601(e)).

But there are limits to this exception:

- The FDA may take action if a harmful coal-tar hair dye product if:
  - it does not have the caution statement on its label or come with adequate directions for a skin test, or
  - an ingredient other than the coal-tar hair dye itself is harmful.

- "Coal-tar hair dyes" are not eyebrow or eyelash dyes. Color additives intended for dyeing the eyebrows or eyelashes need FDA approval for that use. No color additives are approved for dyeing the eyebrows or eyelashes.

Safety Issues

While many people use coal-tar hair dyes, FDA is aware of the following problems:

Eye injuries: Hair dyes have caused eye injuries, including blindness, when used in the eye area. Eyebrow and eyelash dyeing are not permitted uses of coal-tar hair dyes.

Allergic reactions: Some coal-tar hair dyes can cause allergic reactions or sensitization that may result in skin irritation and hair loss. People can develop sensitivities with repeated exposure. In addition, formulations may change over time. So, it's possible to have a reaction even if you have dyed your hair in the past, without a problem. That's why it's important to follow the instructions and do the skin test before every use. Even if you don't see a reaction to the skin test, it's still possible to have a reaction when you dye your hair.

One hair dye ingredient, p-phenylenediamine, or "PPD," has been implicated more prominently in leading to allergic reactions. Some people may become allergic to PPD from other exposures, including occupational exposures. This is called "cross-sensitization." Here are some examples;

- Some temporary tattoo inks, sometimes marketed as "black henna"

- Certain textile dyes, ballpoint pen inks, some color additives used in foods and drugs, and other dyes used in semi-permanent and temporary hair dyes

- Rubber and other latex products

- Benzocaine and procaine, local anesthetics used by doctors and dentists

- Para-aminosalicylic acid, a drug used to treat tuberculosis

- Sulfonamides, sulfones, and sulfa drugs

- Para-aminobenzoic acid (PABA), a naturally occurring compound used in some sunscreens and in some cosmetics.

Temporary tattoo artists who use coal-tar hair dyes to color people's skin are misusing these products and ingredients, because coal tar hair dyes are not intended to be used for staining the skin. While the FDA regulates cosmetics products on the market, professional practice is generally subject to state and local authorities, not the FDA.

If you have a reaction to a hair dye or tattoo, ask your healthcare provider about treatment. If you know what ingredient caused the problem, you may be able to find a product that doesn't contain that ingredient. If you color your hair yourself, check the list of ingredients on the label for any you wish to avoid. If you have your hair colored at a salon, your stylist may be able to tell you the ingredients, or you may wish to check with the manufacturer.

Questions about hair dyes and cancer: In the 1980s, some coal-tar hair dyes were found to cause cancer in animals. The FDA published a regulation requiring a special warning statement for all hair dye products containing these two ingredients:

- 4-methoxy-*m*-phenylenediamine 2,4-diaminoanisole

- 2, 4-methoxy-*m*-phenylenediamine sulfate 2,4-diaminoanisole sulfate

The cosmetic industry has since reformulated coal-tar hair dye products, these two ingredients are no longer seen in hair dyes.

The FDA continues to monitor research on hair dye safety. It does not have reliable evidence showing a link between cancer and coal-tar hair dyes on the market today. The FDA is collecting adverse event data which helps assess the safety of this class of ingredients. If you experience an adverse event or bad reaction, please report that to the FDA.

Other Types of Hair-Coloring Products

- Hair coloring materials made from plant or mineral sources are regulated the same as other color additives. They must be approved by the FDA and listed in the color additive regulations.

Color additives approved for use on hair include henna (from the Lawsonia plant) as well as lead acetate and bismuth citrate, both of which are used in "progressive" hair dyes that darken hair gradually with repeated applications. Of note, temporary tattoos marketed as "black henna" contain PPD and may increase your risk of allergy to hair dyes. Hair dyes are not meant to be used for staining your skin.

Unusual Colors

People sometime ask whether unusual colors such as pink, orange, blue, and green are regulated differently from other hair dyes. How a hair dye is regulated depends on whether it is a coal-tar hair dye or is made from plant or mineral materials, not on the shade.

Coal-Tar Hair Dye Safety Checklist

- Follow all directions on the label and in the package.

- Do a patch test on your skin every time before dyeing your hair.

- Keep hair dyes away from your eyes, and do not dye your eyebrows or eyelashes. This can hurt your eyes and may even cause blindness.

- Wear gloves when applying hair dye.

- Do not leave the product on longer than the directions say you should. Keep track of time using a clock or a timer.

- Rinse your scalp well with water after using hair dye.

- Keep hair dyes out of the reach of children.

- Do not scratch or brush your scalp three days before using hair dyes.

- Do not dye or relax your hair if your scalp is irritated, sunburned, or damaged.

- Wait at least 14 days after bleaching, relaxing, or perming your hair before using dye.

- Read the ingredient statement to make certain that ingredients that may have caused a problem for you in the past, such as p-phenylenediamine (PPD) are not present.

- If you have a problem, tell your healthcare provider. Then, please report it to the FDA.

How to Report a Problem

If you have a reaction to a hair dye—or any other cosmetic—first contact your healthcare provider for any necessary medical help.

Then, please tell the FDA. The law doesn't require cosmetic companies, including hair dye manufacturers, to share their safety data or consumer complaints with the FDA. So, the information you report is very important to help the FDA monitor the safety of cosmetics on the market.

You can report a problem with a cosmetic to the FDA in either of these ways:

1. Contact MedWatch, the FDA's problem-reporting program, at 800-332-1088, or file a MedWatch Voluntary report online (www.accessdata.fda.gov/scripts/medwatch/index.cfm?action=reporting.home).

2. Contact the consumer complaint coordinator in your area.

Chapter 28

Air Quality and Your Health

Why Is Air Quality Important?

Local air quality affects how you live and breathe. Like the weather, it can change from day to day or even hour to hour. The U.S. Environmental Protection Agency (EPA) and your local air quality agency have been working to make information about outdoor air quality as easy to find and understand as weather forecasts. A key tool in this effort is the Air Quality Index, or AQI. The EPA and local officials use the AQI to provide simple information about your local air quality, how unhealthy air may affect you, and how you can protect your health.

What Is the Air Quality Index?

The AQI is an index for reporting daily air quality. It tells you how clean or unhealthy your air is, and what associated health effects might be a concern. The AQI focuses on health effects you may experience within a few hours or days after breathing unhealthy air. The AQI is calculated for four major air pollutants regulated by the Clean Air Act: ground-level ozone, particle pollution, carbon monoxide (CO), and sulfur dioxide (SO_2). For each of these pollutants, the EPA has established national air quality standards to protect public health. The EPA is currently reviewing the national air quality standard for

This chapter includes text excerpted from "Air Quality Index—A Guide to Air Quality and Your Health," AirNow, U.S. Environmental Protection Agency (EPA), July 27, 2017.

nitrogen dioxide. If the standard is revised, the AQI will be revised as well.

How Does the Air Quality Index Work?

Think of the AQI as a yardstick that runs from 0–500. The higher the AQI value, the greater the level of air pollution and the greater the health concern. For example, an AQI value of 50 represents good air quality with little or no potential to affect public health, while an AQI value over 300 represents air quality so hazardous that everyone may experience serious effects.

An AQI value of 100 generally corresponds to the national air quality standard for the pollutant, which is the level the EPA has set to protect public health. AQI values at or below 100 are generally thought of as satisfactory. When AQI values are above 100, air quality is considered to be unhealthy—at first for certain sensitive groups of people, then for everyone as AQI values increase.

What Do the Air Quality Index Values Mean?

The purpose of the AQI is to help you understand what local air quality means to your health. To make it easier to understand, the AQI is divided into six levels of health concern:

Table 28.1. Air Quality Index (AQI) Values

Air Quality Index (AQI) Values	Levels of Health Concern	Colors
When the AQI is in this range:	*...air quality conditions are:*	*...as symbolized by this color:*
0–50	Good	Green
51–100	Moderate	Yellow
101–150	Unhealthy for Sensitive Groups	Orange
151–200	Unhealthy	Red
201–300	Very Unhealthy	Purple
301–500	Hazardous	Maroon

Values above 500 are considered beyond the AQI. Follow recommendations for the hazardous category

Each category corresponds to a different level of health concern:

• **Good.** The AQI value for your community is between 0 and 50. Air quality is satisfactory and poses little or no health risk.

- **Moderate.** The AQI is between 51 and 100. Air quality is acceptable; however, pollution in this range may pose a moderate health concern for a very small number of individuals. People who are unusually sensitive to ozone or particle pollution may experience respiratory symptoms.

- **Unhealthy for sensitive groups.** When AQI values are between 101 and 150, members of sensitive groups may experience health effects, but the general public is unlikely to be affected.

  - *Ozone:* People with lung disease, children, older adults, and people who are active outdoors are considered sensitive, and therefore, at greater risk.

  - *Particle pollution:* People with heart or lung disease, older adults, and children are considered sensitive, and therefore, at greater risk.

- **Unhealthy.** Everyone may begin to experience health effects when AQI values are between 151 and 200. Members of sensitive groups may experience more serious health effects.

- **Very unhealthy.** AQI values between 201 and 300 trigger a health alert, meaning everyone may experience more serious health effects.

- **Hazardous.** AQI values over 300 trigger health warnings of emergency conditions. The entire population is even more likely to be affected by serious health effects.

How Is a Community's Air Quality Index Calculated and Reported?

Each day, monitors record concentrations of the major pollutants at more than a thousand locations across the country. These raw measurements are converted into a separate AQI value for each pollutant (ground-level ozone, particle pollution, carbon monoxide (CO), and sulfur dioxide (SO_2)) using standard formulas developed by the EPA. The highest of these AQI values is reported as the AQI value for that day. In large cities (more than 350,000 people), state and local agencies are required to report the AQI to the public daily. Many smaller communities also report the AQI as a public health service.

When the AQI is above 100, agencies must also report which groups, such as children or people with asthma or heart disease, may be sensitive to that pollutant. If two or more pollutants have AQI values above 100 on a given day, agencies must report all the groups that are sensitive to those pollutants. For example, if a community's AQI is 130 for ozone and 101 for particle pollution, the AQI value for that day would be announced as 130 for ozone. The announcements would note that particle pollution levels were also high and would alert groups sensitive to ozone or particle pollution about how to protect their health. Many cities also provide forecasts for the next day's AQI. These forecasts help local residents protect their health by alerting them to plan their strenuous outdoor activities for a time when air quality is better.

Where Can I Find the Air Quality Index?

Checking local air quality is as easy as checking the weather. You can find the latest AQI values on the Internet, in your local media, and on many state and local telephone hotlines. You can also sign up to receive AQI forecasts by e-mail:

- **AQI on the Internet.** The EPA and its federal, tribal, state, and local partners have developed an AirNow website to provide the public with easy access to national air quality information. On the website, you will find daily AQI forecasts and real-time AQI conditions for over 300 cities across the United States, with links to more detailed state and local air quality websites. AIRNow's reports are displayed as maps you can use to quickly determine if the air quality is unhealthy near you.

- **AQI via e-mail.** Sign up for EnviroFlash (www.enviroflash. info), a free service that will alert you via e-mail when air quality is forecast to be a concern in your area.

- **AQI in the media.** Many local media—television, radio, and newspapers—and some national media (such as USA Today, The Weather Channel, and Cable News Network (CNN)) provide daily air quality reports, often as part of the weather forecast.

What Are Typical Air Quality Index Values in Most Communities?

In many U.S. communities, AQI values are usually below 100, with higher values occurring just a few times a year. Larger cities typically have more air pollution than smaller cities, so their AQI values may exceed 100 more often. AQI values higher than 200 are infrequent, and

AQI values above 300 are extremely rare—they generally occur only during events such as forest fires. You can compare the air quality of U.S. cities and find out about quality trends in your area by visiting "AirCompare" at www.epa.gov/aircompare.

AQI values can vary from one season to another. In winter, carbon monoxide (CO) may be high in some areas because cold weather makes it difficult for car emission control systems to operate effectively. Ozone is often higher in warmer months, because heat and sunlight increase ozone formation. Particle pollution can be elevated any time of the year.

AQI values also can vary depending on the time of day. Ozone levels often peak in the afternoon to early evening. Carbon monoxide (CO) may be a problem during morning or evening rush hours. And particle pollution can be high any time of day, and is often elevated near busy roadways, especially during morning or evening rush hours.

How Can I Avoid Being Exposed to Unhealthy Air?

You can take simple steps to reduce your exposure to unhealthy air. First, you need to find out whether AQI levels are a concern in your area. You can do this, as described previously, by visiting the AIRNow website, signing up for EnviroFlash, or checking your local media. If the AQI for ozone, particle pollution, carbon monoxide (CO), or sulfur dioxide (SO_2) is a concern in your area, you can learn what steps to take to protect your health by checking the charts on the following pages. Two important terms you will need to understand are:

Heavy exertion means an intense activity that causes you to breathe hard.

- **Prolonged exertion.** This means any outdoor activity that you'll be doing intermittently for several hours and that makes you breathe slightly harder than normal. A good example of this is working in the yard for part of a day. When air quality is unhealthy, you can protect your health by reducing how much time you spend on this type of activity.

- **Heavy exertion.** This means intense outdoor activities that cause you to breathe hard. When air quality is unhealthy, you can protect your health by reducing how much time you spend on this type of activity, or by substituting a less intense activity—for example, go for a walk instead of a jog. Be sure to reduce your activity level if you experience any unusual coughing, chest discomfort, wheezing, breathing difficulty, or unusual fatigue.

Chapter 29

Climate Change and Respiratory Allergies

Allergy

An allergy is a reaction of your immune system to something that, for most people, is essentially harmless, such as pet dander, nuts, or pollen. For most seasonal allergy sufferers, the diagnosis is hay fever, or—as your doctor would write it down in your medical chart—allergic rhinitis. Reactions range from annoying—sneezing, itching, watery eyes, stuffy nose—to dangerous: in some people, allergies can trigger asthma attacks.

Seasonal allergies afflict up to 30 percent of the world's human population, studies have found, and the Cleveland Clinic reports a rising allergy prevalence. For most people, allergies aren't life threatening, but they can hamper one's enjoyment of life—for months at a stretch. Tree pollen strikes in the spring, grass pollen in the summer, and weed pollen in the summer and fall.

This chapter contains text excerpted from the following sources: Text under the heading "Allergy" is excerpted from "Climate and Allergies," Climate.gov, National Oceanic and Atmospheric Administration (NOAA), June 7, 2018; Text beginning with the heading "Aeroallergens and Rates of Allergic Diseases in the United States" is excerpted from "Climate Impacts on Aeroallergens and Respiratory Diseases," U.S. Global Change Research Program (USGCRP), 2016; Text under the heading "Climate and Human Health" is excerpted from "Asthma, Respiratory Allergies and Airway Diseases," National Institute of Environmental Health Sciences (NIEHS), August 24, 2017.

If you have hay fever, your worst enemy is probably ragweed—common ragweed, giant ragweed, lanceleaf ragweed, or western ragweed. Ragweed likely causes more hay fever than all other plants put together, according to the U.S. Department of Agriculture (USDA) plant physiologist Lewis Ziska, and a single ragweed plant can produce a billion pollen grains. Those grains contain a protein that excels in annoying the human immune system.

It's Getting Worse . . .

Multiple studies indicate that, as climate warms, pollen seasons will start sooner, last longer, and produce more pollen than in the past. In fact, it's already happening. A 2014 study led by Rutgers University's Yong Zhang found that between 2001 and 2010, pollen season in the contiguous United States started on average three days earlier than it did in the 1990s, and the annual total of daily airborne pollen increased more than 40 percent.

Longer pollen seasons mean more time for the human body to become sensitized to allergens and to produce an inappropriate response. Warming climate also means a higher number of frost-free days, which especially benefit allergen-producing weeds.

The climate and allergy connection isn't just about longer growing seasons, however. Part of the pollen problem is directly down to more carbon dioxide. In the 1990s, Ziska conducted studies of the effect of carbon dioxide levels on ragweed. In his experiment, plants exposed to rising levels of carbon dioxide grew to greater size and produced more pollen. Most irritating of all, ragweed plants exposed to more of the gas produced more of the protein that specifically nags human noses.

But worsening hay fever isn't entirely the fault of carbon dioxide and pollen. The 2014 U.S. National Climate Assessment (NCA 2014) warned that simultaneous exposure to allergens and toxic air pollutants can amplify allergic responses. Meanwhile, the assessment reports, extreme rainfall and rising temperatures can lead to growth of indoor fungi and molds—another category of allergy triggers for some people.

As a further complication, thunderstorms often coincide with spikes in emergency room visits for asthma attacks. A review paper published in the *World Allergy Organization* Journal describes a possible mechanism for the connection: thunderstorms carry pollen grains at ground level, and updrafts sweep those grains into the humid bases of storm clouds; the grains rupture and release allergy-inducing starch granules; the pollen fragments can be inhaled much more deeply into human airways than whole pollen grains would have been.

Identifying the impact of climate change on specific types of extreme weather events will require more research, the NCA2014 says, especially since these events occur over small scales that are hard to predict. But where thunderstorms do strike, they pose a risk to people with allergic asthma. Most climate models project that heavy precipitation is likely to increase in a warmer world. If that increase in heavy rain comes via more thunderstorms, the risk of allergic asthma attacks may also rise.

. . . But Not Everywhere

Ziska's 2011 study, which found a lengthening pollen season in North America, didn't see the same changes everywhere. Ziska's team examined measurements of airborne pollen collected by 10 National Allergy Bureau (NAB) pollen-counting stations between 1995 and 2009, on a path stretching from east Texas northward to Saskatoon, Saskatchewan. The team found that pollen season lengthened more at higher latitudes, anywhere from 13–27 days north of roughly 44°N (roughly the latitude of Minneapolis). At the southernmost station (Georgetown, Texas), pollen season actually decreased by one day.

Ziska's team's finding was not unique; multiple studies have uncovered the same phenomenon, and it's in keeping with broader findings that climate change is more pronounced at higher latitudes. As reported in *Environmental Health Perspectives*, the geographic differences in allergy season impacts can probably be attributed to water vapor. In more humid, rainier southern latitudes, water vapor likely increases cloud cover, moderating the warming. Furthermore, rain washes pollen out of the air, at least for a little while. So, pollen-triggered allergies may not worsen as much in the southern United States as the north—assuming there's no climate-driven increase in thunderstorms picking on asthmatics.

Predicting future changes, as well as fully understanding changes that have already occurred, is complicated by the United States' uneven distribution of NAB pollen-sampling stations. The contiguous United States is divided into nine climate regions: Northeast, Southeast, South, Central, East North Central, West North Central, Southwest, West, and Northwest. While the Northeast region enjoys a relative abundance of NAB stations, the West North Central region has only two—and they sit along the border with the East North Central region. Matching pollen counts with weather statistics is also a challenge in some regions. In the 2014 study headed by Zhang, the distance between the NAB pollen station and the nearest National Oceanic and Atmospheric Administration (NOAA) weather station was sometimes just a few kilometers, but other times tens of kilometers. The uneven distribution of NAB stations remains a source of uncertainty in pollen-climate predictions.

You Can't Cure It, but You Can Try to Avoid It

If your nose is already driving you crazy, what can you do? The *World Allergy Organization Journal* has a few suggestions, including educating yourself on when pollen season peaks in your area, and avoiding extended outdoor activities during those times; protecting your face with closed-visor helmets when biking; keeping car windows rolled up while driving; and staying indoors on windy days and during thunderstorms.

If you want to move someplace where pollen seasons are shortening rather than lengthening, you can always head to the United States' Southern or Southeastern climate regions.

Climate change may alter the production, allergenicity, distribution, and timing of airborne allergens (aeroallergens). These changes contribute to the severity and prevalence of allergic disease in humans. The very young, those with compromised immune systems, and the medically uninsured bear the brunt of asthma and other allergic illnesses. While aeroallergen exposure is not the sole, or even necessarily the most significant factor associated with allergic illnesses, that relationship is part of a complex pathway that links aeroallergen exposure to the prevalence of allergic illnesses, including asthma episodes. On the other hand, climate change may reduce adverse allergic and asthmatic responses in some areas. For example, as some areas become drier, there is the potential for a shortening of the pollen season due to plant stress.

Aeroallergens and Rates of Allergic Diseases in the United States

Aeroallergens are substances present in the air that, once inhaled, stimulate an allergic response in sensitized individuals. Aeroallergens include tree, grass, and weed pollen; indoor and outdoor molds; and other allergenic proteins associated with animal dander, dust mites, and cockroaches. Ragweed is the aeroallergen that most commonly affects persons in the United States.

Allergic diseases develop in response to complex and multiple inter-actions among both genetic and nongenetic factors, including a developing immune system, environmental exposures (such as ambient air pollution or weather conditions), and socioeconomic and demographic factors. Aeroallergen exposure contributes to the occurrence of asthma episodes, allergic rhinitis or hay fever, sinusitis, conjunctivitis, urticaria (hives), atopic dermatitis or eczema, and anaphylaxis (a severe, whole-body allergic reaction that can be life-threatening). Allergic illnesses, including hay fever, affect about one-third of the U.S. population, and more than 34 million Americans have been diagnosed with asthma. These diseases have increased in the United States over the past 30 years. The prevalence of hay fever has increased from 10 percent of the population in 1970 to 30 percent in 2000. Asthma rates have increased from approximately 8–55 cases per 1,000 persons to approximately 55–90 cases per 1,000 persons over that same time period; however, there is variation in reports of active cases of asthma as a function of geography and demographics.

Climate Impacts on Aeroallergen Characteristics

Climate change contributes to changes in allergic illnesses as greater concentrations of CO_2, together with higher temperatures and changes in precipitation, extend the start or duration of the growing season, increase the quantity and allergenicity of pollen, and expand the spatial distribution of pollens.

Historical trends show that climate change has led to changes in the length of the growing season for certain allergenic pollens. For instance, the duration of pollen release for common ragweed (*Ambrosia artemisiifolia*) has been increasing as a function of latitude in recent decades in the midwestern region of North America. Latitudinal effects on increasing season length were associated primarily with a delay in first frost during the fall season and lengthening of the frost-free period. Studies in controlled indoor environments find that increases in temperature and CO_2 result in earlier flowering, greater floral numbers, greater pollen production, and increased allergenicity in common ragweed. In addition, studies using urban areas as proxies for both higher CO_2 and higher temperatures demonstrate earlier flowering of pollen species, which may lead to a longer total pollen season.

For trees, earlier flowering associated with higher winter and spring temperatures has been observed over a 50-year period for oak. Research on loblolly pine (*Pinus taeda*) also demonstrates that elevated CO_2

could induce earlier and greater seasonal pollen production. Annual birch (*Betula*) pollen production and peak values from 2020–2100 are projected to be 1.3–2.3 times higher, relative to average values for 2000, with the start and peak dates of pollen release advancing by two to four weeks.

Climate Variability and Effects on Allergic Diseases

Climate change related alterations in local weather patterns, including changes in minimum and maximum temperatures and rainfall, affect the burden of allergic diseases. The role of weather on the initiation or exacerbation of allergic symptoms in sensitive persons is not well understood. So-called "thunderstorm asthma" results as allergenic particles are dispersed through osmotic rupture, a phenomenon where cell membranes burst. Pollen grains may, after contact with rain, release part of their cellular contents, including allergen-laced fine particles. Increases in the intensity and frequency of heavy rainfall and storminess over the coming decades is likely to be associated with spikes in aeroallergen concentrations and the potential for related increases in the number and severity of allergic illnesses.

Potential nonlinear interactions between aeroallergens and ambient air pollutants (including ozone (O_3), nitrogen dioxide (NO_2), sulfur dioxide (SO_2), and fine particulate matter) may increase health risks for people who are simultaneously exposed. In particular, preexposure to air pollution (especially ozone or fine particulate matter) may magnify the effects of aeroallergens, as prior damage to airways may increase the permeability of mucous membranes to the penetration of allergens, although existing evidence suggests greater sensitivity but not necessarily a direct link with ozone exposure. A report noted remaining uncertainties across the epidemiologic, controlled human exposure, and toxicology studies on this emerging topic.

Climate and Human Health

Climate change is expected to affect air quality through several pathways, including production and allergenicity of allergens and increase regional concentrations of ozone, fine particles, and dust. Some of these pollutants can directly cause respiratory disease or exacerbate existing conditions in susceptible populations, such as children or the elderly.

Some of the impacts that climate change can have on air quality include:

Health Impacts

- Increase in ground level ozone and fine particle concentrations, which can trigger a variety of reactions including chest pains, coughing, throat irritation, and congestion, as well as reduce lung function and cause inflammation of the lungs

- Increase in carbon dioxide concentrations and temperatures, thereby affecting the timing of aeroallergen distribution and amplifying the allergenicity of pollen and mold spores

- Increase in precipitation in some areas leading to an increase in mold spores

- Increase in rate of ozone formation due to higher temperatures and increased sunlight

- Increase in frequency of droughts, leading to increased dust and particulate matter

Adaptation and Mitigation

- Mitigating short-lived contamination species that both air pollutants and greenhouse gases, such as ozone or black carbon. Examples include urban tree covers or rooftop gardens in urban settings.

- Decreasing the use of vehicle miles traveled to reduce ozone precursors

- Utilizing alternative transportation options, such as walking or biking, which have the cobenefit of reducing emissions while increasing cardiovascular fitness and contributing to weight-loss. However, these activities also have the potential to increase exposure to harmful outdoor air pollutants, particularly in urban areas.

- Increasing the use of air conditioning can alleviate the health effects of exposure to chronic or acute heat. However, this can potentially result in higher greenhouse gas emissions depending on the method of power generation.

Chapter 30

Smoking

Cigarette smoke contains a number of toxic chemicals and irritants. People with allergies may be more sensitive to cigarette smoke than others and research studies indicate that smoking may aggravate allergies.

Smoking does not just harm smokers but also those around them. Research has shown that children and spouses of smokers tend to have more respiratory infections and asthma than those of nonsmokers. In addition, exposure to secondhand smoke can increase the risk of allergic complications such as sinusitis and bronchitis.

Common symptoms of smoke irritation are burning or watery eyes, nasal congestion, coughing, hoarseness, and shortness of breath presenting as a wheeze.

Preventive Strategies

- Don't smoke and if you do, seek support to quit smoking.

- Seek smoke-free environments in restaurants, theaters, and hotel rooms.

This chapter contains text excerpted from the following sources: Text in this chapter begins with excerpts from "Cigarette Smoke," National Institute of Environmental Health Sciences (NIEHS), May 1, 2018; Text beginning with the heading "Secondhand Smoke Facts" is excerpted from "Secondhand Smoke (SHS) Facts—Smoking and Tobacco Use," Centers for Disease Control and Prevention (CDC), January 17, 2018.

- Avoid smoking in closed areas like homes or cars where others may be exposed to secondhand smoke.

Secondhand Smoke Facts

Secondhand smoke (SHS) harms children and adults, and the only way to fully protect nonsmokers is to eliminate smoking in all homes, worksites, and public places. You can take steps to protect yourself and your family from secondhand smoke, such as making your home and vehicles smoke-free.

Separating smokers from nonsmokers, opening windows, or using air filters does not prevent people from breathing secondhand smoke. Most exposure to secondhand smoke occurs in homes and workplaces.

People are also exposed to secondhand smoke in public places—such as in restaurants, bars, and casinos—as well as in cars and other vehicles. People with lower income and lower education are less likely to be covered by smoke-free laws in worksites, restaurants, and bars.

Secondhand Smoke Harms Children and Adults

- There is no risk-free level of secondhand smoke exposure; even brief exposure can be harmful to health.
- Since 1964, approximately 2,500,000 nonsmokers have died from health problems caused by exposure to secondhand smoke.

Health Effects in Children

In children, secondhand smoke causes the following:

- Ear infections
- More frequent and severe asthma attacks
- Respiratory symptoms (for example, coughing, sneezing, and shortness of breath)
- Respiratory infections (bronchitis and pneumonia)
- A greater risk for sudden infant death syndrome (SIDS)

Health Effects in Adults

In adults who have never smoked, secondhand smoke can cause:

- Heart disease
  - For nonsmokers, breathing secondhand smoke has immediate harmful effects on the heart and blood vessels.

- It is estimated that secondhand smoke caused nearly 34,000 heart disease deaths each year during 2005–2009 among adult nonsmokers in the United States.

- Lung cancer

  - Secondhand smoke exposure caused more than 7,300 lung cancer deaths each year during 2005–2009 among adult nonsmokers in the United States.

- Stroke

  Smoke-free laws can reduce the risk for heart disease and lung cancer among nonsmokers.

Patterns of Secondhand Smoke Exposure

Exposure to secondhand smoke can be measured by testing saliva, urine, or blood to see if it contains cotinine. Cotinine is created when the body breaks down the nicotine found in tobacco smoke.

Secondhand Smoke Exposure Has Decreased in Recent Years

- Measurements of cotinine show that exposure to secondhand smoke has steadily decreased in the United States over time.

  - During 1988–1991, almost 90 of every 100 (87.9%) nonsmokers had measurable levels of cotinine.

  - During 2007–2008, about 40 of every 100 (40.1%) nonsmokers had measurable levels of cotinine.

  - During 2011–2012, about 25 of every 100 (25.3%) nonsmokers had measurable levels of cotinine.

- The decrease in exposure to secondhand smoke is likely due to:

  - The growing number of states and communities with laws that do not allow smoking in indoor areas of workplaces and public places, including restaurants, bars, and casinos

  - The growing number of households with voluntary smoke-free home rules

  - Significant declines in cigarette smoking rates

  - The fact that smoking around nonsmokers has become much less socially acceptable

Many People in the United States Are Still Exposed to Secondhand Smoke

- During 2011–2012, about 58 million nonsmokers in the United States were exposed to secondhand smoke.

- Among children who live in homes in which no one smokes indoors, those who live in multi-unit housing (for example, apartments or condos) have 45 percent higher cotinine levels (or almost half the amount) than children who live in single-family homes.

- During 2011–2012, 2 out of every 5 children ages 3–11—including 7 out of every 10 Black children—in the United States were exposed to secondhand smoke regularly.

- During 2011–2012, more than 1 in 3 (36.8%) nonsmokers who lived in rental housing were exposed to secondhand smoke.

Differences in Secondhand Smoke Exposure

Racial and Ethnic Groups

Cotinine levels have declined in all racial and ethnic groups, but cotinine levels continue to be higher among non-Hispanic Black Americans than non-Hispanic White Americans and Mexican Americans. During 2011–2012:

- Nearly half (46.8%) of Black nonsmokers in the United States were exposed to secondhand smoke.

- About 22 of every 100 (21.8%) non-Hispanic White nonsmokers were exposed to secondhand smoke.

- Nearly a quarter (23.9%) of Mexican American nonsmokers were exposed to secondhand smoke.

Income

- Secondhand smoke exposure is higher among people with low incomes.

- During 2011–2012, more than 2 out of every 5 (43.2%) nonsmokers who lived below the poverty level were exposed to secondhand smoke.

Occupation

- Differences in secondhand smoke exposure related to people's jobs decreased over the past 20 years, but large Smoke-free still exist.

- Some groups continue to have high levels of secondhand smoke exposure. These include:

  - Blue-collar workers and service workers

  - Construction workers

What You Can Do

You can protect yourself and your family from secondhand smoke by:

- Quitting smoking if you are not already a smoke-free

- Not allowing anyone to smoke anywhere in or near your home

- Not allowing anyone to smoke in your car, even with the windows down

- Making sure your children's daycare center and schools are tobacco-free

- Seeking out restaurants and other places that do not allow smoking (if your state still allows smoking in public areas)

- Teaching your children to stay away from secondhand smoke

- Being a good role model by not smoking or using any other type of tobacco

Chapter 31

Multiple Chemical Sensitivity

The condition now most commonly known as multiple chemical sensitivity (MCS) was brought to the attention of the U.S. medical establishment when the late Theron Randolph, a physician trained in allergy and immunology, reported that a number of his patients reacted adversely to chemicals in their environment. He compared the condition to Selye's stress-oriented general adaptation syndrome and linked the adverse effects of this "petrochemical problem" to contact with chemicals found in commonly encountered substances such as cosmetics, auto fuels, exhaust fumes, and food additives. He also observed that many of his patients reacted to many industrial solvents found in small amounts in manufactured products such as construction materials, newspaper and other ink-related products, furniture, and carpet.

Although Randolph and other physicians who shared his theories published articles in the medical literature during the 1950s and early 1960s, his views were not widely accepted among physicians,

This chapter contains text excerpted from the following sources: Text in this chapter begins with excerpts from "A Report on Multiple Chemical Sensitivity (MCS)," Office of Disease Prevention and Health Promotion (ODPHP), U.S. Department of Health and Human Services (HHS), December 1, 2017; Text under the heading "Fragrance-Free Environment" is excerpted from "Fragrance-Free Environment," U.S. Access Board, July 26, 2000. Reviewed August 2018; Text beginning with the heading "Fragrances in Cosmetics" is excerpted from "Fragrances in Cosmetics," U.S. Food and Drug Administration (FDA), August 8, 2018.

particularly those trained in allergy and immunology. In 1965, in response to this lack of acceptance within his specialty, he founded the Society for Human Ecology (SHE) and invited physicians of all specialties (who were later often referred to as clinical ecologists) to take part. In 1985, the Society changed its name to the American Academy of Environmental Medicine (AAEM). Members are referred to as environmental physicians. However, the term clinical ecologist remains in use.

The American Academy of Environmental Medicine has stated that a wide variety of symptoms, stemming from many different organs, "[m]ay all be the result of biologic system dysfunctions triggered by environmental stressors in susceptible patients." AAEM supports the application of a comprehensive model of environmental medicine to elucidate the nature of these system dysfunctions. The model states the following:

Environmentally triggered illnesses (EI) result from a disruption of homeostasis by environmental stressors. This disruption may result from a wide range of possible exposures, ranging from a severe acute exposure to a single stressor to cumulative relatively low-grade exposures to many stressors over time. The disruption can affect any part of the body via dysfunctioning of any number of the body's many biologic mechanisms and systems. The ongoing manifestations of environmentally triggered illnesses are shaped by the nature of stressors and the timing of exposures to them, by the biochemical individuality of the patient, and by the dynamic interactions over time resulting from various governing principles such as the total load, the level of adaptation, the bipolarity of responses, the spreading phenomenon, the switch phenomenon, and individual susceptibility (biochemical individuality) (AAEM emphasis).

There has been increasing debate over MCS in the years since Randolph's publications. A wide variety of symptoms have been reported, including fatigue, malaise, difficulty concentrating, loss of memory, weakness, headaches, nausea, mucous membrane irritation, and dizziness. MCS patients have associated their symptoms with many substances, including colognes and perfumes, aerosol air freshener, laundry detergent, gasoline exhaust, cleaners, insecticide sprays, and cigarette smoke. MCS has been associated with exposure to many kinds of substances. These exposures may occur in workplaces, homes, and outdoors.

Topics that have been debated include: whether MCS is a distinct disease entity, its etiology (or etiologies), its pathophysiology, how to define the condition, how it should be treated, and how it should be approached in the legal and legislative arenas. The condition has become more visible through increased media attention. One result of this visibility has been an increase in the number of scientists and physicians taking part in the debate. The discussions have, at times, become contentious, and there have been calls for governmental action by MCS patients, advocacy groups, and legislators.

The federal agencies have increased their interagency cooperation on MCS issues through sharing of current knowledge, development of research recommendations, and cosponsorship of workshops and conferences.

Terminology

Many other names have been applied to the condition called MCS. Among them are environmental illness (EI), ecological illness, total allergy syndrome, the 20th Century disease, and idiopathic environmental intolerances (IPCS). The last term, which is discussed in Section VI, was recommended by a MCS workshop that was organized by the International Program on Chemical Safety (a program cosponsored by the United Nations Environmental Program (UNEP), the International Labor Office (ILO), and the World Health Organization (WHO)).

Until more is known about the etiology of the condition, it is not possible to determine what name would be both descriptive and physiologically correct.

Definitions

The most basic disagreement surrounding the study of MCS has been how to define the condition in ways acceptable to the many interested parties. In 1987, Mark Cullen, M.D., a professor of medicine and epidemiology at Yale University, edited an issue of *Occupational Medicine State of the Art Reviews* entitled "Workers With Multiple Chemical Sensitivities." He described the case of a middle-aged man who had developed sensitivities to a wide variety of chemicals, including common household products. This occurred after the patient had developed pneumonia following exposure to a chemical spilled at work. Cullen reported his lack of success in treating the patient and noted that there were other patients in whom the same symptoms developed following similar situations. From this experience, Cullen proposed a definition that has become the one most commonly referenced, and is, for some, the de facto definition of MCS.

Public Health Issues in Medical Evaluation and Care of Multiple Chemical Sensitivity Patients

Many physicians are uncertain how to approach the evaluation and care of persons who have multiple symptoms that attribute to low-level chemical exposure. Although medical approaches and therapies differ considerably because of differing beliefs about MCS by physicians, all individuals who report suffering from chemical sensitivities should receive a competent, complete medical evaluation and compassionate, understanding care. The goal of this care should be to promote health without causing additional harm. Individuals should not be subjected to ineffective, costly, or potentially dangerous treatments. Appropriate care for well-characterized medical and psychological illnesses should not be withheld or delayed. The ramifications of recommending functional changes in workplace or home settings should be carefully considered.

Medical Evaluation

The identification of MCS is based largely on the patient's description of the symptoms and the relationship of these symptoms to environmental exposures. The evaluation of an individual for MCS should, therefore, begin a complete and detailed history, including a comprehensive exposure history. The *Agency for Toxic Substances and Disease Registry (ATSDR)/National Institute for Occupational Safety and Health (NIOSH) Case Study in Environmental Medicine—Taking An Exposure History* is a useful guide for physicians unfamiliar with taking an environmental exposure history.

MCS patients often report that their symptoms began after an accidental overexposure to a chemical, typically a solvent or a pesticide, and that their symptoms recurred following exposure to lower levels of the same chemical. Symptoms then began to occur in response to low-level exposure to an increasing number of other chemicals, often unrelated to the initiating compound. Commonly reported symptoms are listed alphabetically, therefore, are not in any order of frequency of occurrence.

Commonly Reported MCS Symptoms

- Breathing difficulty
- Headache
- Chest pain

- Inability to concentrate

- Depression

- Joint and muscle pain

- Eye, ear, nose, throat irritation

- Malaise

- Fatigue

- Memory loss, confusion, dizziness

- Gastrointestinal problems

- Skin disorders

MCS patients often associate symptoms with such substances as colognes and perfumes, aerosol air freshener, laundry detergent, gasoline exhaust, cleaners, insecticide sprays, and cigarette smoke. Miller (1995) reported that an acquired, self-identified intolerance to alcohol is notably frequent among MCS patients.

Although physical findings and the results of laboratory tests in MCS patients are typically within normal limits, the physical examination, laboratory evaluation, and psychological assessment should be sufficiently comprehensive to establish or exclude underlying and coexisting medical conditions that are amenable to treatment. Physicians should be careful not to overlook other medical conditions that are amenable to treatment in an MCS patient.

No test result or panel of results can currently identify MCS. A number of tests have been suggested for evaluating MCS or have been used in studies of patients with MCS or chemical sensitivities; such tests include immunologic assays, quantitative electroencephalography, brain electrical activity mapping, evoked potentials, positron emission tomography, and single photon emission computed tomography. However, no laboratory test has been validated for sensitivity or specificity as a diagnostic predictor of MCS.

Physicians should recognize that classifying a condition as MCS does not explain the pathogenesis of the disorder. NRC's Subcommittee on Immunotoxicology advised that, "[w]henever possible, the term multiple chemical sensitivity should be replaced with a specific diagnosis to avoid the confusion between diagnosis and etiology that is inherent in the term." Some clinicians do not believe that MCS is a distinct disease and will not diagnose MCS under any circumstances.

Treatment

Different treatment approaches for MCS have been described that parallel the proposed mechanisms. Treatment modalities that include avoidance of chemicals, megavitamins, restricted or rotation diets, provocation-neutralization, sauna detoxification, and psychiatric treatment have been suggested. The effectiveness of these treatments has not been demonstrated. Because the etiology of MCS is unknown, the primary goals of most physicians are aimed at relieving symptoms and improving function. With an absence of data from definitive clinical trials, no conclusions about the optimal choice of treatment modalities can currently be made. However, aggressive therapies of unproven benefit that are potentially harmful cannot be recommended.

Healthcare providers must recognize the fundamental obligation to "First, do no harm." Ill persons must not be subjected to costly, time-consuming, ineffective, or dangerous therapeutic regimens. Caregivers must ensure that their treatment methods meet the standards of peer review and tests of efficacy, and offer reports on such treatment methods in the open and critically reviewed literature.

Persons identified as having MCS also need to be educated about what is known and not known about MCS. MCS patients should be informed about the lack of proven efficacy for various treatments and cautioned about costly and potentially harmful treatments. Avoidance of some exposures may be warranted, but recommendations of complete avoidance of chemical exposures should not be made without considering the impact of such restrictions. Major lifestyle modifications can have substantial consequences, including the loss of social support and employment. Because some individuals who have symptoms of MCS suffer social and psychological consequences of their condition, healthcare should be supportive.

Fragrance-Free Environments

There are many people who experience unpleasant physical effects from scented products, such as perfumes and colognes. Sometimes, it might be a headache or nausea when passing by a department store's fragrance counter or riding in an elevator with someone wearing a certain fragrance. However, there is a growing number of people who suffer more severe reactions to these and many other types of products and chemicals. This condition is known as multiple chemical sensitivities (MCS) and involves people who have developed an acute sensitivity to various chemicals in the environment. People with MCS experience a range of debilitating physical reactions, some even life-threatening, to chemicals used in a variety of products, including fragrances and personal care products, deodorizers and cleaners, pesticides, wall and floor coverings, and building materials.

It's a complex issue with a variety of triggering agents and physical reactions. Different people are affected by different products in different ways. The common factor is that the reaction, whatever the type, is very strong and disabling. Information needs to be developed on exactly what brings about such an acute sensitivity to certain chemicals, how and why this happens, and what can be done about it.

Fragrances in Cosmetics

Many products we use everyday contain fragrances. Some of these products are regulated as cosmetics by U.S. Food and Drug Administration (FDA). Some belong to other product categories and are regulated differently, depending on how the product is intended to be used.

How to Know If a Fragrance Product Is Regulated as a Cosmetic

If a product is intended to be applied to a person's body to make the person more attractive, it's a cosmetic under the law. Here are some examples of fragrance products that are regulated as cosmetics:

- Perfume

- Cologne

- Aftershave

Fragrance ingredients are also commonly used in other products, such as shampoos, shower gels, shaving creams, and body lotions. Even some products labeled "unscented" may contain fragrance ingredients. This is because the manufacturer may add just enough fragrance to mask the unpleasant smell of other ingredients, without giving the product a noticeable scent.

Some fragrance products that are applied to the body are intended for therapeutic uses, such as treating or preventing disease, or affecting the structure or function of the body. Products intended for this type of use are treated as drugs under the law, or sometimes as both cosmetics and drugs. Here are some examples of labeling statements that will cause a product containing fragrances to be treated as a drug:

- Easing muscle aches
- Soothing headaches
- Helping people sleep
- Treating colic

Many other products that may contain fragrance ingredients, but are not applied to the body, are regulated by the Consumer Product Safety Commission (CPSC). Here are some examples:

- Laundry detergents
- Fabric softeners
- Dryer sheets
- Room fresheners
- Carpet fresheners

Statements on labels, marketing claims, consumer expectations, and even some ingredients may determine a product's intended use.

"Essential Oils" and "Aromatherapy"

There is no regulatory definition for "essential oils," although people commonly use the term to refer to certain oils extracted from plants. The law treats Ingredients from plants the same as those from any other source.

For example, "essential oils" are commonly used in so-called aromatherapy products. If an "aromatherapy" product is intended to treat or prevent disease, or to affect the structure or function of the body, it's a drug.

Similarly, a massage oil intended to lubricate the skin is a cosmetic. But if claims are made that a massage oil relieves aches or relaxes muscles, apart from the action of the massage itself, it's a drug, or possibly both a cosmetic and a drug.

Safety Requirements

Fragrance ingredients in cosmetics must meet the same requirement for safety as other cosmetic ingredients. The law does not require

FDA approval before they go on the market, but they must be safe for consumers when they are used according to labeled directions, or as people customarily use them. Companies and individuals who manufacture or market cosmetics have a legal responsibility for ensuring that their products are safe and properly labeled.

If a cosmetic is marketed on a retail basis to consumers, such as in stores, on the Internet, or person-to-person, it must have a list of ingredients. In most cases, each ingredient must be listed individually. But under U.S. regulations, fragrance and flavor ingredients can be listed simply as "Fragrance" or "Flavor."

Here's why: The FDA requires the list of ingredients under the Fair Packaging and Labeling Act (FPLA). This law is not allowed to be used to force a company to tell "trade secrets." Fragrance and flavor formulas are complex mixtures of many different natural and synthetic chemical ingredients, and they are the kinds of cosmetic components that are most likely to be "trade secrets."

Fragrance Allergies and Sensitivities

Some individuals may be allergic or sensitive to certain ingredients in cosmetics, food, or other products, even if those ingredients are safe for most people. Some components of fragrance formulas may have a potential to cause allergic reactions or sensitivities for some people.

The FDA does not have the same legal authority to require allergen labeling for cosmetics as for food. So, if you are concerned about fragrance sensitivities, you may want to choose products that are fragrance free, and check the ingredient list carefully. If consumers have questions, they may choose to contact the manufacturer directly.

Phthalates as Fragrance Ingredients

Phthalates are a group of chemicals used in hundreds of products. The phthalate commonly used in fragrance products is diethyl phthalate, or DEP. DEP does not pose known risks for human health as it is currently used in cosmetics and fragrances.

313

Chapter 32

Lanolin Allergy

What Is Lanolin?

Lanolin, a natural product most commonly extracted from the fleece of sheep, is widely used in cosmetic and pharmaceutical products. It is sometimes also referred to as wool fat, wool wax, and wool grease. About 50 percent of lanolin is made up of wool alcohol, a substance containing allergens that can cause skin rashes and itching. A good emulsifier and excellent emollient, lanolin is frequently used in lotions, hair products, and toiletries.

The use of lanolin traces its roots to ancient Greece, where it was first discovered that the water in which sheep's wool was washed contained an oily substance that proved to be a good emollient or moisturizer. The substance was refined through various treatments and became lanolin. Despite improved purification processes, some impurities still remain, some of which include the allergens.

Types of Lanolin Allergy

Skin reactions to lanolin-based products are usually mild, but in some cases may be more extreme. Most often, a rash will appear after the application of a lanolin product on the skin, generally on the hands, legs, neck, and face, areas on which these products are commonly used. Small red itchy bumps or scaly patches of skin may denote a mild

---

allergic reaction to lanolin, but more serious reactions can result in swelling and blisters.

Symptoms of Lanolin Allergy

Symptoms of lanolin allergy often occur during the teen years, although they can go undiagnosed for a long time. Common symptoms include red bumpy rashes or scaly patches on the skin. Some people experience nasal congestion and, in extreme cases, lips or other body parts may swell up. Itchy rashes can also form blisters, which can sometimes be quite painful. Constant overall itchiness may also develop. Skin reactions to lanolin products on the body can appear from few hours to few days. The rashes are usually found in a single area, but over time, they may spread to other parts of the body.

Testing and Prevention of Lanolin Allergy

Testing can be done by a healthcare professional, or you can try a simple test yourself. Dermatologists typically administer a patch test using 30-percent wool alcohol and then monitor for a lanolin reaction. In a self-test, small amounts of lanolin can be applied over a small patch of skin and observed for five to seven days to see if the skin changes color or a rash develops. However, self-test is recommended only after consultation with a healthcare provider.

Allergies caused by lanolin products can be prevented by testing cosmetic and skin products on a small patch of skin before use. Products that contain wool alcohol should be avoided unless a dermatologist is consulted before the products are used on skin. A dermatologist should also be informed before ointments or creams are prescribed to a person with a lanolin allergy, since many of these products contain lanolin or related substances.

Treatment for Lanolin Allergy

Lanolin allergy can cause rashes or breakouts on skin that are annoying and unsightly, as well as more serious symptoms, like painful blisters. The best possible treatment is prevention itself; however, if a person has used a lanolin-based product and an allergic reaction results, then the first step of treatment would be to stop using that product or any substance that contains such ingredients as wool and wool alcohol or its derivatives. The next step would be to consult a professional healthcare provider. Topical steroids and oral antihistamines are most often used for the treatment of lanolin allergies, although if the reaction is extreme, the doctor may recommend a longer course of treatment with oral steroids and possibly antibiotics to treat secondary skin infections.

References

1. Cooley, Andrea. "Skin Reaction to Lanolin," Livestrong.com, July 18, 2012.

2. Cynia. "Lanolin Allergy," Instah.com, September 6, 2014.

3. Jacob, Sharon, M.D. "The Lanolin-Wool Wax Alcohol Update," The Dermatologist, February 18, 2014.

4. Ngan, Vanessa. "Allergy to Wood Alcohols," DermNet New Zealand, 2002.

Chapter 33

Sick Building Syndrome

The term "sick building syndrome" (SBS) is used to describe situations in which building occupants experience acute health and comfort effects that appear to be linked to time spent in a building, but no specific illness or cause can be identified. The complaints may be localized in a particular room or zone, or may be widespread throughout the building. In contrast, the term "building related illness" (BRI) is used when symptoms of diagnosable illness are identified and can be attributed directly to airborne building contaminants. A 1984 World Health Organization (WHO) Committee report suggested that up to 30 percent of new and remodeled buildings worldwide may be the subject of excessive complaints related to indoor air quality (IAQ). Often this condition is temporary, but some buildings have long-term problems. Frequently, problems result when a building is operated or maintained in a manner that is inconsistent with its original design or prescribed operating procedures. Sometimes indoor air problems are a result of poor building design or occupant activities.

Indicators of SBS include:

- Building occupants complain of symptoms associated with acute discomfort, e.g., headache; eye, nose, or throat irritation; dry cough; dry or itchy skin; dizziness and nausea; difficulty in concentrating; fatigue; and sensitivity to odors.

This chapter includes text excerpted from "Indoor Air Facts No. 4 (Revised) Sick Building Syndrome," U.S. Environmental Protection Agency (EPA), October 14, 2015.

- The cause of the symptoms is not known.

- Most of the complainants report relief soon after leaving the building.

  Indicators of BRI include:

- Building occupants complain of symptoms such as cough; chest tightness; fever, chills; and muscle aches.

- The symptoms can be clinically defined and have clearly identifiable causes.

- Complainants may require prolonged recovery times after leaving the building.

It is important to note that complaints may result from other causes. These may include an illness contracted outside the building, acute sensitivity (e.g., allergies), job-related stress or dissatisfaction, and other psychosocial factors. Nevertheless, studies show that symptoms may be caused or exacerbated by indoor air quality problems.

Causes of Sick Building Syndrome

The following have been cited causes of or contributing factors to sick building syndrome (SBS):

Inadequate ventilation: In the early and mid-1900's, building ventilation standards called for approximately 15 cubic feet per minute (CFM) of outside air for each building occupant, primarily to dilute and remove body odors. As a result of the 1973 oil embargo, however, national energy conservation measures called for a reduction in the amount of outdoor air provided for ventilation to 5 CFM per occupant. In many cases, these reduced outdoor air ventilation rates were found to be inadequate to maintain the health and comfort of building occupants. Inadequate ventilation, which may also occur if heating, ventilating, and air conditioning (HVAC) systems do not effectively distribute air to people in the building, is thought to be an important factor in SBS. In an effort to achieve acceptable IAQ while minimizing energy consumption, the American Society of Heating, Refrigerating and Air-Conditioning Engineers (ASHRAE) revised its ventilation standard to provide a minimum of 15 CFM of outdoor air per person (20 CFM/person in office spaces). Up to 60 CFM/person may be required in some spaces (such as smoking lounges) depending on the activities that normally occur in that space.

Chemical contaminants from indoor sources: Most indoor air pollution comes from sources inside the building. For example, adhesives, carpeting, upholstery, manufactured wood products, copy machines, pesticides, and cleaning agents may emit volatile organic compounds (VOCs), including formaldehyde. Environmental tobacco smoke contributes high levels of VOCs, other toxic compounds, and respirable particulate matter. Research shows that some VOCs can cause chronic and acute health effects at high concentrations, and some are known carcinogens. Low to moderate levels of multiple VOCs may also produce acute reactions. Combustion products such as carbon monoxide (CO), nitrogen dioxide (NO_2), as well as respirable particles, can come from unvented kerosene and gas space heaters, woodstoves, fireplaces, and gas stoves.

Chemical contaminants from outdoor sources: The outdoor air that enters a building can be a source of indoor air pollution. For example, pollutants from motor vehicle exhausts; plumbing vents, and building exhausts (e.g., bathrooms and kitchens) can enter the building through poorly located air intake vents, windows, and other openings. In addition, combustion products can enter a building from a nearby garage.

Biological contaminants: Bacteria, molds, pollen, and viruses are types of biological contaminants. These contaminants may breed in stagnant water that has accumulated in ducts, humidifiers and drain pans, or where water has collected on ceiling tiles, carpeting, or insulation. Sometimes insects or bird droppings can be a source of biological contaminants. Physical symptoms related to biological contamination include cough, chest tightness, fever, chills, muscle aches, and allergic responses such as mucous membrane irritation and upper respiratory congestion. One indoor bacterium, legionella, has caused both Legionnaires' Disease and Pontiac Fever.

These elements may act in combination, and may supplement other complaints such as inadequate temperature, humidity, or lighting. Even after a building investigation, however, the specific causes of the complaints may remain unknown.

Building Investigation Procedures

The goal of a building investigation is to identify and solve indoor air quality complaints in a way that prevents them from recurring and which avoids the creation of other problems. To achieve this goal,

321

it is necessary for the investigator(s) to discover whether a complaint is actually related to indoor air quality, identify the cause of the complaint, and determine the most appropriate corrective actions. An indoor air quality investigation procedure is best characterized as a cycle of information gathering, hypothesis formation, and hypothesis testing. It generally begins with a walkthrough inspection of the problem area to provide information about the four basic factors that influence indoor air quality:

- the occupants
- the heating, ventilation, and air conditioning (HVAC) system
- possible pollutant pathways
- possible contaminant sources

Preparation for a walkthrough should include documenting easily obtainable information about the history of the building and of the complaints; identifying known HVAC zones and complaint areas; notifying occupants of the upcoming investigation; and, identifying key individuals needed for information and access. The walkthrough itself entails visual inspection of critical building areas and consultation with occupants and staff.

The initial walkthrough should allow the investigator to develop some possible explanations for the complaint. At this point, the investigator may have sufficient information to formulate a hypothesis, test the hypothesis, and see if the problem is solved. If it is, steps should be taken to ensure that it does not recur. However, if insufficient information is obtained from the walkthrough to construct a hypothesis, or if initial tests fail to reveal the problem, the investigator should move on to collect additional information to allow formulation of additional hypotheses. The process of formulating hypotheses, testing them, and evaluating them continues until the problem is solved.

Although air sampling for contaminants might seem to be the logical response to occupant complaints, it seldom provides information about possible causes. While certain basic measurements, e.g., temperature, relative humidity, carbon dioxide (CO_2), and air movement, can provide a useful "snapshot" of current building conditions, sampling for specific pollutant concentrations is often not required to solve the problem and can even be misleading. Contaminant concentration levels rarely exceed existing standards and guidelines even when occupants continue to report health complaints. Air sampling should not be undertaken until considerable information on the factors listed above has been collected, and any sampling strategy should be based on a comprehensive understanding of how the building operates and the nature of the complaints.

Solutions to Sick Building Syndrome

Solutions to sick building syndrome usually include combinations of the following:

- **Pollutant source removal or modification** is an effective approach to resolving an IAQ problem when sources are known and control is feasible. Examples include routine maintenance of HVAC systems, e.g., periodic cleaning or replacement of filters; replacement of water-stained ceiling tile and carpeting; institution of smoking restrictions; venting contaminant source emissions to the outdoors; storage and use of paints, adhesives, solvents, and pesticides in well-ventilated areas, and use of these pollutant sources during periods of nonoccupancy; and allowing time for building materials in new or remodeled areas to off-gas pollutants before occupancy. Several of these options may be exercised at one time.

- **Increasing ventilation rates** and air distribution often can be a cost-effective means of reducing indoor pollutant levels. HVAC systems should be designed, at a minimum, to meet ventilation standards in local building codes; however, many systems are not operated or maintained to ensure that these design ventilation rates mid-1900's. In many buildings, IAQ can be improved by, the HVAC system to at least its design standard, and to ASHRAE Standard 62-1989 if possible. When there are strong pollutant sources, local exhaust ventilation may be appropriate to exhaust contaminated air directly from the building. Local exhaust ventilation is particularly recommended to remove pollutants that accumulate in specific areas such as restrooms, copy rooms, and printing facilities.

- **Air cleaning** can be a useful adjunct to source control and ventilation but has certain limitations. Particle control devices such as the typical furnace filter are inexpensive but do not effectively capture small particles; high-performance air filters capture the smaller, respirable particles but are relatively expensive to install and operate. Mechanical filters do not remove gaseous pollutants. Some specific gaseous pollutants may be removed by adsorbent beds, but these devices can be expensive and require frequent replacement of the adsorbent material. In sum, air cleaners can be useful, but have limited application.

- **Education and communication** are important elements in both remedial and preventive indoor air quality management programs. When building occupants, management, and maintenance personnel fully communicate and understand the causes and consequences of IAQ problems, they can work more effectively together to prevent problems from occurring, or to solve them if they do.

Chapter 34

Insect Sting Allergy

Stinging or biting insects or scorpions can be hazardous to outdoor workers. Stinging or biting insects include bees, wasps, hornets, and fire ants.

The health effects of stinging or biting insects or scorpions range from mild discomfort or pain to a lethal reaction for those workers allergic to the insect's venom. Anaphylactic shock is the body's severe allergic reaction to a bite or sting and requires immediate emergency care. Thousands of people are stung by insects each year, and as many as 90–100 people in the United States die as a result of allergic reactions. This number may be underreported as deaths may be mistakenly diagnosed as heart attacks or sunstrokes or may be attributed to other causes.

It is important for employers to train their workers about their risk of exposure to insects and scorpions, how they can prevent and protect themselves from stings and bites, and what they should do if they are stung or bitten.

Bees, Wasps, and Hornets

Bees, wasps, and hornets are most abundant in the warmer months. Nests and hives may be found in trees, under roof eaves, or on equipment such as ladders.

This chapter includes text excerpted from "Insects and Scorpions," Centers for Disease Control and Prevention (CDC), May 31, 2018.

U.S. Geographic Region

Bees, wasps, and hornets are found throughout the United States.

Employer Recommendations

Employers should protect their workers from stinging insects by training them about:

- Their risk of exposure
- Insect identification
- How to prevent exposure
- What to do if stung

Worker Recommendations

Workers should take the following steps to prevent insect stings:

- Wear light-colored, smooth-finished clothing.
- Avoid perfumed soaps, shampoos, and deodorants.
  - Don't wear cologne or perfume.
  - Avoid bananas and banana-scented toiletries.
- Wear clean clothing and bathe daily. (Sweat may anger bees.)
- Wear clothing to cover as much of the body as possible.
- Avoid flowering plants when possible.
- Keep work areas clean. Social wasps thrive in places where humans discard food.
- Remain calm and still if a single stinging insect is flying around. (Swatting at an insect may cause it to sting.)
- If you are attacked by several stinging insects at once, run to get away from them. (Bees release a chemical when they sting, which may attract other bees.)
  - Go indoors.
  - A shaded area is better than an open area to get away from the insects.
  - If you are able to physically move out of the area, do not to attempt to jump into water. Some insects (particularly

Africanized Honey Bees) are known to hover above the water, continuing to sting once you surface for air.

- If a bee comes inside your vehicle, stop the car slowly, and open all the windows.

- Workers with a history of severe allergic reactions to insect bites or stings should consider carrying an epinephrine auto-injector (EpiPen) and should wear a medical identification bracelet or necklace stating their allergy.

First Aid

If a worker is stung by a bee, wasp, or hornet:

- Have someone stay with the worker to be sure that they do not have an allergic reaction.

- Wash the site with soap and water.

- Remove the stinger using gauze wiped over the area or by scraping a fingernail over the area.

  - Never squeeze the stinger or use tweezers.

- Apply ice to reduce swelling.

- Do not scratch the sting as this may increase swelling, itching, and risk of infection.

Fire Ants

Imported fire ants first came to the United States around 1930. Now there are five times more ants per acre in the United States than in their native South America. The fire ants that came to the United States escaped their natural enemies and thrived in the southern landscape.

Fire ants bite and sting. They are aggressive when stinging and inject venom, which causes a burning sensation. Red bumps form at the sting, and within a day or two they become white fluid-filled pustules.

U.S. Geographic Region

Mostly the Southeastern United States, with limited geographic distribution in New Mexico, Arizona, and California.

Employer Recommendations

Employers should protect their workers from fire ants by training them about:

- Their risk of exposure
- How to identify fire ants and their nests
- How to prevent exposure
- What to do if they are bitten or stung

Worker Recommendations

Workers should take the following steps to prevent fire ant stings and bites:

- Do not disturb or stand on or near ant mounds.
- Be careful when lifting items (including animal carcasses) off the ground, as they may be covered in ants.
- Fire ants may also be found on trees or in water, so always look over the area before starting to work.

First Aid

Workers with a history of severe allergic reactions to insect bites or stings should consider carrying an epinephrine auto-injector (EpiPen) and should wear a medical identification bracelet or necklace stating their allergy.

Workers should take the following steps if they are stung or bitten by fire ants:

- Rub off ants briskly, as they will attach to the skin with their jaws.
- Antihistamines may help.
  - Follow directions on packaging.
  - Drowsiness may occur.
- Take the worker to an emergency medical facility immediately if a sting causes severe chest pain, nausea, severe sweating, loss of breath, serious swelling, or slurred speech.

Scorpions

Scorpions usually hide during the day and are active at night. They may be hiding under rocks, wood, or anything else lying on the ground.

Some species may also burrow into the ground. Most scorpions live in dry, desert areas. However, some species can be found in grasslands, forests, and inside caves.

U.S. Geographic Region

Southern and Southwestern United States.

Symptoms

Symptoms of a scorpion sting may include:

- A stinging or burning sensation at the injection site (very little swelling or inflammation)
- Positive "tap test" (i.e., extreme pain when the sting site is tapped with a finger)
- Restlessness
- Convulsions
- Roving eyes
- Staggering gait
- Thick tongue sensation
- Slurred speech
- Drooling
- Muscle twitches
- Abdominal pain and cramps
- Respiratory depression

These symptoms usually subside within 48 hours, although stings from a bark scorpion can be life-threatening.

Employer Recommendations

Employers should protect their workers from scorpions by training them about:

- Their risk of exposure
- Scorpion identification
- How to prevent exposure
- What to do if stung

Worker Recommendations

Workers should take the following steps to prevent scorpion stings:

- Wear long sleeves and pants.

- Wear leather gloves.

- Shake out clothing or shoes before putting them on.

- Workers with a history of severe allergic reactions to insect bites or stings should consider carrying an epinephrine auto-injector (EpiPen) and should wear a medical identification bracelet or necklace stating their allergy.

First Aid

Workers should take the following steps if they are stung by a scorpion:

- Contact a qualified healthcare provider or poison control center for advice and medical instructions.

- Ice may be applied directly to the sting site (never submerge the affected limb in ice water).

- Remain relaxed and calm.

- Do not take any sedatives.

- Capture the scorpion for identification if it is possible to do so safely.

Chapter 35

Allergies to Medicines and Medical Products

Chapter Contents

Section 35.1

Medications and Drug Allergic Reactions

"Medications and Drug Allergic Reactions,"
© 2018 Omnigraphics. Reviewed August 2018.

Drug allergy (also known as medication allergy) refers to the allergic reactions caused by the negative response of the immune system to drugs and medicines. The symptoms and severity of drug allergies may vary from person to person depending upon the genetic makeup.

Causes

The immune system, in general, acts as a protective shield to the human body. It produces antibodies to fight against harmful invaders, such as bacteria, viruses, fungi, and other disease-causing foreign bodies. But, sometimes, the immune system may get triggered by drugs and medicines, as if they were invaders, and produce antibodies such as immunoglobulin E (IgE) to fight against them. An unfavorable response of the immune system to harmless substances such as this is called a hyper-immune response. The chemicals released during this process react to cause various allergic symptoms.

Any kind of drug may cause allergic reactions. However, some commonly known allergy-causing drugs as listed below:

- Antibiotics such as amoxicillin, penicillin, tetracycline, etc.

- Anticonvulsants

- Antiseizure drugs

- Chemotherapy drugs

- Iodine

- Insulin

- Monoclonal antibody therapy

- Nonsteroidal agents such as aspirin, ibuprofen, and naproxen

- Sulfa drugs

Signs and Symptoms

The symptoms of drug allergy can be as mild as skin itching or life threatening (anaphylaxis). The mild and most common symptoms include:

- Congestion
- Itching of skin and eyes
- Runny nose
- Skin flushing
- Skin hives
- Skin rashes
- Sore throat

The more serious symptoms include:

- Abdominal pain
- Diarrhea, nausea, and vomiting
- Dizziness and fainting
- Drop in blood pressure
- Fever
- Increase in pulse rate
- Joint pain
- Loss of consciousness
- Seizure
- Swelling of lips and throat
- Wheezing

In most cases, the symptoms of drug allergy occur soon after the intake of drugs. However, there are cases in which the allergic reactions may take several hours or days to develop.

Diagnosis

If you experience allergy-like symptoms after taking a medicine, contact your healthcare provider. Initially, your healthcare provider will ask a few questions to gain a clear understanding about your personal and medical history. This will be followed by a thorough physical examination. Based on the initial findings, the following tests may be carried out to confirm the allergy.

Skin test: A small amount of suspected drug allergen is injected under the patient's skin to check for a reaction. If the patient develops redness, itching, or bumps, he/she is more likely to be allergic to the particular drug. However, the skin test is available only for a few drugs and the results are not always accurate.

Patch test: This test is used to determine delayed allergic reactions. A small amount of suspected allergen is placed on the patient's skin and covered with a bandage. The doctor will remove the bandage after two to four days and check for rashes on the skin.

Blood test: The blood sample of the patient is collected and a small amount of suspected allergen is added to it. The amount of antibodies produced by the blood to fight against the allergen is measured to determine if the patient is allergic or not. This test is also called as specific immunoglobulin E (sIgE) blood test. Like a skin test, the blood test is available only for only a few drugs and its results are not always accurate.

Graded drug challenge: Occasionally, the doctor may recommend a graded drug challenge in which the patient is given the suspected medication in specific doses under medical supervision.

Prevention and Treatment

Since there is no cure for drug allergy, the only way to prevent it is to avoid the allergic drugs and similar medicines. Treatments are available to relieve the symptoms of allergic reactions, though.

Antihistamines such as diphenhydramine (Benadryl) help to suppress immune system chemicals and can be used to relieve itching and rashes.

Bronchodilators such as Albuterol can be used to reduce coughing, lung congestion, and asthma-like symptoms.

Epinephrine can be injected for anaphylactic symptoms such as breathing difficulty and loss of consciousness.

References

1. "Drug allergies." MedlinePlus, August 2, 2018.

2. "Medication Allergies." Cleveland Clinic, June 15, 2016.

3. "Drug Allergy." Mayo Clinic, December 16, 2017.

4. Omudhome Ogbru. "Drug Allergy (Medication Allergy)." MedicineNet, November 21, 2016.

5. "Allergies." Asthma and Allergy Foundation of America (AAFA), October 2105.

6. Christine B. Cho. "Drug Allergy: Diagnosis and Treatment." National Jewish Health (NJH), December 1, 2016.

Section 35.2

Is It Really a Penicillin Allergy?

This section includes text excerpted from "Evaluation and Diagnosis of Penicillin Allergy for Healthcare Professionals," Centers for Disease Control and Prevention (CDC), October 31, 2017.

Five Facts about Penicillin Allergy (Type 1, Immunoglobulin E (IgE)-Mediated)

1. Approximately 10 percent of all U.S. patients report having an allergic reaction to a penicillin class antibiotic in their past.

2. However, many patients who report penicillin allergies do not have true Immunoglobulin (IgE)-mediated reactions. When evaluated, fewer than 1 percent of the population are truly allergic to penicillins.

3. Approximately 80 percent of patients with IgE-mediated penicillin allergy lose their sensitivity after 10 years.

4. Broad-spectrum antibiotics are often used as an alternative to penicillins. The use of broad-spectrum antibiotics in

patients labeled "penicillin-allergic" is associated with higher healthcare costs, increased risk for antibiotic resistance, and suboptimal antibiotic therapy.

5. Correctly identifying those who are not truly penicillin-allergic can decrease unnecessary use of broad-spectrum antibiotics.

10 percent of the population reports a penicillin allergy but <1 percent of the whole population is truly allergic. Before prescribing broad-spectrum antibiotics to a patient thought to be penicillin-allergic, evaluate the patient for true penicillin allergy (IgE-mediated) by conducting a history and physical, and, when appropriate, a skin test and challenge dose.

Broad-spectrum antibiotics are often used as an alternative to narrow-spectrum penicillins.

- Using broad-spectrum antibiotics can increase healthcare costs and antibiotic resistance, and may mean the patient receives less than the best care.

- Correctly identifying if the patient is actually penicillin-allergic can decrease these risks by reducing unnecessary use of broad-spectrum antibiotics.

History and Physical Examination

The history and physical examination are important components when evaluating a patient's drug reactions.

- Questions to ask during the examination:
  - What medication were you taking when the reaction occurred?
  - What kind of reaction occurred?
  - How long ago did the reaction occur?
  - How was the reaction managed?
  - What was the outcome?
- Characteristics of an IgE-mediated (Type 1) reaction:
  - Reactions that occur immediately or usually within one hour
  - Hives: Multiple pink/red raised areas of skin that are intensely itchy
  - Angioedema: Localized edema without hives affecting the abdomen, face, extremities, genitalia, oropharynx, or larynx

- Wheezing and shortness of breath

- Anaphylaxis

- Anaphylaxis requires signs or symptoms in at least two of the following systems:

  - Skin: Hives, flushing, itching, and/or angioedema

  - Respiratory: Cough, nasal congestion, shortness of breath, chest tightness, wheeze, sensation of throat closure or choking, and/or change in voice-quality (laryngeal edema)

  - Cardiovascular: Hypotension, faintness, tachycardia or less commonly bradycardia, tunnel vision, chest pain, sense of impending doom, and/or loss of consciousness

  - Gastrointestinal: Nausea, vomiting, abdominal cramping, and diarrhea

Penicillin Skin Tests and Challenge Doses

Based on the patient history and physical exam, additional tests may be needed to confirm a penicillin allergy.

Penicillin skin testing and challenge doses are reliable and useful methods for evaluating for IgE-mediated penicillin allergy.

Penicillin Skin Testing

A positive result means the patient is likely to have a penicillin allergy. If negative, the skin test is usually followed by an oral penicillin class challenge (e.g., with amoxicillin) to safely rule out an IgE-mediated penicillin allergy.

- The current standard of care is to perform a skin test with the major determinant penicilloyl-polylysine and commercially-available penicillin G.

- To rule out penicillin allergy, an oral challenge dose can be done after skin testing. The negative predictive value of skin testing with the major and minor determinants is more than 95 percent, but approaches 100 percent when followed by a challenge dose.

A direct oral challenge without prior skin testing may also be performed in selected patients and can rule out penicillin allergy.

Special Considerations

Patients with Severe Hypersensitivity Syndromes

Patients with other severe hypersensitivity syndromes—like Stevens-Johnson syndrome, toxic epidermal necrolysis, serum sickness, acute interstitial nephritis, hemolytic anemia, and drug rash with eosinophilia and systemic symptoms (DRESS)—should not use the offending drug in the future. The skin test and challenge described here are not appropriate for patients with these severe hypersensitivity syndromes.

Cephalosporin Use in Penicillin-Allergic Patients

Many cephalosporins, especially in the later generations, can be safely tolerated despite a penicillin allergy. Patients with anaphylaxis or other severe reactions to penicillin may require further evaluation prior to the use of cephalosporins.

Pediatric Patients

Children who are receiving amoxicillin or ampicillin and have Epstein-Barr virus infection can develop a nonallergic, nonpruritic rash that can appear similar to an allergic reaction.

Section 35.3

Allergies to Vaccines

This section includes text excerpted from "ACIP Adverse Reactions Guidelines for Immunization," Centers for Disease Control and Prevention (CDC), July 12, 2017.

Parents, guardians, legal representatives, and adolescent and adult patients should be informed about the benefits of and risks from vaccines in language that is culturally sensitive and at an appropriate educational level. Opportunity for questions should be provided before each vaccination. Discussion of the benefits of and risks from vaccination is sound medical practice and is required by law.

The National Childhood Vaccine Injury Act (NCVIA) of 1986 requires that vaccine information materials be developed for each vaccine covered by the Act (uscode.house.gov). These materials, known as vaccine information statements (VISs), must be provided by all public and private vaccination providers each time a vaccine is administered. Copies of VISs are available from state health authorities responsible for vaccination and from the Centers for Disease Control and Prevention (CDC). Translations of VISs into languages other than English are available from certain state vaccination programs and from the Immunization Action Coalition (IAC) website (www.immunize.org). The act does not require that a signature be obtained; however, documentation of consent might be recommended or required by certain state or local health authorities or school authorities.

Some parents or patients question the need for or safety of vaccinations and want to discuss the risks from and benefits of certain vaccines. Some refuse certain vaccines or reject all vaccinations for personal or religious reasons. Having a basic understanding of how patients and parents of patients view vaccine risk and developing effective approaches to address vaccine safety concerns are imperative for vaccination providers.

Each person understands and reacts to vaccine information on the basis of different factors, including previous experience, education, personal values, method of data presentation, perceptions of the risk for disease and perceived ability to control these risks, and risk tolerance. In some circumstances, decisions about vaccination are based on inaccurate information about risk provided by the media and certain websites. Websites and other sources of vaccine information may be inaccurate or incomplete. Healthcare providers can be a pivotal source of science-based credible information by discussing with parents and patients the risks from and benefits of vaccines, which helps patients make informed decisions.

When a parent or patient initiates a discussion about a perceived vaccine adverse reaction, the healthcare provider should discuss the specific concerns and provide factual information, using appropriate language. Effective, empathetic vaccine risk communication is essential in responding to misinformation and concerns, with healthcare providers recognizing that risk assessment and decision-making can be difficult and confusing. Certain vaccines might be acceptable to a parent who is resistant to other vaccines. This partial acceptance can be used to facilitate additional communication. Their concerns can be addressed using the VIS and offering other resource materials (e.g., vaccination information from the CDC).

The American Academy of Pediatrics (AAP) does not recommend that providers exclude from their practice patients whose parents or guardians question or refuse vaccination. However, an effective public health strategy is to identify common ground and discuss measures that need to be followed if the decision is to defer vaccination. Healthcare providers should reinforce key points about each vaccine, including safety, and emphasize risks for disease among unvaccinated children. Parents should be advised of state laws regarding entry to schools or child-care facilities, which might require that unvaccinated children be excluded from the facility during outbreaks. These discussions should be documented in the patient's medical record, including the refusal to receive certain vaccines (i.e., informed refusal). When a vaccine is refused when first offered the provider should take the opportunity to offer the vaccine again at the next visit.

Preventing Adverse Allergic Reactions

Vaccines are intended to produce active immunity to specific antigens. An adverse reaction is an undesirable side effect that occurs after a vaccination. Vaccine adverse reactions are classified as:

1. local,

2. systemic, or

3. allergic.

Local reactions (e.g., redness) are usually the least severe and most frequent. Systemic reactions (e.g., fever) occur less frequently than local reactions, and severe allergic reactions (e.g., anaphylaxis) are the least frequent reactions. Severe adverse reactions are rare.

Some of the systemic reactions may be complicated by the onset of syncope. Syncope (vasovagal or vasodepressor reaction) can occur after vaccination and is most common among adolescents and young adults. In 2005, the Vaccine Adverse Event Reporting System (VAERS) began detecting a trend of increasing syncope reports that coincided with the licensure of 3 vaccines for adolescents: human papillomavirus (HPV), Meningococcal group A, C, W-135 and Y conjugate (MenACWY), and Tetanus, diphtheria, and pertussis (Tdap). Of particular concern among adolescents has been the risk for serious secondary injuries, including skull fracture and cerebral hemorrhage. Of 463 VAERS reports of syncope during January 1, 2005, to July 31, 2007, a total of 41 listed syncope with secondary injury with information on the timing after vaccination, and the majority of these syncope reports

(76%) occurred among adolescents. Among all age groups, 80 percent of reported syncope episodes occur within 15 minutes of vaccine administration (additional information). Providers should take appropriate measures to prevent injuries if a patient becomes weak or dizzy or loses consciousness. Adolescents and adults should be seated or lying down during vaccination. Vaccine providers, particularly when vaccinating adolescents, should consider observing patients (with patients seated or lying down) for 15 minutes after vaccination to decrease the risk for injury should they faint. If syncope develops, patients should be observed until the symptoms resolve.

Although allergic reactions are a common concern for vaccine providers, these reactions are uncommon and anaphylaxis following vaccines is rare, occurring at a rate of approximately one per million doses for many vaccines. Epinephrine and equipment for managing an airway should be available for immediate use. The best practice to prevent allergic reactions is to identify individuals at increased risk by obtaining a history of allergy to previous vaccinations and vaccine components that might indicate an underlying hypersensitivity. Acute allergic reactions following vaccinations might be caused by the vaccine antigen, residual animal protein, antimicrobial agents, preservatives, stabilizers, or other vaccine components. Components of each vaccine are listed in the respective package insert. An extensive list of vaccine components and their use, as well as the vaccines that contain each component, has been published and also is available from the CDC. Additional information and tables of potential allergens in different vaccines are available. The allergens identified in the history can be cross-checked against the allergens identified in package inserts.

Managing Acute Vaccine Reactions

Vaccine providers should be familiar with identifying immediate-type allergic reactions, including anaphylaxis, and be competent in treating these events at the time of vaccine administration. Providers should also have a plan in place to contact emergency medical services immediately in the event of a severe acute vaccine reaction.

Allergic reactions can include: local or generalized urticaria (hives) or angioedema; respiratory compromise due to wheezing or swelling of the throat; hypotension; and shock. Immediate-immunoglobulin E (IgE)–mediated (type 1) immune reactions, such as anaphylaxis, usually occur within minutes of parenteral administration and involve specific IgE interactions with discrete antigens. Rapid recognition and initiation of treatment are required to prevent possible progression to respiratory failure or cardiovascular collapse. It is important to note that urticaria may not be present in all cases of anaphylaxis. For respiratory or cardiovascular symptoms, or other signs or symptoms of anaphylaxis, immediate intramuscular epinephrine is the treatment of choice. Additional doses of epinephrine as well as other drugs also might be indicated. If hypotension is present, the patient should be placed in a recumbent position with the legs elevated. Maintenance of the airway, oxygen administration, and intravenous normal saline might be necessary. After the patient is stabilized, arrangements should be made for immediate transfer to an emergency facility for additional evaluation and treatment. Because anaphylaxis may recur after patients begin to recover, monitoring in a medical facility for several hours is advised, even after complete resolution of symptoms and signs. Additional information on management of patients with anaphylaxis has been published.

Persons Who Have Had an Allergic Reaction Following a Previous Immunization

For an individual patient who has experienced an immediate reaction to immunization, it is important to identify the type of reaction that occurred, obtain a history of prior allergic reactions, and try to identify the particular agent responsible. An algorithm approach to these patients has been published and additional advice is available for allergists on the evaluation of these adverse events. In general, a history of a severe allergic reaction to a vaccine should be considered a contraindication to additional doses of the same vaccine. Referral of the individual to an allergist for evaluation is usually indicated to possibly determine the component responsible, before making decisions regarding administration of the additional doses of the same vaccine or other vaccines that have the same components. Patients who have not had a severe allergic reaction following a vaccine, but who have a history of possible allergy to a vaccine component can often be vaccinated safely after careful evaluation.

Influenza Vaccination of Persons with a History of Egg Allergy

Severe allergic and anaphylactic reactions can occur in response to a number of influenza vaccine components, but such reactions are rare. All but the recombinant inactivated influenza vaccine may have come into contact with egg protein. The use of influenza vaccines for persons with a history of egg allergy has been reviewed by ACIP. VAERS data mining did not identify a higher than expected proportion of serious allergic events after influenza vaccination during the 2011–2012 season, relative to all other reported vaccines and adverse events in the database. Persons with a history of egg allergy should receive recombinant inactivated vaccine (if 18 years or older), or IIV.

Other measures, such as dividing and administering the vaccine by a two-step approach and skin testing with vaccine, are not recommended.

All vaccines should be administered in settings in which personnel and equipment for rapid recognition and treatment of anaphylaxis are available. ACIP recommends that all vaccination providers be certified in cardiopulmonary resuscitation (CPR), have an office emergency plan, and ensure that all staff are familiar with the plan. Some persons who report allergy to egg might not be egg-allergic. Those who are able to eat lightly cooked egg (e.g., scrambled egg) without reaction are unlikely to be allergic.

Egg-allergic persons might tolerate egg in baked products (e.g., bread or cake). Tolerance to egg-containing foods does not exclude the possibility of egg allergy. Egg allergy can be confirmed by a consistent medical history of adverse reactions to eggs and egg-containing foods, plus skin and/or blood testing for IgE antibodies to egg proteins.

A previous severe allergic reaction to influenza vaccine, regardless of the component suspected to be responsible for the reaction, is a contraindication to future receipt of the vaccine.

Yellow Fever Vaccination of Persons with a History of Egg Allergy

Yellow fever vaccine contains egg protein. There have been insufficient studies to determine which patients with egg allergy may be able to receive yellow fever vaccine, but there are reports of patients with true egg allergy safely receiving yellow fever vaccine after evaluation by specialists with expertise in the management of allergic reactions. According to the manufacturer, persons who are able to eat eggs or egg products may receive the vaccine. However, potential hypersensitivity reactions might occur in persons with a history of minor reactions to eggs. For egg-sensitive persons, a scratch test or intradermal test can be performed before administering the vaccine to check for reactivity. If a person has a severe egg-sensitivity or has a positive skin test to the vaccine, but the vaccination is recommended because of their travel destination-specific risk, desensitization can be performed under direct supervision of a physician experienced in the management of anaphylaxis. The desensitization procedure is detailed in the product insert.

Vaccines with Measles, Mumps and Rubella or Varicella Components and Persons with a History of Egg Allergy

Varicella vaccine is grown in human diploid cell cultures and can safely be administered to persons with a severe allergy to eggs or egg proteins. Measles and mumps vaccine viruses are grown in chick embryo fibroblast tissue culture. However, persons with a severe egg allergy can receive measles- or mumps-containing vaccines in the usual manner because the content of these proteins is extremely low. The rare severe allergic reactions after measles- or mumps-containing vaccines or varicella are thought to be caused by other components of the vaccine (e.g., gelatin). measles, mumps and rubella (MMR), measles, mumps, rubella, and varicella (MMRV), varicella and other vaccines contain hydrolyzed gelatin as a stabilizer.

Vaccines and Persons with a History of Allergy to Substances Other than Eggs

Persons who have had an anaphylactic reaction to gelatin or gelatin-containing products should be evaluated by an allergist prior to receiving gelatin-containing vaccines.

Certain vaccines contain trace amounts of antimicrobial agents or other preservatives (e.g., neomycin or thimerosal), although allergies to these are rare. No licensed vaccine contains penicillin or penicillin derivatives.

Most often, neomycin hypersensitivity manifests as contact dermatitis, a delayed-type (cell-mediated) immune response rather than immediate-hypersensitivity (IgE-mediated allergy)–type response. A history of delayed-type reactions to neomycin is not a contraindication for administration of neomycin-containing vaccines. There has only been 1 reported case of immediate hypersensitivity reaction following a neomycin-containing vaccine. Persons who have had anaphylactic reactions to neomycin should be evaluated by an allergist prior to receiving vaccines containing neomycin.

Thimerosal, an organic mercurial compound in use since the 1930s, is added to certain immunobiologics as a preservative. Since mid-2001, vaccines routinely recommended for infants younger than six months of age have been manufactured without thimerosal as a preservative. Live, attenuated vaccines have never contained thimerosal. Thimerosal-free formulations of inactivated influenza vaccine are available. Inactivated influenza vaccine also is available in formulations with only trace amounts of thimerosal, which remains as a manufacturing residual but is not added at the higher concentration that would be necessary for it to function as a preservative. Thimerosal at a preservative concentration is present in certain other vaccines that can be administered to children (e.g., Td and DT). Information about the thimerosal content of vaccines is available from the FDA.

Reactions to thimerosal have been described as local delayed-type hypersensitivity reactions with only rare reports of immediate reactions. Thimerosal elicits positive delayed-type hypersensitivity patch tests in 1–18 percent of persons tested; however, these tests have no relevance to acute allergic reactions that might occur within minutes or hours after immunization. The majority of persons do not experience reactions to thimerosal administered as a component of vaccines even when patch or intradermal tests for thimerosal indicate hypersensitivity. A local or delayed-type hypersensitivity reaction to thimerosal is not a contraindication to receipt of a vaccine that contains thimerosal.

Latex is sap from the rubber tree. Latex contains naturally occurring plant proteins that can be responsible for immediate-type allergic reactions. Latex is processed to form either natural rubber latex products such as gloves or dry, natural rubber products such as syringe plunger tips and vial stoppers. Synthetic rubber is also used in gloves, syringe plungers, and vial stoppers but does not contain the latex proteins linked to immediate-type allergic reactions. Natural rubber latex or dry, natural rubber used in vaccine packaging generally is noted in the manufacturers' package inserts.

Immediate-type allergic reactions due to latex allergy have been described after vaccination, but such reactions are rare.

If a person reports a severe anaphylactic allergy to latex, vaccines supplied in vials or syringes that contain natural rubber latex should be avoided if possible. If not, if the decision is made to vaccinate, providers should be prepared to treat immediate allergic reactions due to latex, including anaphylaxis. The most common type of latex hypersensitivity is a delayed-type (type 4, cell-mediated) allergic contact dermatitis. For patients with a history of contact allergy to latex, vaccines supplied in vials or syringes that contain dry natural rubber or natural rubber latex may be administered.

Reporting Adverse Events after Vaccination

Modern vaccines are safe and effective; however, adverse events have been reported after administration of all vaccines. More complete information about adverse reactions to a specific vaccine is available in the package insert for each vaccine and from the CDC. An adverse event is an untoward event that occurs after a vaccination that might be caused by the vaccine product or vaccination process. These events range from common, minor, local reactions to rare, severe, allergic reactions (e.g., anaphylaxis). Reporting to VAERS helps establish trends, identify clusters of adverse events, or generate hypotheses. However, establishing evidence for cause and effect on the basis of case reports and case series alone is usually not possible, because health problems that have a temporal association with vaccination do not necessarily indicate causality.

Many adverse events require more detailed epidemiologic studies to compare the incidence of the event among vaccines with the incidence among unvaccinated persons. Potential causal associations between reported adverse events after vaccination can be assessed through epidemiologic or clinical studies.

The National Childhood Vaccine Injury Act of 1986 requires health-care personnel and vaccine manufacturers to report to VAERS specific adverse events that occur after vaccination. The reporting requirements are different for manufacturers and healthcare personnel. Manufacturers are required to report all adverse events that occur after vaccination to VAERS, whereas healthcare providers are required to report events that appear in the reportable events table on the VAERS website.

In addition to the mandated reporting of events listed on the reportable events table, healthcare personnel should report to VAERS all events listed in product inserts as contraindications, as well as all clinically significant adverse events, even if they are uncertain that the adverse event is related causally to vaccination. Persons other than healthcare personnel also can report adverse events to VAERS.

Part Five

Diagnosing and Treating Allergies

Chapter 36

When You Should See an Allergist

Allergy/immunology is the field of medicine that deals with the human body's immune system. The immune system is a network of cells, tissues, and organs that defends the body against potentially harmful foreign organisms and particles. Normally, the spleen, lymph nodes, T and B lymphocytes, mast cells, dendritic cells, platelets, bone marrow, and thymus are some important organs or cells that take part. A physician specializing in this field of medicine is called an allergist/immunologist.

The human body is well equipped to defend itself against disease-causing organisms such as bacteria, viruses, or fungi. It also defends itself from foreign particles such as dust or mold. When the body encounters substances that it recognizes as potentially harmful, the immune system produces antibodies to eliminate them or by engulfing and destroying by macrophages phagocytosis, etc.

Under normal circumstances, this defense mechanism does a good job of protecting the body and keeping it healthy. Sometimes, the immune system overreacts to harmless substances—like a certain food or pollen—by releasing chemicals and triggering changes in the body to destroy the invaders. This process is called an allergic reaction. When the reaction is severe enough to require medical care, an allergist/immunologist is usually involved in diagnosing and treating the patient's condition.

Types of Allergic Reactions

Allergic reactions tend to happen in locations where the immune system has concentrated its defenses to protect against foreign substances entering the body. They frequently affect the skin, the eyes, the respiratory system (nose, sinuses, throat, lungs), and the digestive system (stomach, intestines). Some common types of allergic reactions include contact dermatitis or skin allergies, allergic rhinitis (inflammation of the lining of the nose and sinuses), and asthma. Anaphylaxis is a sudden, severe, whole-body allergic reaction that can be life threatening without immediate medical attention.

In contact dermatitis, the reaction may take hours or days to develop in case of poison ivy. For example, in allergic rhinitis there will be sneezing, running nose, and itching in nose, eyes, and throat.

Causes of Allergic Reactions

People can develop allergies to a variety of ordinary substances that they are exposed to daily. Common types of allergens include: foods such as milk, wheat, nuts, fish, soy, and eggs; airborne particles such as dust, pollen, mold, and pet dander; insect bites and stings; certain chemicals and medications; and substances like latex. Certain plants, like poison ivy, can also trigger severe allergic reactions.

Seeing an Allergist/Immunologist

The symptoms of allergic reactions can range from a mild runny nose or skin rash to diarrhea and vomiting or anaphylaxis. Sometimes the symptoms can be controlled with occasional doses of over-the-counter (OTC) allergy medications, and sometimes they get worse over time and detract from the person's quality of life. Generally speaking, patients should consider seeing an allergist/immunologist under the following circumstances:

- an abnormal reaction to inhaling, ingesting, or coming into contact with something;

- symptoms of asthma such as wheezing, difficulty in breathing, or chest pressure;

- more than three infections of the ear, nose, throat, or lungs per year;

- skin conditions like rashes or hives that appear frequently or without a known cause;

- a severe reaction to a bee sting or an insect bite;

- allergic reactions that interfere with performing activities of daily living;

- symptoms that do not improve with the use of OTC medications.

Who Is an Allergist?

An allergist/immunologist has to undergo a minimum of nine years of medical education and training, including four years of medical school, three years of residency training as an internist or pediatrician, and two years of specialized study in the field of allergy/immunology. The physician then has to pass a certification examination conducted by the American Board of Allergy and Immunology (ACAAI).

What Are All the Common Allergic Tests?

An allergist will conduct a medical history and physical examination and perform certain tests to identify the allergen responsible for the patient's reaction. One of the most common tests is the skin-prick test, in which the allergist uses a small needle to prick the patient's skin and insert tiny quantities of allergy-causing substances. If the patient is allergic to a specific substance, they will develop a bump on the skin similar to a mosquito bite. Another test that is often performed by allergists is a challenge test, in which the patient inhales or ingests a very small quantity of allergen under medical supervision to see if they have a reaction. Finally, an allergist may conduct blood tests to check for immunoglobulin E (IgE) antibodies, which are indicators of an allergic reaction.

To prepare for a visit to an allergist, it may be helpful to keep a diary of allergic reactions, recording details about symptoms, exposure to potential allergens, and timing. This information makes it easier for the allergist to diagnose and treat the condition. Prompt diagnosis and identification of allergens will help the patient avoid exposure to these substances or control their reactions if they are exposed to them. Patients with severe allergies may be required to carry emergency medication, like an epinephrine auto-injector or an inhaler, with them at all times.

References

1. "Allergy Testing," American College of Allergy, Asthma, and Immunology (ACAAI), 2015.

2. "When to See an Allergist," American College of Allergy, Asthma, and Immunology (ACAAI), 2014.

Chapter 37

Cold, Flu, or Allergy?

Know the Difference for Best Treatment

You're feeling pretty lousy. You've got sniffles, sneezing, and a sore throat. Is it a cold, flu, or allergies? It can be hard to tell them apart because they share so many symptoms. But understanding the differences will help you choose the best treatment.

"If you know what you have, you won't take medications that you don't need, that aren't effective, or that might even make your symptoms worse," says National Institutes of Health's (NIH) Dr. Teresa Hauguel, an expert on infectious diseases that affect breathing.

Cold, flu, and allergy all affect your respiratory system, which can make it hard to breathe. Each condition has key symptoms that set them apart.

Colds and flu are caused by different viruses. "As a rule of thumb, the symptoms associated with the flu are more severe," says Hauguel. Both illnesses can lead to a runny, stuffy nose; congestion; cough; and sore throat. But the flu can also cause high fever that lasts for three to four days, along with a headache, fatigue, and general aches and pain. These symptoms are less common when you have a cold.

"Allergies are a little different, because they aren't caused by a virus," Hauguel explains. "Instead, it's your body's immune system reacting to a trigger, or allergen, which is something you're allergic to." If you have allergies and breathe in things like pollen or pet dander,

This chapter includes text excerpted from "Cold, Flu, or Allergy?" *NIH News in Health*, National Institutes of Health (NIH), October 2014. Reviewed August 2018.

the immune cells in your nose and airways may overreact to these harmless substances. Your delicate respiratory tissues may then swell, and your nose may become stuffed up or runny.

"Allergies can also cause itchy, watery eyes, which you don't normally have with a cold or flu," Hauguel adds.

Allergy symptoms usually last as long as you're exposed to the allergen, which may be about six weeks during pollen seasons in the spring, summer, or fall. Colds and flu rarely last beyond two weeks.

Most people with a cold or flu recover on their own without medical care. But check with a healthcare provider if symptoms last beyond 10 days or if symptoms aren't relieved by over-the-counter (OTC) medicines.

To treat colds or flu, get plenty of rest and drink lots of fluids. If you have the flu, pain relievers such as aspirin, acetaminophen, or ibuprofen can reduce fever or aches. Allergies can be treated with antihistamines or decongestants.

Be careful to avoid "drug overlap" when taking medicines that list two or more active ingredients on the label. For example, if you take two different drugs that contain acetaminophen—one for a stuffy nose and the other for headache—you may be getting too much acetaminophen.

"Read medicine labels carefully—the warnings, side effects, dosages. If you have questions, talk to your doctor or pharmacist, especially if you have children who are sick," Hauguel says. "You don't want to overmedicate, and you don't want to risk taking a medication that may interact with another."

Table 37.1. Cold, Flu, and Airborne Allergy

Symptoms	Cold	Flu	Airborne Allergy
Fever	Rare	Usual, high (100–102°F), sometimes higher, especially in young children); lasts 3–4 days	Never
Headache	Uncommon	Common	Uncommon
General aches, Pains	Slight	Usual; often severe	Never
Fatigue, weakness	Sometimes	Usual, can last up to 3 weeks	Sometimes
Extreme exhaustion	Never	Usual, at the beginning of the illness	Never

Table 37.1. Continued

Symptoms	Cold	Flu	Airborne Allergy
Stuffy, runny nose	Common	Sometimes	Common
Sneezing	Usual	Sometimes	Usual
Sore throat	Common	Sometimes	Sometimes
Cough	Common	Common, can become severe	Sometimes
Chest discomfort	Mild to moderate	Common	Rare, except for those with allergic asthma
Treatment	Get plenty of rest. Stay hydrated. (Drink plenty of fluids.) Decongestants. Aspirin (ages 18 and up), acetaminophen, or ibuprofen for aches and pains	Get plenty of rest. Stay hydrated. Aspirin (ages 18 and up), acetaminophen, or ibuprofen for aches, pains, and fever Antiviral medicines (see your doctor)	Avoid allergens (things that you're allergic to) Antihistamines Nasal steroids Decongestants
Prevention	Wash your hands often. Avoid close contact with anyone who has a cold.	Get the flu vaccine each year. Wash your hands often. Avoid close contact with anyone who has the flu.	Avoid allergens, such as pollen, house dust mites, mold, pet dander, cockroaches.
Complications	Sinus infection middle ear infection, asthma	Bronchitis, pneumonia; can be life-threatening	Sinus infection, middle ear infection, asthma

Treatment Choices

Treatment depends on which you have. A health professional can help you choose the best therapy.

Airborne Allergy

- Lasts as long as allergens (such as pollen, pet dander) are present

- Stuffy, runny nose; itchy, watery eyes

- Treated with antihistamines, decongestants, nasal steroids

Common Cold

- Symptoms last up to two weeks

- Stuffy, runny nose; sore throat; cough

- Treated with rest, fluids, OTC medicines to ease symptoms

Seasonal Flu

- Symptoms usually last 1–2 weeks

- High fever (100–102°F, or higher in youngsters), headache, aches and pains, weakness, exhaustion, cough, chest discomfort

- Treated with rest, fluids, OTC medicines, prescription antiviral drugs

Chapter 38

Health Insurance Issues for People with Allergies and Asthma

Your kids can get the care they need for allergies, asthma, or just a common cold. And you can breathe easier knowing that coverage is just a click or phone call away.

Medicaid and the Children's Health Insurance Program (CHIP) offer free or low-cost health coverage for kids and teens up to age 19. Parents may be eligible for Medicaid too.

These programs cover routine check-ups, immunizations, doctor visits, lab services, prescriptions, dental and vision care for kids, hospital care, and emergency services.

You can apply for and enroll in Medicaid or CHIP any time of year. If you qualify, your coverage can begin immediately.

This chapter contains text excerpted from the following sources: Text in this chapter begins with excerpts from "Breathe Easier with Medicaid and Chip Coverage," Centers for Medicare & Medicaid Services (CMS), August 5, 2014. Reviewed August 2018; Text beginning with the heading "Medicaid and Children's Health Insurance Program Basics" is excerpted from "Medicaid and CHIP," Centers for Medicare and Medicaid Services (CMS), October 9, 2015.

Medicaid and Children's Health Insurance Program Basics

Medicaid and the Children's Health Insurance Program (CHIP) provide free or low-cost health coverage to millions of Americans, including some low-income people, families and children, pregnant women, the elderly, and people with disabilities.

Some states have expanded their Medicaid programs to cover all people below certain income levels.

Even if you don't qualify for Medicaid based on income, you should apply. You may qualify for your state's program, especially if you have children, are pregnant, or have a disability. You can apply for Medicaid any time of year—Medicaid and CHIP do not have open enrollment periods.

How to Apply for Medicaid and Children's Health Insurance Program

1. Through the Health Insurance Marketplace

    Fill out an application through the Health Insurance Marketplace.

    *   If it looks like anyone in your household qualifies for Medicaid or CHIP, information will be sent to your state agency. They'll contact you about enrollment.

    *   When you submit your Marketplace application, you'll also find out if you qualify for an individual insurance plan with savings based on your income instead. Plans may be more affordable than you think.

2. Through your state Medicaid agency

    You can also apply directly to your state Medicaid agency.

Medicaid Expansion and What It Means for You

Some states have expanded their Medicaid programs to cover all people with household incomes below a certain level. Others haven't.

Whether you qualify for Medicaid coverage depends partly on whether your state has expanded its program.

*   In all states: You can qualify for Medicaid based on income, household size, disability, family status, and other factors. Eligibility rules differ between states.

- In states that have expanded Medicaid coverage: You can qualify based on your income alone. If your household income is below 133 percent of the federal poverty level, you qualify. (Because of the way this is calculated, it turns out to be 138 percent of the federal poverty level. A few states use a different income limit.)

If Your Income Is Low and Your State Hasn't Expanded Medicaid

If your state hasn't expanded Medicaid, your income is below the federal poverty level, and you don't qualify for Medicaid under your state's current rules, you won't qualify for either health insurance savings program: Medicaid coverage or savings on a private health plan bought through the Marketplace.

Apply for Medicaid Coverage, Even If Your State Hasn't Expanded

Even if your state hasn't expanded Medicaid and it looks like your income is below the level to qualify for financial help with a Marketplace plan, you should fill out a Marketplace application.

Each state has coverage options that could work for you—particularly if you have children, are pregnant, or have a disability. And when you provide more detailed income information you may fall into the range to save.

If You Don't Qualify for Either Medicaid or Marketplace Savings

- You can get care at a nearby community health center. The healthcare law has expanded funding to community health centers, which provide primary care for millions of Americans. These centers provide services on a sliding scale based on your income. See how to get low-cost care in your community.

- If you don't have any coverage, you don't have to pay the fee. Under the law, most people must have health coverage or pay a fee. But you won't have to pay this fee if you live in a state that hasn't expanded Medicaid and you would have qualified if it had. This is called having an exemption from the fee. You can get an exemption when you apply for coverage in the Marketplace. Or you can apply for the exemption without having to fill out a Marketplace application.

- If your expected yearly income increases so it's between 100 percent and 400 percent of the federal poverty level, you become eligible for a Marketplace plan with advance payments of the premium tax credit (APTC). In this case, you may qualify for a Special Enrollment Period (SEP) that allows you to enroll in a Marketplace plan any time of year. You must contact the Marketplace Call Center within 60 days from the date your income changed to request this SEP. When you call, you'll need to attest that you:

  - Weren't eligible for Medicaid when you first applied because you live in a state that hasn't expanded Medicaid

  - Weren't eligible for a Marketplace plan with tax credits when you first applied because your income was too low

  - Had an increase in expected yearly income that now qualifies you for a Marketplace plan with tax credits

The Children's Health Insurance Program

If your children need health coverage, they may be eligible for the Children's Health Insurance Program (CHIP).

CHIP provides low-cost health coverage to children in families that earn too much money to qualify for Medicaid. In some states, CHIP covers pregnant women. Each state offers CHIP coverage, and works closely with its state Medicaid program.

See If Your Children Qualify and Apply for Children's Health Insurance Program

Each state program has its own rules about who qualifies for CHIP. You can apply right now, any time of year, and find out if you qualify. If you apply for Medicaid coverage to your state agency, you'll also find out if your children qualify for CHIP. If they qualify, you won't have to buy an insurance plan to cover them.

Two Ways to Apply for Children's Health Insurance Program

- Call 800-318-2596 (TTY: 855-889-4325).

- Fill out an application through the Health Insurance Marketplace. If it looks like anyone in your household qualifies for Medicaid or CHIP, information will be sent to your state agency. They'll contact you about enrollment. When you submit your Marketplace application, you'll also find out if you qualify for an individual insurance plan with savings based on your income instead. Create an account or log in to an existing account to get started.

What Children's Health Insurance Program Covers

CHIP benefits are different in each state. But all states provide comprehensive coverage, including:

- Routine check-ups
- Immunizations
- Doctor visits
- Prescriptions
- Dental and vision care
- Inpatient and outpatient hospital care
- Laboratory and X-ray services
- Emergency services

What Children's Health Insurance Program Costs

Routine "well child" doctor and dental visits are free under CHIP. But there may be copayments for other services. Some states charge a monthly premium for CHIP coverage. The costs are different in each state, but you won't have to pay more than 5 percent of your family's income for the year.

Using Your New Medicaid or Children's Health Insurance Program Coverage

If you're enrolled in Medicaid or the Children's Health Insurance Program (CHIP), here are some things to know about coverage and care.

Using Your Coverage

For most questions, contact your state Medicaid or CHIP agency.

- If you're enrolled in a health plan through Medicaid or CHIP, contact the member services phone number on your eligibility letter or the back of your enrollment card. This information should also be on the websites of your health plan or Medicaid or CHIP agency.

- Talk to your doctor or pharmacist. They may be able to answer questions about what services are covered.

When to Contact Your State Medicaid or Children's Health Insurance Program Agency

Issues to take to your state Medicaid or CHIP agency include:

- You didn't get an enrollment card and aren't sure you're covered

- You can't find a doctor who accepts Medicaid or CHIP, or you can't get an appointment

- You want to know if a service or product is covered

- You have a life change that may affect if you're eligible for Medicaid or CHIP—like getting a job that increases your income, your dependent reaching an age where they no longer qualify, or getting married or divorced.

If they don't have enough information, most pharmacies can give you enough medicine for three days. Call your Medicaid or CHIP agency or health plan for help getting the rest of your medicine.

If your pharmacy doesn't accept Medicaid, CHIP, or your health plan, call the number in your eligibility letter to find a pharmacy you can use. You can usually find this information on the state Medicaid or CHIP agency website too.

Chapter 39

Allergy Tests

Chapter Contents

Section 39.1

Allergy Blood Test

This section includes text excerpted from "Allergy Blood Test,"
MedlinePlus, National Institutes of Health (NIH), July 18, 2018.

What Is an Allergy Blood Test?

Allergies are a common and chronic condition that involves the
body's immune system. Normally, your immune system works to fight
off viruses, bacteria, and other infectious agents. When you have an
allergy, your immune system treats a harmless substance, like dust or
pollen, as a threat. To fight this perceived threat, your immune system
makes antibodies called immunoglobulin E (IgE).

Substances that cause an allergic reaction are called allergens.
Besides dust and pollen, other common allergens include animal dander, foods, including nuts and shellfish, and certain medicines, such as
penicillin. Allergy symptoms can range from sneezing and a stuffy nose
to a life-threatening complication called anaphylactic shock. Allergy
blood tests measure the amount of IgE antibodies in the blood. A small
amount of IgE antibodies is normal. A larger amount of IgE may mean
you have an allergy.

Other names: IgE allergy test, Quantitative IgE, Immunoglobulin
E, Total IgE, Specific IgE.

What Is It Used For?

Allergy blood tests are used to find out if you have an allergy. One
type of test called a total IgE test measures the overall number of IgE
antibodies in your blood. Another type of allergy blood test called a
specific IgE test measures the level of IgE antibodies in response to
individual allergens.

Why Do I Need an Allergy Blood Test?

Your healthcare provider may order allergy testing if you have
symptoms of an allergy. These include:

- Stuffy or runny nose

- Sneezing

- Itchy, watery eyes

- Hives (a rash with raised red patches)
- Diarrhea
- Vomiting
- Shortness of breath
- Coughing
- Wheezing

What Happens during an Allergy Blood Test?

A healthcare professional will take a blood sample from a vein in your arm, using a small needle. After the needle is inserted, a small amount of blood will be collected into a test tube or vial. You may feel a little sting when the needle goes in or out. This usually takes less than five minutes.

Will I Need to Do Anything to Prepare for the Test?

You don't need any special preparations for an allergy blood test.

Are There Any Risks to the Test?

There is very little risk to having an allergy blood test. You may have slight pain or bruising at the spot where the needle was put in, but most symptoms go away quickly.

What Do the Results Mean?

If your total IgE levels are higher than normal, it likely means you have some kind of allergy. But it does not reveal what you are allergic to. A specific IgE test will help identify your particular allergy. If your results indicate an allergy, your healthcare provider may refer you to an allergy specialist or recommend a treatment plan.

Your treatment plan will depend on the type and severity of your allergy. People at risk for anaphylactic shock, a severe allergic reaction that can cause death, need to take extra care to avoid the allergy-causing substance. They may need to carry an emergency epinephrine treatment with them at all times.

Be sure to talk to your healthcare provider if you have questions about your test results and/or your allergy treatment plan.

Is There Anything Else I Need to Know about an Allergy Blood Test?

An IgE skin test is another way to detect allergies, by measuring IgE levels and looking for a reaction directly on the skin. Your healthcare provider may order an IgE skin test instead of, or in addition to, an IgE allergy blood test.

Section 39.2

Allergenics

This section includes text excerpted from "Allergenics,"
U.S. Food and Drug Administration (FDA), May 2, 2018.

The Center for Biologics Evaluation and Research (CBER) regulates allergenic products. There are three types of allergenic products licensed for use:

1. Allergen extracts

2. Allergen patch tests

3. Antigen skin tests

Allergen Extracts

Allergen extracts are used for the diagnosis and/or treatment of allergic diseases such as allergic rhinitis ("hay fever"), allergic sinusitis, allergic conjunctivitis, bee venom allergy, and food allergy. Currently, there are two types of licensed allergen extracts:

- Injectable allergen extracts are used for both diagnosis and treatment and are sterile liquids that are manufactured from natural substances (such as molds, pollens, insects, insect venoms, and animal hair) known to elicit allergic reactions in susceptible individuals. Injectable allergen extracts for food allergies are used only for diagnostic purposes. Among the injectable allergen extracts, some are standardized; for these products there is an established method to determine the potency (or strength) of the product on a lot-by-lot basis. For the other injectable allergen extracts there is no measure of potency, and these are called "nonstandardized."

- Injectable Allergen Extracts—Standardized
- Injectable Allergen Extracts—Nonstandardized

- Sublingual allergen extract tablets are used for treatment only and are also derived from natural substances known to elicit allergic reactions in susceptible individuals, and are intended for the treatment of allergic rhinitis with or without allergic conjunctivitis.

  - GRASTEK

  - Oralair

  - RAGWITEK

Allergen Patch Tests

Allergen patch tests are diagnostic tests applied to the surface of the skin. Patch tests are used by healthcare providers to determine the specific cause of contact dermatitis, and are manufactured from natural substances or chemicals (such as nickel, rubber, and fragrance mixes) that are known to cause contact dermatitis.

- T.R.U.E. Test
- Rubber Panel T.R.U.E. TEST

Antigen Skin Tests

Antigen skin tests are diagnostic tests injected into the skin to aid in the diagnosis of infection with certain pathogens.

- Candin

- Spherusol

- Tuberculin, Purified Protein Derivative—Tubersol

- Tuberculin, Purified Protein Derivative—Aplisol

Section 39.3

Elimination Diet and Food Challenge Test

This section contains text excerpted from the following
sources: Text in this section begins with excerpts from "Food
Allergy Awareness and Action," Foodsafety.gov, U.S. Department of
Health and Human Services (HHS), May 14, 2018; Text beginning
with the heading "Elimination Diet" is excerpted from "Guidelines for
the Diagnosis and Management of Food Allergy in the
United States," National Institute of Allergy and Infectious
Diseases (NIAID), May 2011. Reviewed August 2018.

For two percent of adults and four to eight percent of children, in
the United States, food allergies are a continuous concern. For these
individuals, the immune response their body produces to normally safe
items—in this case food—can lead to serious illness and even death.
About 90 percent of allergic food reactions are caused by eight foods:
milk, eggs, fish, crustacean shellfish, tree nuts, peanuts, wheat, and
soybeans.

The only way to prevent these reactions is by completely avoiding
foods that contain allergens you are allergic to; however, this can be
challenging because we as Americans eat many foods that comprise
of multiple ingredients, and we often eat foods prepared outside our
homes by other individuals. Reading and understanding labels along
with effectively communicating food allergy risks can be paramount
in protecting those with food allergies.

Reading Ingredient Statements on Labels

All food products containing two or more ingredients are required
by federal regulations to have an ingredients statement listing all
ingredients by common or usual name in descending order of predominance. Reading ingredient statements on labels is the best
way to avoid foods that may contain allergens. For example, some
processed meat and poultry products (e.g., hot dogs, chicken nug-
gets, and canned soup) may be formulated with known allergenic
ingredients, such as nonfat dry milk or hydrolyzed wheat protein.
If the U.S. Department of Agriculture's (USDA) Food Safety and
Inspection Service (FSIS) discovers an allergen in a meat or poultry
product that is not listed in the ingredient statement, the product
is recalled.

Elimination Diet

Your healthcare professional can suggest eliminating specific foods from your diet to help diagnose food allergy. Food elimination may identify foods responsible for some non-IgE-mediated and some mixed IgE- and non- IgE-mediated food allergy disorders.

What Else You Should Know

If your symptoms disappear when you eliminate a food from your diet, you may have food allergy. Your healthcare professional should perform additional tests to confirm the diagnosis.

For non-IgE-mediated food allergy disorders, your medical history and the results of a food elimination diet may provide a diagnosis.

Oral Food Challenge Test

The *Guidelines for the Diagnosis and Management of Food Allergy in the United States* recommend that your healthcare professional use the oral food challenge test to diagnose food allergy.

Note: Because an oral food challenge test always carries a risk, it must be performed by a healthcare professional trained in how to conduct this test and at a medical facility that has appropriate medicines and devices to treat potential severe allergic reactions.

An oral food challenge test includes the following steps:

- You are given doses of various foods, some of which are suspected of triggering an allergic reaction.

- Initially, the dose of food is very small, but the amount is gradually increased during the challenge.

- You swallow each dose.

- You are watched to see whether a reaction occurs.

There are three types of oral food challenge tests:

1. A double-blind placebo-controlled food challenge (DBPCFC) test is considered the best one. In this test, the patient receives increasing doses of the suspected food allergen or a harmless substance (placebo).

2. Neither the patient nor the healthcare professional knows which one the patient receives. A single-blind food challenge is

the next best option. In this test, the healthcare professional knows what the patient is receiving, but the patient does not.

3. An open-food challenge test may be sufficient to diagnose food allergy under certain circumstances. In this test, both the patient and the healthcare professional know whether a food allergen is received.

If an oral food challenge test results in no symptoms, then food allergy can be ruled out. If the challenge results in symptoms and these symptoms are consistent with your medical history and laboratory tests, then a diagnosis of food allergy is confirmed.

What Else You Should Know

The DBPCFC is the most specific test for diagnosing food allergy, but it can be expensive and inconvenient. Your healthcare professional may consider using a single-blind or open-food challenge as an alternative.

Chapter 40

Lung Function Tests

Breathing Tests

Spirometry

Spirometry measures how much air you breathe in and out and how fast you blow it out. This is measured two ways:

1. Peak expiratory flow rate (PEFR)—PEFR is the fastest rate at which you can blow air out of your lungs

2. Forced expiratory volume in one second (FEV1)—FEV1 refers to the amount of air you can blow out in one second

During the test, a technician will ask you to take a deep breath in. Then, you'll blow as hard as you can into a tube connected to a small machine. The machine is called a spirometer.

Your doctor may have you inhale a medicine that helps open your airways. He or she will want to see whether the medicine changes or improves the test results.

Spirometry helps check for conditions that affect how much air you can breathe in, such as pulmonary fibrosis (scarring of the lung tissue). The test also helps detect diseases that affect how fast you can breathe air out, like asthma and COPD (chronic obstructive pulmonary disease).

This chapter includes text excerpted from "Types of Lung Function Tests," National Heart, Lung, and Blood Institute (NHLBI), April 23, 2018.

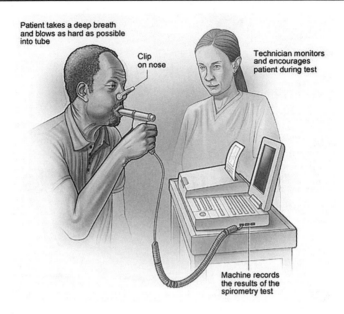

Patient takes a deep breath and blows as hard as possible into tube

Clip on nose

Technician monitors and encourages patient during test

Machine records the results of the spirometry test

Figure 40.1. *Spirometer*

The image shows how spirometry is done. The patient takes a deep breath and blows as hard as possible into a tube connected to a spirometer. The spirometer measures the amount of air breathed out. It also measures how fast the air was blown out.

Lung Volume Measurement

Body plethysmography is a test that measures how much air is present in your lungs when you take a deep breath. It also measures how much air remains in your lungs after you breathe out fully.

During the test, you sit inside a glass booth and breathe into a tube that's attached to a computer. For other lung function tests, you might breathe in nitrogen or helium gas and then blow it out. The gas you breathe out is measured to show how much air your lungs can hold.

Lung volume measurement can help diagnose pulmonary fibrosis or a stiff or weak chest wall.

Lung Diffusion Capacity

This test measures how well oxygen passes from your lungs to your bloodstream. During this test, you breathe in a type of gas through a tube. You hold your breath for a brief moment and then blow out the gas.

Abnormal test results may suggest loss of lung tissue, emphysema (a type of COPD), very bad scarring of the lung tissue, or problems with blood flow through the body's arteries.

Tests to Measure Oxygen Level

Pulse oximetry and arterial blood gas tests show how much oxygen is in your blood. During pulse oximetry, a small sensor is attached to your finger or ear. The sensor uses light to estimate how much oxygen is in your blood. This test is painless and no needles are used.

For an arterial blood gas test, a blood sample is taken from an artery, usually in your wrist. The sample is sent to a laboratory, where its oxygen level is measured. You may feel some discomfort during an arterial blood gas test because a needle is used to take the blood sample.

Testing in Infants and Young Children

Spirometry and other measures of lung function usually can be done for children older than six years, if they can follow directions well. Spirometry might be tried in children as young as five years. However, technicians who have special training with young children may need to do the testing.

Instead of spirometry, a growing number of medical centers measure respiratory system resistance. This is another way to test lung function in young children.

The child wears nose clips and has his or her cheeks supported with an adult's hands. The child breathes in and out quietly on a mouthpiece, while the technician measures changes in pressure at the mouth. During these lung function tests, parents can help comfort their children and encourage them to cooperate.

Very young children (younger than two years) may need an infant lung function test. This requires special equipment and medical staff. This type of test is available only at a few medical centers.

The doctor gives the child medicine to help him or her sleep through the test. A technician places a mask over the child's nose and mouth and a vest around the child's chest.

The mask and vest are attached to a lung function machine. The machine gently pushes air into the child's lungs through the mask. As the child exhales, the vest slightly squeezes his or her chest. This helps push more air out of the lungs. The exhaled air is then measured.

In children younger than five years, doctors likely will use signs and symptoms, medical history, and a physical exam to diagnose lung problems.

Doctors can use pulse oximetry and arterial blood gas tests for children of all ages.

Chapter 41

Allergy Medications and Therapies

Chapter Contents

Section 41.1

Allergy Medications Overview

This section contains text excerpted from the following sources: Text in this section begins with excerpts from "Enjoy the Season: Manage Your Allergies," U.S. Department of Veterans Affairs (VA), May 29, 2012. Reviewed August 2018; Text beginning with the heading "Allergy Medicines: Antihistamines and More" is excerpted from "Seasonal Allergies: Which Medication Is Right for You?" U.S. Food and Drug Administration (FDA), March 29, 2018.

Seasonal allergies are no fun. But the good news is there are ways to manage them. Dr. Joseph Yusin, Chief of Allergy and Immunology at the Greater Los Angeles U.S. Department of Veterans Affairs (VA) Medical Center, suggests several ways to keep allergy symptoms in check.

Natural Remedies

Some of the following natural remedies work for people with allergies. Yusin advises Veterans to discuss these remedies with their healthcare providers before using them.

- **Nasal irrigation.** Flushing the nasal passages with a salt and water solution can help unclog stuffy noses that could cause headaches and face pain. Yusin recommends using a neti pot—a small, ceramic pot with a spout—with distilled water.

- **Herbal supplements.** While some Chinese herbs have been shown to help people with allergies, they could have side effects. These herbs also could interact with certain medicines. Since many Veterans take a lot of different medications, it is especially important that they consult their providers about supplements.

- **Acupuncture.** No good studies show that acupuncture works for allergies, according to Yusin. He recommends trying avoidance measures and other treatments before acupuncture.

Over-the-Counter (OTC) Solutions

Medicines you can buy without a prescription are okay for mild allergies and symptoms, such as a runny nose, according to Yusin. But some products, like those that relieve clogged nasal passages, can bump up blood pressure if overused.

Prescription Medicines

Nasal steroid sprays are among the best prescription medicines for allergies, according to Yusin. If your healthcare provider prescribes one of these sprays, be sure to learn how to use it properly and read about possible side effects. Yusin said he prescribes allergy shots as a last resort.

When to See a Doctor

How do you know when to treat your allergies on your own and when to see your healthcare provider? Consider these criteria:

- **Frequency.** If your allergies do not act up too often, you can try to manage them on your own with over-the-counter (OTC) products.

- **Severity.** You also can try to manage your symptoms if they are mild. However, see a doctor if your allergy symptoms are severe or become severe. Severe symptoms are more extreme and may interfere with your ability to function normally. Some people have to cut back on their usual daily activities, while others just stay home.

Allergy Medicines: Antihistamines and More

Seasonal allergies are usually caused by plant pollen, which can come from trees, weeds and grasses in the spring, and by ragweed and other weeds in late summer and early fall.

Since you can't always stay indoors when pollen counts are high, your healthcare provider may recommend prescription or OTC medications to relieve symptoms. The U.S. Food and Drug Administration (FDA) regulates a number of medications that offer allergy relief.

Antihistamines reduce or block symptom-causing histamines and are available in many forms, including tablets and liquids. Many oral antihistamines are available OTC and in generic form.

When choosing an OTC antihistamine, patients should read the Drug Facts label closely and follow dosing instructions, says Jenny Kelty, M.D., a pediatric pulmonologist at the FDA. Some antihistamines can cause drowsiness and interfere with the ability to drive or operate heavy machinery, like a car. There are other antihistamines that do not have this side effect; they are nonsedating. Some nonsedating antihistamines are available by prescription.

Nasal corticosteroids are typically sprayed into the nose once or twice a day to treat inflammation. Side effects may include stinging in the nose.

Decongestants are drugs available both by prescription and OTC and come in oral and nasal spray forms. They are sometimes recommended in combination with antihistamines, which used alone do not have an effect on nasal congestion.

Drugs that contain pseudoephedrine are available without a prescription but are kept behind the pharmacy counter to prevent their use in making methamphetamine—a powerful, highly addictive stimulant often produced illegally in home laboratories. You will need to ask your pharmacist and show identification to purchase drugs that contain pseudoephedrine.

Using decongestant nose sprays and drops more than a few days may give you a "rebound" effect—your nasal congestion could get worse. These drugs are more useful for short-term use to relieve nasal congestion.

Immunotherapy is another option. One form of allergen immunotherapy is allergy shots in which your body responds to injected amounts of a particular allergen, given in gradually increasing doses, by developing immunity or tolerance to that allergen.

Patients can receive injections from a healthcare provider; a common course of treatment would begin with weekly injections for two to three months until the maximum dose is reached. After that, treatment could continue monthly for three to five years.

Another form of allergen immunotherapy therapy involves administering the allergens in a tablet form under the tongue (sublingual) and is intended for daily use, before and during the pollen season. These medications are available by prescription for the treatment of hay fever caused by certain pollens and have the potential for dialing down the immune response to allergens. However, they are not meant for immediate symptom relief, says Jay Slater, M.D., an allergist with the FDA. Sublingual therapy should start three to four months before allergy season. Although they are intended for at-home use, the first doses are to be taken in the presence of a healthcare provider.

A Word about Over-the-Counter (OTC) Products and Kids

Always read the label before buying an OTC product for you or your children, says Kelty. "Some products can be used in children as young as two years, but others are not appropriate for children of any age."

Talk to your healthcare professional if your child needs to use nasal steroid spray for more than two months a year.

Section 41.2

Antihistamines

This section includes text excerpted from "Antihistamines," LiverTox®, National Institutes of Health (NIH), July 5, 2018.

Histamine is an important mediator of immediate hypersensitivity reactions acting locally and causing smooth muscle contraction, vasodilation, increased vascular permeability, edema and inflammation. Histamine acts through specific cellular receptors which have been categorized into four types, H1 through H4. Antihistamines represent a class of medications that block the histamine type 1 (H1) receptors. Importantly, antihistamines do not block or decrease the release of histamine, but rather ameliorate its local actions. Agents that specially block other H2 receptors are generally referred to as H2 blockers rather than antihistamines.

H1 receptors are widely distributed and are particularly common on smooth muscle of the bronchi, gastrointestinal (GI) tract, uterus and large blood vessels. H1 receptors are also found in the central nervous system. The antihistamines are widely used to treat symptoms of allergic conditions including itching, nasal stuffiness, runny nose, teary eyes, urticaria, dizziness, nausea and cough. Their most common use alone or in combination with other agents is for symptoms of upper respiratory illnesses such as the common cold. The central nervous system effects of antihistamines include sedation and decrease in anxiety, tension, and adventitious movements.

Antihistamines are typically separated into sedating (first generation) and nonsedating (second generation) forms, based upon their central nervous system effects, the nonsedating agents being less likely to cross the blood–brain barrier (BBB). In addition, some antihistamines have additional anticholinergic, antimuscarinic or other actions. The antihistamines are some of the most commonly used drugs in medicine, and most are available in multiple forms, both by prescription and in over-the-counter (OTC) products, alone or combined with analgesics or sympathomimetic agents. Common uses include short-term treatment of symptoms of the common cold, seasonal allergic rhinitis (hay fever), motion sickness, nausea, vertigo, cough, urticaria, pruritus, and anaphylaxis. The sedating antihistamines are also used as mild sleeping aids and to alleviate tension and anxiety. Many antihistamines are also available in topical forms, as creams, nasal sprays and eye drops for local use in alleviating allergic symptoms. The nonsedating antihistamines are typically used in extended or long-term treatment of allergic disorders, including allergic rhinitis (hay fever), sinusitis, atopic dermatitis, and chronic urticaria.

The antihistamines have several adverse side effects which are related to their antihistaminic actions. Side effects are, however, usually mild and rapidly reversed with stopping therapy or decreasing the dose. These common side effects include sedation, impaired motor function, dizziness, dry mouth and throat, blurred vision, urinary retention and constipation. Antihistamines can worsen urinary retention and narrow-angle glaucoma.

The antihistamines rarely cause liver injury. Their relative safety probably relates to their use in low doses for a short time only. The nonsedating antihistamines, however, are often used for an extended period and several forms have been linked to rare instances of clinically apparent acute liver injury which has generally been mild and self-limiting; the antihistamines most commonly linked to liver injury have been cyproheptadine, cetirizine, and terfenadine (which is no longer in clinical use).

The first generation oral antihistamines in clinical use (with common brand name(s) and year of approval in the United States, if available) include brompheniramine (Bromphen, Dimetapp), chlorpheniramine, carbinoxamine (Palgic), clemastine, cyclizine, cyproheptadine, diphenhydramine, dimenhydrinate (Dramamine), doxylamine, hydroxyzine, meclizine, phenyltoloxamine (Acuflex), promethazine, and triprolidine (Triafed). Second generation antihistamines in general use and used orally include acrivastine (Semprex-D), cetirizine, levocetirizine, loratadine, desloratadine, and fexofenadine.

First generation antihistamines

- Brompheniramine
- Carbinoxamine
- Chlorcyclizine
- Chlorpheniramine

- Clemastine
- Cyclizine
- Cyproheptadine
- Dexbrompheniramine
- Dexchlorpheniramine
- Dimenhydrinate
- Diphenhydramine

- Doxylamine
- Hydroxyzine
- Meclizine
- Phenyltoloxamine
- Promethazine
- Triprolidine

Second generation antihistamines

- Acrivastine
- Cetirizine
- Fexofenadine

- Levocetirizine
- Loratadine
- Desloratadine

Section 41.3

Decongestants

This section contains text excerpted from the following sources: Text in this section begins with excerpts from "Effective Healthcare Program," Effective Health Care Program, Agency for Healthcare Research and Quality (AHRQ), July 2013. Reviewed August 2018; Text under the heading "Safety Information for Parents and Caregivers" is excerpted from "Use Caution When Giving Cough and Cold Products to Kids," U.S. Food and Drug Administration (FDA), February 8, 2018; Text beginning with the heading "Misuse of Decongestants" is excerpted from "Legal Requirements for the Sale and Purchase of Drug Products Containing Pseudoephedrine, Ephedrine, and Phenylpropanolamine," U.S. Food and Drug Administration (FDA), November 24, 2017.

Decongestants stimulate the sympathetic nervous system to produce vasoconstriction, which results in decreased nasal swelling and decreased congestion. After several days of nasal decongestant use, rebound congestion (rhinitis medicamentosa) may occur. Other local adverse effects may include nosebleeds, stinging, burning, and dryness. Oral decongestants are used alone and in combination, often with antihistamines. Systemic adverse effects of decongestants may include hypertension, tachycardia, insomnia, headaches, and irritability. Decongestants are used with caution, if at all, in patients with diabetes mellitus, ischemic heart disease (IHD), unstable hypertension, prostatic hypertrophy, hyperthyroidism, and narrow-angle glaucoma. Oral decongestants are contraindicated with coadministered monoamine oxidase inhibitors (MAOIs) and in patients with uncontrolled hypertension or severe coronary artery disease (CAD).

Safety Information for Parents and Caregivers

Children under two years of age should not be given any kind of cough and cold product that contains a decongestant or antihistamine because serious and possibly life-threatening side effects could occur. Reported side effects of these products included convulsions, rapid heart rates, and death. What about older children? When giving cough and cold medicine to children over two years of age, parents, and caregivers should use caution.

Treating Toddlers and Older Children

Cough and cold products for children older than two years of age were not affected by the voluntary removal and these products are still sold in pharmacies and other retail outlets. Manufactures also voluntarily relabeled these cough and cold products to state: "do not use in children under four years of age."

Parents need to be aware that many over-the-counter (OTC) cough and cold products contain multiple ingredients which can lead to accidental overdosing. Reading the Drug Facts label can help parents learn about what drugs (active ingredients) are in a product.

When giving children four years of age and older a cough and cold product, remember, OTC cough and cold products can be harmful if:

- More than the recommended amount is used

- They are given too often

- More than one product containing the same drug is being used

Children should not be given medicines that are packaged and made for adults.

Other Options for Treating Colds

Here are a few alternative treatments for infants to help with cough and cold symptoms:

- A cool mist humidifier helps nasal passages shrink and allow easier breathing. Do not use warm mist humidifiers. They can cause nasal passages to swell and make breathing more difficult.

- Saline nose drops or spray keep nasal passages moist and helps avoid stuffiness.

- Nasal suctioning with a bulb syringe—with or without saline nose drops—works very well for infants less than a year old. Older children often resist the use of a bulb syringe.

- Acetaminophen or ibuprofen can be used to reduce fever, aches, and pains. Parents should carefully read and follow the product's instructions for use on the Drug Facts label.

- Drinking plenty of liquids will help children stay hydrated.

Misuse of Decongestants

The Combat Methamphetamine Epidemic Act of 2005 (CMEA) has been incorporated into the Patriot Act signed by President Bush on March 9, 2006. The act bans OTC sales of cold medicines that contain the ingredient pseudoephedrine, which is commonly used to make methamphetamine. The sale of cold medicine containing pseudoephedrine is limited to behind the counter. The amount of pseudoephedrine that an individual can purchase each month is limited and individuals are required to present photo identification to purchase products containing pseudoephedrine. In addition, stores are required to keep personal information about purchasers for at least two years.

What Is Pseudoephedrine?

Pseudoephedrine is a drug found in both prescription and OTC products used to relieve nasal or sinus congestion caused by the common cold, sinusitis, hay fever, and other respiratory allergies. It can also be used illegally to produce methamphetamine.

What Is Methamphetamine?

Methamphetamine is a powerful, highly addictive stimulant. It is manufactured in covert, illegal laboratories throughout the United

States. Methamphetamine can be ingested by swallowing, inhaling, injecting or smoking. The side effects, which arise from the use and abuse of methamphetamine, include irritability, nervousness, insomnia, nausea, depression, and brain damage.

Does This Mean I Need a Prescription from My Doctor to Buy Pseudoephedrine?

No. The Act allows for the sale of pseudoephedrine only from locked cabinets or behind the counter. The law:

- Limits the monthly amount any individual could purchase

- Requires individuals to present photo identification to purchase such medications

- Requires retailers to keep personal information about these customers for at least two years after the purchase of these medicines

I Have Chronic Sinus Problems. Will I Be Limited from Getting the Amount of Pseudoephedrine I Need?

Yes, with this new law there will be limits on the number of tablets of ephedrine, pseudoephedrine, or phenylpropanolamine that can be purchased in a 30-day period. As there a many different dosages and formulations of these products, you should ask your pharmacist how much you will be allowed to purchase over a 30-day period for specific product you use.

Section 41.4

Corticosteroids

This section includes text excerpted from "Corticosteroids," LiverTox®, National Institutes of Health (NIH), July 5, 2018.

The corticosteroids are a group of chemically related natural hormones and synthetic agents that resemble the human adrenal hormone cortisol and have potent anti-inflammatory and immunosuppressive properties and are widely used in medicine. Corticosteroid therapy is associated with several forms of liver injury, some due to exacerbation of an underlying liver disease and some that appear to be caused directly by corticosteroid therapy. This discussion will cover eight agents: betamethasone, cortisone, dexamethasone, hydrocortisone, methylprednisolone, prednisolone, prednisone, and triamcinolone.

The corticosteroids are hormones that have glucocorticoid (cortisol-like) and/or mineralocorticoid (aldosterone-like) activities and which are synthesized predominantly by the adrenal cortex. In clinical practice, the term "corticosteroids" usually refers to the glucocorticoids and are represented by a large group of natural or synthetic steroid compounds that have varying potency, durations of action and relative glucocorticoid (measured by anti-inflammatory activity) versus mineralocorticoid (measured by sodium retention) activities. Cortisol and the corticosteroids act by engagement of the intracellular glucocorticoid receptor (GR), which then is translocated to the cell nucleus where the receptor-ligand complex binds to specific glucocorticoid-response elements on deoxyribonucleic acid (DNA), thus activating genes that mediate glucocorticoid responses. The number of genes modulated by corticosteroids are many and the effects are multiple and interactive with other intracellular pathways. Thus, the effects of corticosteroids on inflammation and the immune system cannot be attributed to a single gene or pathway. The potent anti-inflammatory and immunosuppressive qualities of the corticosteroids have made them important agents in the therapy of many diseases.

Corticosteroids are available in multiple forms, including oral tablets and capsules; powders and solutions for parenteral administration; topical creams and lotions for skin disease; eye, ear and nose liquid drops for local application; aerosol solutions for inhalation and liquids or foams for rectal application. Representative corticosteroids (and the year of their approval for use in the United States) include cortisone, prednisone, prednisolone, methylprednisolone, dexamethasone, betamethasone, and hydrocortisone. All are available in generic forms.

The corticosteroids are used widely in medicine largely for their potent anti-inflammatory and immunosuppressive activities. The clinical conditions for which corticosteroids are used include, but are not limited to: asthma, systemic lupus erythematosus (SLE), rheumatoid arthritis (RA), psoriasis, inflammatory bowel disease (IBD), nephritic syndrome, cancer, leukemia, organ transplantation, autoimmune hepatitis, hypersensitivity reactions, cardiogenic and septic shock, and, of course, glucocorticoid deficiency diseases such as in Addison disease and panhypopituitarism.

Corticosteroids are used in several liver diseases, most commonly in autoimmune hepatitis for which they have been shown to improve outcome and survival. Corticosteroids are also used after liver transplantation to prevent rejection. An important element in managing these liver diseases and conditions is to maintain the dose of corticosteroids at the lowest effective level. The adverse effects of long-term corticosteroid therapy (which are rarely hepatic) are still major causes of morbidity and even mortality in these conditions.

Prednisone, prednisolone, methylprednisone, and triamcinolone are the most commonly used oral agents as they are inexpensive, rapid in onset, intermediate in duration of action and have potent glucocorticoid with minimal mineralocorticoid activities, at least as compared to cortisone and hydrocortisone. Betamethasone and dexamethasone have greater glucocorticoid potency and less aldosterone-like activity than prednisone, but have a longer duration of action, and they are mostly used in topical or liquid forms for local application and in injectable forms for severe hypersensitivity reactions and inflammation. Methylprednisone and hydrocortisone are most commonly used for intravenous administration, typically given in emergency or critical situations in which rapid and profound immunosuppression or anti-inflammatory activity is needed.

The table below provides the major forms of corticosteroids and their relative glucocorticoid and mineralocorticoid activity and equivalent daily doses.

Table 41.1. Relative Potencies of Corticosteroids

Agent	Glucocorticoid Activity	Mineralocorticoid Activity	Equivalent Oral or Intravenous Dose
Cortisol	1	1	20
Cortisone	0.8	0.8	25
Prednisone	4	0.8	5
Prednisolone	4	0.8	5
Methylprednisolone	5	0.5	4
Triamcinolone	5	0	4
Betamethasone	25	0	0.75
Dexamethasone	25	0	0.75

Hydrocortisone is a rapid and short-acting glucocorticoid that is used for therapy of adrenal insufficiency and in treatment of allergic and inflammatory conditions. Hydrocortisone has the same chemical structure as cortisol and thus most closely resembles the human adrenal hormone. Hydrocortisone is available in generic forms in tablets of 5, 10, and 20 mg, with 20 mg being considered a daily physiologic dose in adults. Hydrocortisone is also available in multiple forms in solution for oral, rectal, topical or parenteral administration. A major use of intravenous hydrocortisone is in the acute therapy of severe hypersensitivity reactions and shock. Hydrocortisone has both glucocorticoid and mineralocorticoid properties.

Prednisone is a synthetic, intermediate-acting glucocorticoid that is widely used in the therapy of severe inflammation, autoimmune conditions, hypersensitivity reactions and organ rejection. Prednisone is converted to prednisolone, its active form, in the liver. Prednisone is available in multiple generic forms in tablets of 1, 2.5, 5, 10, 20, and 50 mg and as oral solutions. Four times more potent that cortisol, prednisone is used in varying doses, with 5 mg daily being considered physiologic doses in adults.

Prednisolone is a synthetic, intermediate-acting glucocorticoid that is widely used in the therapy of severe inflammation, autoimmune conditions, hypersensitivity reactions, and organ rejection. Prednisolone is available in multiple generic forms in tablets of 5, 10, 15, and 30 mg and in several forms for systemic administration. Four times more potent that cortisol, prednisolone is used in varying doses, with 5 mg daily being considered physiologic doses in adults.

Methylprednisolone is a synthetic, intermediate acting glucocorticoid that widely used in the therapy of severe inflammation, autoimmune conditions, hypersensitivity reactions, and organ rejection. Methylprednisolone is available in multiple forms in tablets of 2, 4, 8, 16, and 32 mg generically and under the brand name of Medrol and in Medrol Dosepaks (21 tablets of 4 mg each). Injectable forms of methylprednisolone are also available generically and under brand names of Solu-Medrol and Depo-Medrol. Five times more potent that cortisol, methylprednisolone is used in varying doses, with 4 mg daily being considered physiologic doses in adults. Methylprednisolone has minimal mineralocorticoid activity.

Triamcinolone is a synthetic, long-acting glucocorticoid that is used in topical solutions and aerosols for therapy of allergic and hypersensitivity reactions and control of inflammation as well as in parenteral formulations for therapy of hypersensitivity reactions, shock, and severe inflammation. Oral forms of triamcinolone include tablets of 4 and 8 mg and oral syrups. Parenteral forms for injection are available under various generic and trade names including

Aristocort and Kenacort. Triamcinolone is five times more potent than cortisol in its glucocorticoid activity, but has minimal mineralocorticoid activity.

Dexamethasone is a synthetic, long-acting glucocorticoid that is used parenterally as therapy of severe hypersensitivity reactions, shock, and control of severe inflammation as well as in topical, otic, ophthalmologic solutions, aerosols, and lotions or creams for local therapy of allergic reactions and inflammation. Dexamethasone is available in multiple forms for injection under various generic and trade names including Decadron. Dexamethasone is 25 times more potent than cortisol in its glucocorticoid activity, but has minimal mineralocorticoid activity.

Betamethasone is a synthetic, long-acting glucocorticoid that used in parenteral forms for therapy of allergic and hypersensitivity reactions and control of severe inflammation. Betamethasone is available in solution for injection under the trade name of Celestone and in multiple generic forms as syrups and effervescent tablets for oral use, edemas and foams for rectal use, aerosols for nasal and respiratory use, and creams and lotions for topical use. Betamethasone is 25 times more potent than cortisol in glucocorticoid activity, but has minimal mineralocorticoid activity.

Hepatotoxicity, Mechanism of Injury

Corticosteroids have multiple adverse side effects, due to their multiplicity of actions affecting virtually all organs. Long-term use has very profound effects on growth and can lead to cataracts, glaucoma, opportunistic infections, thinning of the skin, weight gain and redistribution of fat, insulin resistance and diabetes, hypertension, headache, psychiatric problems, sodium retention and peripheral edema; all of the clinical features of Cushing syndrome.

Corticosteroids also have major effects on the liver, particularly when given long term and in higher than physiologic doses. Glucocorticoid use can result in hepatic enlargement and steatosis or glycogenosis. Corticosteroids can trigger or worsen nonalcoholic steatohepatitis. Long-term use can also exacerbate chronic viral hepatitis. Importantly, treatment with corticosteroids followed by withdrawal or pulse therapy can cause reactivation of hepatitis B and worsening or de novo induction of autoimmune hepatitis, both of which can be fatal. Finally, high doses of intravenous corticosteroids, largely methylprednisolone, have been associated with acute liver injury which can result in acute liver failure and death. Thus, the hepatic complications of corticosteroids usually represent the worsening or triggering of an underlying liver disease and rarely are the result of drug hepatotoxicity.

Corticosteroid therapy can cause hepatic steatosis and hepatic enlargement, but this is often not clinically apparent, particularly in adults. This effect can occur quite rapidly and is rapidly reversed with discontinuation. High doses and long-term use has been associated with the development or exacerbation of nonalcoholic steatohepatitis with elevations in serum aminotransferase levels and liver histology resembling alcoholic hepatitis with steatosis, chronic inflammation, centrilobular ballooning degeneration and Mallory bodies. However, symptomatic or progressive liver injury from corticosteroid-induced steatohepatitis is uncommon. Furthermore, corticosteroids may act to worsen an underlying nonalcoholic fatty liver disease rather than causing the condition de novo. The worsening may be due to direct effects of glucocorticoids on insulin resistance or fatty acid metabolism or may be the result of weight gain which is common with long-term corticosteroid therapy. While simple steatosis induced by corticosteroids is rapidly reversible, steatohepatitis can be slow to resolve upon withdrawal of corticosteroids.

Corticosteroids in high doses can also cause hepatic glycogenosis, in which liver cells exhibit a homogenous appearance and stain strongly for glycogen (using Periodic acid–Schiff (PAS) staining with and without diastase). Glycogenosis can also be associated with hepatomegaly (in children) and elevations in serum aminotransferase levels with minimal or no change in alkaline phosphatase or bilirubin levels. Glycogenosis is usually asymptomatic and does not appear to progress to chronic liver injury, cirrhosis or acute liver failure. While glycogenosis has been described largely in patients with poorly controlled type 1 diabetes, it also can occur acutely in patients started on high dose corticosteroids.

An important complication of corticosteroid therapy is the worsening of an underlying chronic viral hepatitis. In chronic hepatitis B, corticosteroids can induce increases in viral replication and serum hepatitis B virus (HBV) DNA levels while decreasing serum aminotransferase levels. Eventually, however, the increase in viral replication can worsen the underlying liver disease. Exacerbation of hepatitis becomes particularly evident when corticosteroids are withdrawn or lowered to physiological levels. As the immune system recovers, hepatitis worsens and serum aminotransferase levels can rise to greater than 10- to 20-fold elevated usually accompanied by a prompt decrease in HBV DNA levels. This flare of disease following withdrawal of corticosteroids can be severe and result in acute liver failure or significant worsening of chronic hepatitis and development of cirrhosis. Indeed, even patients with the "inactive carrier states" (as shown by the presence of HBsAg in serum without HBeAg or detectable HBV DNA or any elevation in serum aminotransferase levels) can suffer severe reactivation of disease and acute liver failure as a result of a short course of high dose corticosteroids as occurs with cancer chemotherapy or with treatment of severe autoimmune conditions or even asthma, hay fever or allergic dermatitis. Reactivation of hepatitis B can be prevented by prophylactic use of antiviral therapy during the period of immunosuppression, but even this may not prevent some degree of liver injury.

Corticosteroids also appear to worsen the course of chronic hepatitis C, although in a less dramatic fashion than in chronic hepatitis B. Corticosteroid therapy leads to a rise in hepatitis C virus (HCV) ribonucleic acid (RNA) levels which may eventually cause worsening of the underlying liver disease. Chronic hepatitis C appears to be more severe and is particularly difficult to manage in patients receiving chemotherapy or immunosuppression, and corticosteroids are believed to be a major factor in this effect. Thus, corticosteroids should be avoided if possible in patients with underlying chronic viral hepatitis.

Corticosteroids are used in the therapy of autoimmune hepatitis and, therefore, are likely to be beneficial rather than harmful in patients with this disease. The difficulty arises when corticosteroids are stopped, which can cause a rebound exacerbation of the autoimmune hepatitis that is often severe and can be fatal. Importantly, there have been multiple reported instances of de novo appearance of severe autoimmune hepatitis in patients who received a short course or pulse of corticosteroids for another, unrelated condition (such as asthma or allergic reactions). In these situations, a mild and subclinical autoimmune hepatitis was likely present before corticosteroids were started, and the suppression of the disease followed by immune rebound caused the clinical presentation of the condition. These patients generally respond to restarting corticosteroids, but may require long term if not lifelong immunosuppressive treatment thereafter.

Finally, there have been several reports of an acute hepatitis-like liver injury arising after a short, high dose course of intravenous methylprednisolone that can be severe and even fatal, and in which viral hepatitis and autoimmune hepatitis cannot be clearly implicated. The cause of this apparent hepatotoxicity is not known, but it may represent severe autoimmune hepatitis triggered by the sudden profound immunosuppression and subsequent immune reconstitution. Importantly, symptoms and jaundice develop two to four weeks after stopping methylprednisolone and the pattern of serum enzyme elevations is typically hepatocellular. These episodes are usually symptomatic and can be severe. Immunoallergic manifestations are uncommon and autoantibodies may not be present. Several instances have resulted in acute liver failure resulting in death or need for emergency liver transplantation. Restarting corticosteroids may be appropriate in this situation, but it has not been evaluated systematically and many instances have resolved spontaneously. Recurrence of injury, often in a more rapid and severe form, arises upon reexposure to high dose pulse methylprednisolone.

Section 41.5

Leukotriene Modifiers

This section includes text excerpted from "Leukotriene
Receptor Antagonists," LiverTox®, National Institutes of
Health (NIH), July 5, 2018.

The leukotriene receptor antagonists are among the most prescribed drugs for the management of asthma, used both for treatment and prevention of acute asthmatic attacks. This class of drugs acts by binding to cysteinyl leukotriene (CysLT) receptors and blocking their activation and the subsequent inflammatory cascade which cause the symptoms commonly associated with asthma and allergic rhinitis.

The cysteinyl leukotrienes (C4, D4, and E4) are products of arachidonic acid metabolism and are released from various cells, including mast cells and eosinophils. These eicosanoids bind to CysLT receptors. The CysLT type-1 receptor is found in the human airway smooth muscle cells and airway macrophages and on other proinflammatory cells. In asthmatic patients, leukotriene-mediated effects include airway edema, smooth muscle contraction, and altered cellular activity associated with the inflammatory process. In allergic rhinitis, CysLTs are released from the nasal mucosa after allergen exposure and precipitate the symptoms of allergic rhinitis.

Two leukotriene receptor antagonists are available in the United States, zafirlukast and montelukast. Both are oral agents used in management of asthma and allergic rhinitis. Both have been associated with rare cases of acute liver injury. While they have similar mechanisms of action, these two agents are structurally distinct, and the liver injury they cause does not appear to be similar in pattern of presentation or outcome. Indeed, several instances of hepatotoxicity due to one agent have been described in which the patient has tolerated the other agent without recurrence.

Section 41.6

Treatment for Living with Food Allergy

This section includes text excerpted from "Treatment for Living with Food Allergy," National Institute of Allergy and Infectious Diseases (NIAID), April 19, 2016.

There is presently no cure for many food allergies. Healthcare providers can manage patients' food allergies by encouraging them to avoid foods that may cause an allergic reaction and by treating severe reactions when they arise. But the rate of food allergic reactions are high—about one each year for allergic children, according to a National Institute of Allergy and Infectious Diseases (NIAID)-funded study.

To address this high rate of events, scientists are working to develop immunotherapy approaches to prevent and treat food allergy. Immunotherapy involves exposing the immune system to an allergen in a controlled way in order to eventually lessen the immune response to that allergen. This basic approach can take many forms, all of which are experimental. Immunotherapy is not currently approved by the U.S. Food and Drug Administration (FDA) for use to treat food allergy. However, research to investigate different approaches to immunotherapy in food allergy is ongoing.

NIAID-funded researchers have implemented several clinical trials to assess the effectiveness of different forms of immunotherapy for the treatment of food allergy.

Oral Immunotherapy

Oral immunotherapy (OIT) is being tested in several NIAID-funded clinical trials to evaluate the role of OIT in treating and managing food allergy. OIT involves eating small doses of the food that causes the allergy—usually in the form of a powder mixed with a harmless food—and gradually increasing these doses every day. A study from the NIAID-funded Consortium of Food Allergy Research (CoFAR) suggested that egg OIT can benefit children with egg allergy. Most of the study participants could be safely exposed to egg while on egg OIT, and some were able to safely eat egg after stopping OIT. Most of the study participants could be safely exposed to egg while on egg OIT, and some were able to safely eat egg after stopping OIT.

Another ongoing NIAID-funded study called MAP-X is testing whether using an additional medication, an injectable antibody called omalizumab, taken during OIT could improve the safety of the therapy or make it more effective in individuals with allergies to several different foods. Omalizumab blocks IgE activity, so researchers believe the medication may reduce allergic reactions during OIT.

Other OIT trials include the IMPACT study, conducted by the NIAID-sponsored Immune Tolerance Network. In this ongoing study, investigators are testing the ability of peanut OIT to elicit tolerance to peanut among young children with peanut allergy.

In small clinical trials, OIT has been shown to provide some benefits to patients with milk, egg, or peanut allergies. However, many issues still need to be addressed before this therapy can be broadly applied to food allergy sufferers. Researchers are working to improve the safety and effectiveness of OIT for a wider variety of food allergies.

Epicutaneous Immunotherapy

In epicutaneous immunotherapy, or EPIT, an allergen is delivered to the skin's surface by a wearable patch. The NIAID-funded Consortium of Food Allergy Research completed a study to evaluate the safety and efficacy of EPIT for peanut allergy. The therapy enabled recipients of the patch to tolerate larger amounts of peanut in a blinded oral food challenge after one year of treatment compared to the amounts they could tolerate in an oral food challenge at the start of the study. The patch was associated with skin reactions, but these were mostly mild, local reactions that did not interfere with use. Patients are now receiving longer term administration of the patch and follow up within the study.

Subcutaneous Immunotherapy

For several allergy problems, like hay fever, healthcare providers may recommend subcutaneous immunotherapy, or allergy shots, in which allergens are injected directly into a person's body. Researchers are no longer pursuing this approach as a treatment for food allergy because initial attempts too frequently caused severe allergic reactions.

Baked Milk and Egg Therapy

Consumption of food that includes baked milk or egg products is a potential alternative to OIT for treatment of milk and egg allergies. Temperature-associated changes in certain milk and egg proteins may render baked versions of these foods less allergenic. However, the same does not hold true for all allergy-triggering foods. For example, roasting peanuts can make them even more likely to cause allergic reactions.

Studies have suggested that some children who are allergic to uncooked egg and milk can tolerate small amounts of these foods in fully cooked products such as muffins. One NIAID-funded study in 2011 found that more than half of baked-milk-tolerant children were able to tolerate foods containing uncooked milk after caregivers followed specific instructions to include baked milk products into their diets. The results also suggested that children who consumed baked milk outgrew their milk allergies more quickly than children who did not. However, many of the children treated with baked products were never able to eat unheated milk without allergic reactions. Additional studies are needed to determine how beneficial the baked food approach can be for certain people with food allergy.

Section 41.7

Therapies for Seasonal Allergic Rhinitis

This section includes text excerpted from "Treatments for
Seasonal Allergic Rhinitis," Effective Health Care Program, Agency
for Healthcare Research and Quality (AHRQ), July 2013.
Reviewed August 2018.

Seasonal allergic rhinitis (SAR), also known as hay fever, is an
allergic reaction in the upper airways that occurs when sensitized
individuals encounter airborne allergens (typically tree, grass, and
weed pollens and some molds). SAR afflicts approximately 10 percent
of the U.S. population, or 30 million individuals. Although pollen seasons vary across the United States, generally, tree pollens emerge in
the spring, grass pollens in the summer, and weed pollens in the fall.
Outdoor molds generally are prevalent in the summer and fall. SAR
is distinguished from perennial allergic rhinitis (PAR), which is triggered by continuous exposure to house dust mites, animal dander, and
other allergens generally found in an individual's indoor environment.
Patients may have either SAR or PAR or both (i.e., PAR with seasonal
exacerbations). The four defining symptoms of allergic rhinitis are
nasal congestion, nasal discharge (rhinorrhea), sneezing, and/or nasal
itch. Many patients also experience eye symptoms, such as itching,
tearing, and redness. Additional signs of rhinitis include the "allergic
salute" (rubbing the hand against the nose in response to itching and
rhinorrhea), "allergic shiner"(bruised appearance of the skin under
one or both eyes), and "allergic crease" (a wrinkle across the bridge of
the nose caused by repeated allergic salute). SAR can adversely affect
quality of life, sleep, cognition, emotional life, and work or school performance. Treatment improves symptoms and quality of life.

Treatments for SAR include allergen avoidance, pharmacotherapy, and immunotherapy. Although allergen avoidance may be the
preferred treatment, for SAR, total allergen avoidance may be an
unrealistic approach, as it may require limiting time spent outdoors.
Thus, pharmacotherapy is preferable to allergen avoidance for SAR
symptom relief.

Six classes of drugs and nasal saline are used to treat SAR.

- Antihistamines used to treat allergic rhinitis bind peripheral H1
histamine receptor selectively or nonselectively. Nonselective
binding to other receptor types can cause dry mouth, dry eyes,
urinary retention, constipation, and tachycardia. Sedation

results from the nonselective binding to central H1 receptors. In Contrast, selective antihistamines may have reduced incidence of adverse effects. Both selective and nonselective antihistamines interact with drugs that inhibit cytochrome P450 isoenzymes, which may impact patient selection. Two nasal antihistamines—azelastine and olopatadine—are approved by the U.S. Food and Drug Administration (FDA) for the treatment of SAR. Adverse effects of nasal antihistamines may include a bitter aftertaste.

- Corticosteroids are potent anti-inflammatory drugs. Intranasal corticosteroids are recommended as first-line treatment for moderate/severe or persistent allergic rhinitis. However, their efficacy for the symptom of nasal congestion compared with nasal antihistamine is uncertain, particularly in patients with mild allergic rhinitis. For patients with unresponsive symptoms, it is unclear whether adding oral or nasal antihistamine provides any additional benefit. Little is known about cumulative corticosteroid effects in patients who take concomitant oral or inhaled formulations for other diseases. Intranasal corticosteroids do not appear to cause adverse events associated with systemic absorption (e.g., adrenal suppression, bone fracture among the elderly, and reduced bone growth and height in children). Adverse local effects may include increased intraocular pressure and nasal stinging, burning, bleeding, and dryness.

- Decongestants stimulate the sympathetic nervous system to produce vasoconstriction, which results in decreased nasal swelling and decreased congestion. After several days of nasal decongestant use, rebound congestion (rhinitis medicamentosa) may occur. Other local adverse effects may include nosebleeds, stinging, burning, and dryness. Oral decongestants are used alone and in combination, often with antihistamines. Systemic adverse effects of decongestants may include hypertension, tachycardia, insomnia, headaches, and irritability. Decongestants are used with caution, if at all, in patients with diabetes mellitus, ischemic heart disease, unstable hypertension, prostatic hypertrophy, hyperthyroidism, and narrow-angle glaucoma. Oral decongestants are contraindicated with coadministered monoamine oxidase inhibitors and in patients with uncontrolled hypertension or severe coronary artery disease.

- Ipratropium nasal spray is an anticholinergic drug approved by the FDA for treating rhinorrhea associated with SAR. Postmarketing experience suggests that there may be some systemic absorption. Cautious uses advised for patients with narrow-angle glaucoma, prostatic hypertrophy, or bladder neck obstruction, particularly if another anticholinergic is coadministered. Local adverse effects may include nosebleeds and nasal and oral dryness.

- Nasal mast cell stabilizers are commonly administered prophylactically, before an allergic reaction is triggered, although as-needed use has been described and maybe of benefit. Cromolyn is the only mast cell stabilizer approved by the FDA for the treatment of SAR. For Prophylaxis, it requires a loading period during which it is applied four times daily for several weeks. Systemic absorption is minimal. Local adverse effects may include nasal irritation, sneezing, and an unpleasant taste.

- Leukotriene receptor antagonists (LTRAs) are oral medications that reduce allergy symptoms by reducing inflammation. Montelukast is the only leukotriene receptor antagonist approved by the FDA for the treatment of SAR. Potential adverse effects include upper respiratory tract infection and headache.

Nasal saline has been shown to be beneficial in treating nasal SAR symptoms. Because it is associated with few adverse effects, nasal saline may be particularly well suited for treating SAR symptoms during pregnancy, in children, and in those whose treatment choices are restricted due to comorbidities, such as hypertension and urinary retention.

The optimal treatment of SAR during pregnancy is unknown. Drugs effective before pregnancy may be effective during pregnancy, but their use may be restricted because of concerns about maternal and fetal safety.

Preferred treatments are Pregnancy Category B drugs (nasal cromolyn, budesonide, and ipratropium; several oral selective and non-selective antihistamines; and the oral leukotriene receptor antagonist montelukast) commencing in the second trimester, after organogenesis.

Section 41.8

Epinephrine Injections for Life-Threatening Allergic Reactions

"Epinephrine Injections for Life-Threatening Allergic Reactions," © 2018 Omnigraphics. Reviewed August 2018.

What Are Epinephrine Injections?

Epinephrine injections are used to treat severe allergic reactions or anaphylaxis. Insect bites or stings, food, latex, medicines, or other allergens can cause life-threatening allergic reactions that require immediate medical treatment. The chemical epinephrine helps relax airways and narrows blood vessels to reverse wheezing, hives, skin itching, severe low blood pressure, and other serious allergic reactions. The medication is only available with a doctor's prescription and can be ordered in injectable or solution form. For individuals with a history of allergic attacks, epinephrine is most conveniently available in an auto-injector.

How Should Epinephrine Injections Be Used?

Epinephrine injections should always be used under the direction of a qualified healthcare provider. The needle or prefilled automatic injection device can be inserted under the skin or into the muscle, most often into the thigh. Injecting into the hands or feet is not recommended, since this can cause side effects resulting in reduced blood flow to those regions. Young children may squirm or flinch when being given an injection, so it's important to hold their legs firmly in position before and after the shot. After use, some residue may remain in the injector, which is normal, but this liquid should not be reused.

Using an Epinephrine Auto-Injector

An epinephrine auto-injector contains a needle kit and the exact dosage of medicine prescribed by a doctor. The device can be used only once and needs to be discarded properly after use. Here are the steps for using an epinephrine auto-injector:

- The auto-injector comes with a safety cap that should not be removed until the patient is ready to use it. To remove the safety cap, grasp the injector with its tip pointing down and pull off the cap.

- To avoid accidental injection, keep fingers away from the tip while removing the cap.

- After removal of the safety cap, place the auto-injector tip on the thigh.

- Inject the dose into the thigh muscle by pushing on the auto-injector, which will release the needle and deliver the medication. Hold the auto-injector in place for about 10 seconds.

- After the injection, remove the auto-injector, and gently massage the area.

- Recap the device and place it into its carrying tube. Then take it to the healthcare provider, who will record how much epinephrine has been used and dispose of the injector properly.

Precautions about the Use of Epinephrine Injections

A number of precautions must be taken while using epinephrine injections, especially if the patient needs to use the medication frequently:

- Be sure to inject doses at regular time intervals as prescribed by a healthcare provider.

- The medication should never be injected into the buttocks muscle or into a vein.

- If a family member is helping the patient with epinephrine injections, that individual needs to understand how to administrate the drug properly.

- To avoid accidental injection, the safety release or end caps should not be removed prior to use.

- Epinephrine auto-injectors come with a "trainer pen," which contains no medicine or needle. The trainer pen is used for practice so that the patient or caregiver can be prepared before an emergency.

- The effects of the medication generally last from 10–20 minutes, and since epinephrine is only a first line of treatment, further observation and consultation with a medical professional is required.

- If the patient does not respond to the first shot of epinephrine, then a second dose could be administered, but only under medical supervision.

- Patients who are prone to allergic reactions should always carry an epinephrine injector with them.

- If the liquid changes color, or if there are solids present in it, the medication should be discarded. Regularly checking the liquid for discoloration or other signs of deterioration is essential.

- The medicine needs to be kept at normal temperature; it should not be refrigerated or allowed to be in direct sunlight or heat.

- The expired medicine should be discarded properly.

- The injection should be kept out of children's reach. They should never be allowed to use it on their own.

- Dosages differ from person to person. The dosage should not be changed by the patient unless advised by a healthcare provider.

Discussion with a Healthcare Provider before Using Epinephrine Injections

A healthcare provider needs to know the detailed health condition of a patient before prescribing epinephrine injections. The following are some of the topics that will be covered:

- If the patient is allergic to sulfites or to any medications.

- All the prescribed and over-the-counter (OTC) medicines the patient is currently taking.

- Whether the patient has associated illnesses, such as Parkinson disease, asthma, diabetes, heart disease, high blood pressure, hyperthyroidism, depression, or irregular heartbeat.

- If the patient is pregnant or breastfeeding.

Side Effects of Epinephrine Injection

Some common side effects include pounding heartbeats, dizziness, feeling weak or tired, pale skin, shivering, headache, or vomiting. If the patient experiences certain side effects like redness of the skin, infection around the injection site, swelling, pain, or warmth, a healthcare provider should be contacted immediately.

References

1. "Epinephrine Injection," U.S. National Library of Medicine (NLM), September 21, 2017.

2. "Epinephrine (Injection Route)," Mayo Clinic, March 1, 2017.

3. "Epinephrine Injection," Drugs.com, September 1, 2017.

4. Wood, Joseph P., MD, Stephen J. Traub, MD, and Christopher Lipinski, MD. "Safety of Epinephrine for Anaphylaxis in the Emergency Setting," U.S. National Library of Medicine (NLM), 2013.

Section 41.9

Anti Immunoglobulin E Therapy

This section contains text excerpted from the following sources: Text beginning with the heading "Monoclonal Antibodies" is excerpted from "Monoclonal Antibodies," LiverTox®, National Institutes of Health (NIH), July 4, 2015; Text under the heading "Omalizumab" is excerpted from "Omalizumab," LiverTox®, National Institutes of Health (NIH), July 5, 2018; Text under the heading "Omalizumab Improves Efficacy of Oral Immunotherapy for Multiple Food Allergies" is excerpted from "Omalizumab Improves Efficacy of Oral Immunotherapy for Multiple Food Allergies," National Institutes of Health (NIH), December 11, 2017.

Monoclonal Antibodies

Monoclonal antibodies (mAb) are antibodies that have a high degree of specificity (mono-specificity) for an antigen or epitope. Monoclonal antibodies are typically derived from a clonal expansion of antibody producing malignant human plasma cells. The initial monoclonal antibodies were created by fusing spleen cells from an immunized mouse with human or mouse myeloma cells (malignant self-perpetuating antibody producing cells), and selecting out and cloning the hybrid cells (hybridomas) that produced the desired antibody reactivity. Initial monoclonal antibodies were mouse antibodies and were very valuable in laboratory and animal research and diagnostic assays, but were problematic as therapeutic agents because of immune reactions to the foreign, mouse protein. Subsequently, production of chimeric mouse-human monoclonal antibodies and means of further "humanizing" them and producing fully human recombinant monoclonal antibodies were developed. The conventions used in the nomenclature of monoclonal antibodies indicate whether they are mouse (-omab), chimeric (-ximab), humanized (-zumab), or fully human (-umab).

Use of Monoclonal Antibodies in Autoimmune Diseases

Monoclonal antibodies have broad clinical and experimental medical uses. Many of the initial monoclonal antibodies used in clinical medicine were immunomodulatory agents with activity against specific immune cells, such as CD4 or CD3 lymphocytes, which are important in the pathogenesis of rejection after solid organ transplantation. Subsequently, monoclonal antibodies were prepared against specific cytokines (anti-cytokines), which were believed to play a role in cell and tissue damage in immunologically mediated diseases such as rheumatoid arthritis, ankylosing spondylitis, inflammatory bowel disease, multiple sclerosis and psoriasis, among others. In addition, therapeutic monoclonal antibodies were developed, aimed at blocking or inhibiting the activity of specific enzymes, cell surface transporters or signaling molecules and have been used in cancer chemotherapy and to treat severe viral infections. Use of monoclonal antibodies is currently broadening to therapy of other severe, nonmalignant conditions including asthma, atopic dermatitis, migraine headaches, hypercholesterolemia, osteoporosis, and viral or bacterial infections. Thus, the therapeutic monoclonal antibodies do not fall into a single class and have broad therapeutic uses. As of 2018, more than 60 therapeutic monoclonal antibodies are approved and in current use in the United States.

Omalizumab

Omalizumab is a recombinant, human monoclonal antibody to IgE which binds avidly to circulating immunoglobulin E, preventing its attachment to high-affinity receptors on mast cells and basophils. This receptor inhibition prevents the release of histamine and other mediators of the allergic immune response, reducing airway inflammation and spasm and alleviating symptoms of asthma and allergic rhinitis. Therapy with omalizumab has been shown to reduce the requirement for inhaled corticosteroids and lower the frequency of exacerbations of asthma and to decrease the severity and symptoms of chronic urticaria of unknown cause. Omalizumab was approved for use in the United States in 2003 for therapy of patients with severe and persistent asthma despite corticosteroid inhalation therapy. The indications were extended in 2014 to include chronic idiopathic urticaria. Omalizumab has been evaluated in patients with seasonal rhinitis, but has yet to be approved for that use. Omalizumab is available in single use vials of 150 mg under the brand name Xolair. The recommended dose is 150–300 mg intravenously every 4 weeks or 225–375 mg every 2 weeks based upon body weight and IgE levels. Common side effects include injection site reactions, rash, diarrhea, nausea and vomiting and epistaxis. Rarely, omalizumab can cause serious acute anaphylaxis or anaphylactoid reactions (~ 0.1%) and should be given under close medical supervision.

Omalizumab Improves Efficacy of Oral Immunotherapy for Multiple Food Allergies

Combining a 16-week initial course of the medication omalizumab with oral immunotherapy (OIT) greatly improves the efficacy of OIT for children with allergies to multiple foods, new clinical trial findings show. After 36 weeks, more than 80 percent of children who received omalizumab and OIT could safely consume two-gram portions of at least two foods to which they were allergic, compared with only a third of children who received placebo and OIT.

Approximately 30 percent of people with food allergy are allergic to multiple foods. Results from the Phase 2 study, funded by the National Institute of Allergy and Infectious Diseases (NIAID), part of the National Institutes of Health (NIH), build on previous work suggesting that omalizumab, an injectable antibody drug approved to treat moderate to severe allergic asthma, can improve the safety and efficacy of OIT for allergies to a single food. Omalizumab blocks the activity of IgE, an immune system molecule central to the allergic response.

Researchers at the Stanford University School of Medicine enrolled 48 participants aged 4–15 years with confirmed allergy to multiple foods, including milk, egg, wheat, soy, sesame seeds, peanut or tree nuts. Participants were randomly assigned to receive omalizumab or placebo injections for the first 16 weeks of the study. At week eight, all participants began daily OIT, an investigational treatment that involves eating small, gradually increasing doses of an allergenic food. They continued OIT until week 36 of the study, at which point they underwent an oral food challenge. Among the 36 children who received omalizumab, 30 (83%) were able to eat at least two grams of two or more foods to which they were allergic, compared with only 4 out of 12 children (33%) who received placebo. Those who received omalizumab also experienced fewer adverse events from OIT during weeks 8–16 of the study.

The findings suggest the potential benefits of using omalizumab to safely and rapidly facilitate desensitization to multiple food allergens. Additional, larger studies will be needed to confirm and expand on these promising results. Neither OIT nor omalizumab (trade name Xolair) currently is approved for the treatment of food allergy.

Section 41.10

Allergy Shots (Immunotherapy) and Allergy Drops for Adults and Children

This section includes text excerpted from "Allergy Shots and Allergy Drops for Adults and Children—A Review of the Research," Agency for Healthcare Research and Quality (AHRQ), U.S. Department of Health and Human Services (HHS), August 2013. Reviewed August 2018.

Allergy Shots or Allergy Drops

This type of treatment works differently than allergy medicines. Allergy shots and drops work to lessen your body's reaction to an allergen. Your doctor may suggest allergy shots or drops to make your symptoms happen less often or to make them less severe.

- **Allergy shots:** shots that are given under the skin (often in the upper arm) usually at the doctor's office.

- **Allergy drops:** a liquid you put under your tongue that you can take at home (this is called "sublingual immunotherapy.")

Table 41.2. Comparing Allergy Shots and Allergy Drops

Conditions	Allergy Shots	Allergy Drops
How are they taken?	The shots are given under the skin (often in the upper arm) usually at the doctor's office.	The liquid drops are placed under the tongue and are usually taken at home.
How often do you take them?	One or more shots each time you go to the doctor's office: • Once or twice a week for the first few months • Once or twice a month after that	A few times a week or every day
How long do you take them?	3–5 years (or sometimes longer)	Typically 3–5 years (or sometimes longer)
Are they approved by the U.S. Food and Drug Administration (FDA) to treat allergies and asthma caused by allergies?	Yes	No, allergy drops are not yet approved by the FDA.* But they are approved and commonly used in Europe and other parts of the world. Allergy drops are available in the United States, and doctors are starting to prescribe them.

* Because allergy drops are not yet approved by the FDA, they may not be covered by your health insurance.

What Are Allergy Shots and Allergy Drops?

Allergy shots and allergy drops help your immune system become less sensitive to allergens. The shots and drops contain a tiny amount of the allergens that cause your allergies. For example, if you are allergic to oak tree pollen, your shots or drops will have a tiny amount of oak tree pollen in them. Allergy shots and drops both contain the allergens that cause your allergies. The difference between them is simply in how they are given.

The amount of the allergen in allergy shots or drops is so small that your immune system likely will not react strongly to it. Your doctor will talk with you about what to do if you have a strong reaction.

Your doctor will slowly put more of the allergen into your shots or drops until your immune system becomes less sensitive to the allergen. This means your immune system will not react strongly when you breathe in the allergen. Over time, your immune system will start to tolerate the allergen, and your allergy symptoms will get better.

Note:

Some people may not be able to take allergy shots or drops. You should talk with your doctor if:

- You (or your child) have severe asthma
- You (or your child) take a type of medicine called a "beta-blocker," used to treat high blood pressure
- You (or your child) have heart problems
- You are pregnant or are thinking of becoming pregnant
- You are considering allergy shots or allergy drops for a child under five years of age

What Have Researchers Found about How Well Allergy Shots and Allergy Drops Work?

In adults:

- Both allergy shots and allergy drops improve allergy and mild asthma symptoms
- Both allergy shots and allergy drops lessen the need to take allergy and asthma medicines
- Both allergy shots and allergy drops improve quality of life

In children:

- Both allergy shots and allergy drops improve allergy and mild asthma symptoms
- Allergy drops lessen the need to take allergy and asthma medicines
- Allergy shots also appear to lessen the need to take allergy and asthma medicines, but more research is needed to know this for sure

Researchers also found:

- There is not enough research to know if allergy shots or allergy drops work better.

What Are the Possible Side Effects of Allergy Shots and Allergy Drops?

Allergy shots and allergy drops are safe, and side effects are usually mild.

Common side effects of allergy shots include:

- Itching, swelling, and redness at the place where the shot was given
- Headache
- Coughing
- Tiredness
- Mucus dripping down your
- Throat
- Sneezing

Common side effects of allergy drops include:

- Throat irritation
- Itching or mild swelling in the mouth

Note: Although it is rare, allergy shots and allergy drops could cause a life-threatening allergic reaction called "anaphylaxis." Symptoms of anaphylaxis can include severe swelling of the face, throat, or tongue; itching; a skin rash; trouble breathing; tightness in the chest; wheezing; dizziness; nausea; diarrhea; or loss of consciousness. If you or your child has any of these symptoms after getting an allergy shot or taking allergy drops, call the doctor right away. Anaphylaxis must be treated immediately with a shot of epinephrine, a type of hormone that regulates your heart rate and breathing passages.

What Are the Costs of Allergy Shots and Allergy Drops?

The costs to you for allergy shots and allergy drops depend on your health insurance. Because allergy drops are not yet approved by the U.S. Food and Drug Administration (FDA), they may not be covered by your health insurance. The costs also depend on how many allergens are in your allergy shots or allergy drops. Because allergy shots are usually given at the doctor's office, you may have to pay for an office visit each time you go for a shot.

Chapter 42

Complementary and Alternative Medicine (CAM) for Allergies

Chapter Contents

Section 42.1

CAM to Treat Allergies

This section contains text excerpted from the following sources:
Text in this section begins with excerpts from "Complementary and
Integrative Medicine," MedlinePlus, National Institutes of Health
(NIH), March 6, 2018; Text under the heading "Six Things to Know
About Complementary Health Approaches for Seasonal Allergy
Relief" is excerpted from "6 Things To Know about Complementary
Health Approaches for Seasonal Allergy Relief," National Center for
Complementary and Integrative Health (NCCIH), March 21, 2017.

Many Americans use medical treatments that are not part of mainstream medicine. When you are using these types of care, it may be called complementary, integrative, or alternative medicine.

Complementary medicine is used together with mainstream medical care. An example is using acupuncture to help with side effects of cancer treatment. When healthcare providers and facilities offer both types of care, it is called integrative medicine. Alternative medicine is used instead of mainstream medical care.

The claims that nonmainstream practitioners make can sound promising. However, researchers do not know how safe many of these treatments are or how well they work. Studies are underway to determine the safety and usefulness of many of these practices.

To minimize the health risks of a nonmainstream treatment:

- Discuss it with your doctor. It might have side effects or interact with other medicines.

- Find out what the research says about it

- Choose practitioners carefully

- Tell all of your doctors and practitioners about all of the different types of treatments you use

Complementary Health Approaches for Seasonal Allergy Relief

Seasonal allergies, also called hay fever or allergic rhinitis, are triggered each spring, summer, and fall when trees, weeds, and grasses release pollen into the air. When the pollen ends up in your nose and throat, it can bring on sneezing, runny nose, coughing, and itchy eyes and throat. People manage seasonal allergies by taking medication, avoiding exposure to the substances that trigger their allergic reactions, or having a series of "allergy shots" (a form of immunotherapy).

People also try various complementary approaches to manage their allergies. If you are considering any complementary health approach for the relief of seasonal allergy symptoms, here are some things you need to know.

1. **Nasal saline irrigation.** There is some good evidence that saline nasal irrigation (putting salt water into one nostril and draining it out the other) can be useful for modest improvement of allergy symptoms. Nasal irrigation is generally safe; however, neti pots and other rinsing devices must be used and cleaned properly. According to the U.S. Food and Drug Administration (FDA), tap water that is not filtered, treated, or processed in specific ways is not safe for use as a nasal rinse.

2. **Butterbur extract.** There are hints that the herb butterbur may decrease the symptoms associated with nasal allergies. However, there are concerns about its safety.

3. **Honey.** Only a few studies have looked at the effects of honey on seasonal allergy symptoms, and there is no convincing scientific evidence that honey provides symptom relief. Eating honey is generally safe; however, children under one year of age should not eat honey. People who are allergic to pollen or bee stings may also be allergic to honey.

4. **Acupuncture.** A evaluation of 13 studies of acupuncture for allergic rhinitis, involving a total of 2,365 participants, found evidence that this approach may be helpful.

5. **Probiotics.** There is some evidence that suggests that probiotics may improve some symptoms, as well as quality of life, in people with allergic rhinitis, but because probiotic formulations vary from study to study, it's difficult to make firm conclusions about its effectiveness.

6. **Talk to your healthcare provider.** If you suffer from seasonal allergies and are considering a complementary health approach, talk to your healthcare provider about the best ways to manage your symptoms. You may find that when the pollen count is high, staying indoors, wearing a mask, or rinsing off when you come inside can help.

Section 42.2

Probiotics as a Complementary Health Approach

This section includes text excerpted from "Probiotics: In Depth," National Center for Complementary and Integrative Health (NCCIH), July 31, 2018.

What Are Probiotics?

Probiotics are live microorganisms that are intended to have health benefits. Products sold as probiotics include foods (such as yogurt), dietary supplements, and products that aren't used orally, such as skin creams.

Although people often think of bacteria and other microorganisms as harmful "germs," many microorganisms help our bodies function properly. For example, bacteria that are normally present in our intestines help digest food, destroy disease-causing microorganisms, and produce vitamins. Large numbers of microorganisms live on and in our bodies. Many of the microorganisms in probiotic products are the same as or similar to microorganisms that naturally live in our bodies.

What Kinds of Microorganisms Are in Probiotics?

Probiotics may contain a variety of microorganisms. The most common are bacteria that belong to groups called *Lactobacillus* and *Bifidobacterium*. Each of these two broad groups includes many types of bacteria. Other bacteria may also be used as probiotics, and so may yeasts such as *Saccharomyces boulardii*.

Probiotics, Prebiotics, and Synbiotics

Prebiotics are not the same as probiotics. The term "prebiotics" refers to dietary substances that favor the growth of beneficial bacteria over harmful ones. The term "synbiotics" refers to products that combine probiotics and prebiotics.

How Popular Are Probiotics?

Data from the 2012 National Health Interview Survey (NHIS) show that about four million (1.6 percent) U.S. adults had used probiotics or prebiotics in the past 30 days. Among adults, probiotics or prebiotics were the third most commonly used dietary supplement other than vitamins and minerals, and the use of probiotics quadrupled between 2007 and 2012. The 2012 NHIS also showed that 300,000 children age 4—17 (0.5 percent) had used probiotics or prebiotics in the 30 days before the survey.

What the Science Says about the Effectiveness of Probiotics

Researchers have studied probiotics to find out whether they might help prevent or treat a variety of health problems, including:

- Digestive disorders such as diarrhea caused by infections, antibiotic-associated diarrhea, irritable bowel syndrome, and inflammatory bowel disease

- Allergic disorders such as atopic dermatitis (eczema) and allergic rhinitis (hay fever)

- Tooth decay, periodontal disease, and other oral health problems

- Colic in infants

- Liver disease

- The common cold

- Prevention of necrotizing enterocolitis in very low birth weight infants.

There's preliminary evidence that some probiotics are helpful in preventing diarrhea caused by infections and antibiotics and in improving symptoms of irritable bowel syndrome, but more needs to be learned. We still don't know which probiotics are helpful and which are not. We also don't know how much of the probiotic people would have to take or who would most likely benefit from taking probiotics. Even for the conditions that have been studied the most, researchers are still working toward finding the answers to these questions.

Probiotics are not all alike. For example, if a specific kind of *Lactobacillus* helps prevent an illness, that doesn't necessarily mean that another kind of *Lactobacillus* would have the same effect or that any of the *Bifidobacterium* probiotics would do the same thing.

Although some probiotics have shown promise in research studies, strong scientific evidence to support specific uses of probiotics for most health conditions is lacking. The U.S. Food and Drug Administration

(FDA) has not approved any probiotics for preventing or treating any health problem. Some experts have cautioned that the rapid growth in marketing and use of probiotics may have outpaced scientific research for many of their proposed uses and benefits.

Section 42.3

Saline Nasal Sprays and Irrigation

This section contains text excerpted from the following sources: Text in this section begins with excerpts from "The Common Cold and Complementary Health Approaches: What the Science Says," National Center for Complementary and Integrative Health (NCCIH), August 2017; Text beginning with the heading "Rinsing Your Sinuses with Neti Pots" is excerpted from "Is Rinsing Your Sinuses with Neti Pots Safe?" U.S. Food and Drug Administration (FDA), January 24, 2017.

Saline nasal irrigation may have benefits for relieving symptoms of the common cold in children and adults, and may have potential benefits for relieving some symptoms of acute upper respiratory infection.

What Does the Research Show?

Several randomized controlled trials in both children and adults, as well as a Cochrane review, have been conducted to examine the effects of saline nasal irrigation on the common cold.

- A Cochrane review of five randomized controlled trials involving 544 children and 205 adults found that nasal saline irrigation possibly has benefits for relieving the symptoms of acute upper respiratory tract infections; however, the trials included in the review were generally too small and had a high risk of bias.

- A review in children concluded that during acute illness, saline nasal irrigation can help alleviate sore throat, thin nasal secretions, and improve nasal breathing, and can reduce the need for nasal decongestants and mucolytics.

Rinsing Your Sinuses with Neti Pots

Little teapots with long spouts have become a fixture in many homes to flush out clogged nasal passages and help people breathe easier.

Along with other nasal irrigation systems, these devices—commonly called neti pots—use a saline, or saltwater, solution to treat congested sinuses, colds and allergies. They're also used to moisten nasal passages exposed to dry indoor air. But be careful. According to the U.S. Food and Drug Administration (FDA), improper use of these neti pots and other nasal rinsing devices can increase your risk of infection.

These nasal rinse devices—which include bulb syringes, squeeze bottles, and battery-operated pulsed water devices—are usually safe and effective products when used and cleaned properly, says Eric A. Mann, MD, PhD, a doctor at FDA.

What Does Safe Use Mean?

First, rinse only with distilled, sterile or previously boiled water.

Tap water isn't safe for use as a nasal rinse because it's not adequately filtered or treated. Some tap water contains low levels of organisms—such as bacteria and protozoa, including amoebas—that may be safe to swallow because stomach acid kills them. But in your nose, these organisms can stay alive in nasal passages and cause potentially serious infections. They can even be fatal in some rare cases, according to the Centers for Disease Control and Prevention (CDC).

What Types of Water Are Safe to Use?

- Distilled or sterile water, which you can buy in stores. The label will state "distilled" or "sterile."

- Boiled and cooled tap water—boiled for 3–5 minutes, then cooled until it is lukewarm. Previously boiled water can be stored in a clean, closed container for use within 24 hours.

- Water passed through a filter designed to trap potentially infectious organisms.

Safely Use Nasal Irrigation Systems

Second, make sure you follow instructions.

"There are various ways to deliver saline to the nose. Nasal spray bottles deliver a fine mist and might be useful for moisturizing dry nasal passages. But irrigation devices are better at flushing the nose and clearing out mucus, allergens and bacteria," Mann says.

Information included with the irrigation device might give more specific instructions about its use and care. These devices all work in basically the same way:

- Leaning over a sink, tilt your head sideways with your forehead and chin roughly level to avoid liquid flowing into your mouth.

- Breathing through your open mouth, insert the spout of the saline-filled container into your upper nostril so that the liquid drains through the lower nostril.

- Clear your nostrils. Then repeat the procedure, tilting your head sideways, on the other side.

Sinus rinsing can remove dust, pollen and other debris, as well as help to loosen thick mucus. It can also help relieve nasal symptoms of sinus infections, allergies, colds and flu. Plain water can irritate your nose. The saline allows the water to pass through delicate nasal membranes with little or no burning or irritation.

And if your immune system isn't working properly, consult your healthcare provider before using any nasal irrigation systems.

To use and care for your device:

- Wash and dry your hands.

- Check that the device is clean and completely dry.

- Prepare the saline rinse, either with the prepared mixture supplied with the device, or one you make yourself.

- Follow the manufacturer's directions for use.

- Wash the device, and dry the inside with a paper towel or let it air dry between uses.

Talk with a healthcare provider or pharmacist if the instructions on your device do not clearly state how to use it or if you have any questions.

Nasal Rinsing Devices and Children

Finally, make sure the device fits the age of the person using it. Some children are diagnosed with nasal allergies as early as age 2 and could use nasal rinsing devices at that time, if a pediatrician recommends it. But very young children might not tolerate the procedure.

Whether for a child or adult, talk to your healthcare provider to determine whether nasal rinsing will be safe or effective for your condition. If symptoms are not relieved or worsen after nasal rinsing, then return to your healthcare provider, especially if you have fever, nosebleeds or headaches while using the nasal rinse.

Healthcare professionals and patients can report problems about nasal rinsing devices to the FDA's MedWatch Safety Information and Adverse Event Reporting Program.

Part Six

Avoiding Allergy Triggers and Preventing Symptoms

Chapter 43

A Guide to Indoor Air Quality

Section 43.1

Indoor Air Quality in Your Home

This section includes text excerpted from "The Inside Story:
A Guide to Indoor Air Quality," U.S. Environmental
Protection Agency (EPA), April 27, 2018.

All of us face a variety of risks to our health as we go about our day-to-day lives. Driving in cars, flying in planes, engaging in recreational activities, and being exposed to environmental pollutants all pose varying degrees of risk. Some risks are simply unavoidable. Some we choose to accept because to do otherwise would restrict our ability to lead our lives the way we want. And some are risks we might decide to avoid if we had the opportunity to make informed choices. Indoor air pollution is one risk that you can do something about.

In the last several years, a growing body of scientific evidence has indicated that the air within homes and other buildings can be more seriously polluted than the outdoor air in even the largest and most industrialized cities. Other research indicates that people spend approximately 90 percent of their time indoors. Thus, for many people, the risks to health may be greater due to exposure to air pollution indoors than outdoors.

In addition, people who may be exposed to indoor air pollutants for the longest periods of time are often those most susceptible to the effects of indoor air pollution. Such groups include the young, the elderly and the chronically ill, especially those suffering from respiratory or cardiovascular disease.

What Causes Indoor Air Problems?

Indoor pollution sources that release gases or particles into the air are the primary cause of indoor air quality problems in homes. Inadequate ventilation can increase indoor pollutant levels by not bringing in enough outdoor air to dilute emissions from indoor sources and by not carrying indoor air pollutants out of the home. High temperature and humidity levels can also increase concentrations of some pollutants.

Pollutant Sources

There are many sources of indoor air pollution in any home. These include combustion sources such as:

- Oil

- Gas

- Kerosene

- Coal

- Wood

- Tobacco products

- Building materials and furnishings as diverse as deteriorated, asbestos-containing insulation, wet or damp carpet and cabinetry or furniture made of certain pressed wood products

- Products for household cleaning and maintenance, personal care, or hobbies

- Central heating and cooling systems and humidification devices

- Outdoor sources such as radon, pesticides, and outdoor air pollution

The relative importance of any single source depends on how much of a given pollutant it emits and how hazardous those emissions are. In some cases, factors such as how old the source is and whether it is properly maintained are significant. For example, an improperly adjusted gas stove can emit significantly more carbon monoxide (CO) than one that is properly adjusted.

Some sources, such as building materials, furnishings and household products like air fresheners, release pollutants more or less continuously. Other sources, related to activities carried out in the home, release pollutants intermittently. These include smoking, the use of unvented or malfunctioning stoves, furnaces, or space heaters, the use of solvents in cleaning and hobby activities, the use of paint strippers in redecorating activities and the use of cleaning products and pesticides in housekeeping. High pollutant concentrations can remain in the air for long periods after some of these activities.

Amount of Ventilation

If too little outdoor air enters a home, pollutants can accumulate to levels that can pose health and comfort problems. Unless they are built with special mechanical means of ventilation, homes that are designed and constructed to minimize the amount of outdoor air that can "leak" into and out of the home may have higher pollutant levels than other homes. However, because some weather conditions can drastically reduce the amount of outdoor air that enters a home, pollutants can build up even in homes that are normally considered "leaky."

How Does Outdoor Air Enter a House?

Outdoor air enters and leaves a house by: infiltration, natural ventilation and mechanical ventilation. In a process known as infiltration, outdoor air flows into the house through:

• Openings

• Joints

• Cracks in walls, floors, and ceilings

• Around windows and doors

In natural ventilation, air moves through opened windows and doors. Air movement associated with infiltration and natural ventilation is caused by air temperature differences between indoors and outdoors and by wind. Finally, there are a number of mechanical ventilation devices, from outdoor-vented fans that intermittently remove air from a single room, such as bathrooms and kitchen, to air handling systems that use fans and duct work to continuously remove indoor air and distribute filtered and conditioned outdoor air to strategic points throughout the house. The rate at which outdoor air replaces indoor air is described as the air exchange rate. When there is little infiltration, natural ventilation, or mechanical ventilation, the air exchange rate is low and pollutant levels can increase.

What If You Live in an Apartment?

Apartments can have the same indoor air problems as single-family homes because many of the pollution sources, such as the interior building materials, furnishings, and household products, are similar. Indoor air problems similar to those in offices are caused by such sources as contaminated ventilation systems, improperly placed outdoor air intakes, or maintenance activities.

Solutions to air quality problems in apartments, as in homes and offices, involve such actions as eliminating or controlling the sources of pollution, increasing ventilation, and installing air cleaning devices. Often a resident can take the appropriate action to improve the indoor air quality by removing a source, altering an activity, unblocking an air supply vent, or opening a window to temporarily increase the ventilation; in other cases, however, only the building owner or manager is in a position to remedy the problem.

- You can encourage building management to follow guidance in the U.S. Environmental Protection Agency's (EPA) Indoor Air Quality (IAQ) Building Education and Assessment Model (I-BEAM) (www.epa.gov/indoor-air-quality-iaq/ indoor-air-quality-building-education-and-assessment-model).

    - I-BEAM updates and expands the EPA's existing Building Air Quality guidance and is designed to be comprehensive state-of-the-art guidance for managing IAQ in commercial buildings. This guidance was designed to be used by building professionals and others interested in indoor air quality in commercial buildings. I-BEAM contains text, animation/ visual and interactive/calculation components that can be used to perform a number of diverse tasks.

- You can also encourage building management to follow guidance in the *EPA and National Institute for Occupational Safety and Health (NIOSH) Building Air Quality: A Guide for Building Owners and Facility Managers* (www.epa.gov/indoor-air-quality-iaq/building-air-quality-guide-guide-building-owners-and-facility-managers).

Indoor Air and Your Health

Health effects from indoor air pollutants may be experienced soon after exposure or, possibly, years later.

Immediate effects may show up after a single exposure or repeated exposures. These include irritation of the eyes, nose and throat, headaches, dizziness, and fatigue. Such immediate effects are usually short-term and treatable. Sometimes the treatment is simply eliminating the person's exposure to the source of the pollution, if it can be identified. Symptoms of some diseases, including asthma, hypersensitivity pneumonitis (HP), and humidifier fever, may also show up soon after exposure to some indoor air pollutants.

The likelihood of immediate reactions to indoor air pollutants depends on several factors. Age and preexisting medical conditions are two important influences. In other cases, whether a person reacts to a pollutant depends on individual sensitivity, which varies tremendously from person to person. Some people can become sensitized to biological pollutants after repeated exposures, and it appears that some people can become sensitized to chemical pollutants as well.

Certain immediate effects are similar to those from colds or other viral diseases, so it is often difficult to determine if the symptoms are a result of exposure to indoor air pollution. For this reason, it is important to pay attention to the time and place the symptoms occur. If the symptoms fade or go away when a person is away from the home and return when the person returns, an effort should be made to identify indoor air sources that may be possible causes. Some effects may be made worse by an inadequate supply of outdoor air or from the heating, cooling, or humidity conditions prevalent in the home.

Other health effects may show up either years after exposure has occurred or only after long or repeated periods of exposure. These effects, which include some respiratory diseases, heart disease, and cancer, can be severely debilitating or fatal. It is prudent to try to improve the indoor air quality in your home even if symptoms are not noticeable.

While pollutants commonly found in indoor air are responsible for many harmful effects, there is considerable uncertainty about what concentrations or periods of exposure are necessary to produce specific health problems. People also react very differently to exposure to indoor air pollutants. Further research is needed to better understand which health effects occur after exposure to the average pollutant concentrations found in homes and which occur from the higher concentrations that occur for short periods of time.

Identifying Air Quality Problems

Some health effects can be useful indicators of an indoor air quality problem, especially if they appear after a person moves to a new residence, remodels or refurnishes a home, or treats a home with pesticides. If you think that you have symptoms that may be related to your home environment, discuss them with your doctor or your local health department to see if they could be caused by indoor air pollution. You may also want to consult a board-certified allergist or an occupational medicine specialist for answers to your questions.

Another way to judge whether your home has or could develop indoor air problems is to identify potential sources of indoor air pollution. Although the presence of such sources does not necessarily mean that you have an indoor air quality problem, being aware of the type and number of potential sources is an important step toward assessing the air quality in your home.

A third way to decide whether your home may have poor indoor air quality is to look at your lifestyle and activities. Human activities can be significant sources of indoor air pollution. Finally, look for signs of problems with the ventilation in your home. Signs that can indicate your home may not have enough ventilation include moisture condensation on windows or walls, smelly or stuffy air, dirty central heating and air cooling equipment, and areas where books, shoes, or other items become moldy. To detect odors in your home, step outside for a few minutes, and then upon re-entering your home, note whether odors are noticeable.

Measuring Radon Levels

The federal government recommends that you measure the level of radon in your home. Without measurements there is no way to tell whether radon is present because it is a colorless, odorless, radioactive gas. Inexpensive devices are available for measuring radon. EPA provides guidance as to risks associated with different levels of exposure and when the public should consider corrective action. There are specific mitigation techniques that have proven effective in reducing levels of radon in the home.

For pollutants other than radon, measurements are most appropriate when there are either health symptoms or signs of poor ventilation and specific sources or pollutants have been identified as possible causes of indoor air quality problems. Testing for many pollutants can be expensive. Before monitoring your home for pollutants besides radon, consult your state or local health department or professionals who have experience in solving indoor air quality problems in nonindustrial buildings.

Weatherizing Your Home

The federal government recommends that homes be weatherized in order to reduce the amount of energy needed for heating and cooling. While weatherization is underway, however, steps should also be taken to minimize pollution from sources inside the home.

In addition, residents should be alert to the emergence of signs of inadequate ventilation, such as stuffy air, moisture condensation on cold surfaces, or mold and mildew growth.

Additional weatherization measures should not be undertaken until these problems have been corrected.

Weatherization generally does not cause indoor air problems by adding new pollutants to the air. (There are a few exceptions, such as caulking, that can sometimes emit pollutants.) However, measures such as installing storm windows, weather stripping, caulking, and blown-in wall insulation can reduce the amount of outdoor air infiltrating into a home. Consequently, after weatherization, concentrations of indoor air pollutants from sources inside the home can increase.

Three Basic Strategies

Source Control

Usually the most effective way to improve indoor air quality is to eliminate individual sources of pollution or to reduce their emissions. Some sources, like those that contain asbestos, can be sealed or enclosed; others, like gas stoves, can be adjusted to decrease the amount of emissions. In many cases, source control is also a more cost-efficient approach to protecting indoor air quality than increasing ventilation because increasing ventilation can increase energy costs.

Ventilation Improvements

Another approach to lowering the concentrations of indoor air pollutants in your home is to increase the amount of outdoor air coming indoors. Most home heating and cooling systems, including forced air heating systems, do not mechanically bring fresh air into the house. Opening windows and doors, operating window or attic fans, when the weather permits, or running a window air conditioner with the vent control open increases the outdoor ventilation rate. Local bathroom or kitchen fans that exhaust outdoors remove contaminants directly from the room where the fan is located and also increase the outdoor air ventilation rate.

It is particularly important to take as many of these steps as possible while you are involved in short-term activities that can generate high levels of pollutants—for example, painting, paint stripping, heating with kerosene heaters, cooking, or engaging in maintenance and hobby activities such as welding, soldering, or sanding. You might also choose to do some of these activities outdoors, if you can and if weather permits.

Advanced designs of new homes are starting to feature mechanical systems that bring outdoor air into the home. Some of these designs include energy-efficient heat recovery ventilators (also known as air-to-air heat exchangers).

Air Cleaners

There are many types and sizes of air cleaners on the market, ranging from relatively inexpensive tabletop models to sophisticated and expensive whole-house systems. Some air cleaners are highly effective at particle removal, while others, including most tabletop models, are much less so. Air cleaners are generally not designed to remove gaseous pollutants.

The effectiveness of an air cleaner depends on how well it collects pollutants from indoor air (expressed as a percentage efficiency rate) and how much air it draws through the cleaning or filtering element (expressed in cubic feet per minute). A very efficient collector with a low air-circulation rate will not be effective, nor will a cleaner with a high air-circulation rate but a less efficient collector. The long-term performance of any air cleaner depends on maintaining it according to the manufacturer's directions.

Another important factor in determining the effectiveness of an air cleaner is the strength of the pollutant source. Tabletop air cleaners, in particular, may not remove satisfactory amounts of pollutants from strong nearby sources. People with a sensitivity to particular sources may find that air cleaners are helpful only in conjunction with concerted efforts to remove the source.

Over the past few years, there has been some publicity suggesting that houseplants have been shown to reduce levels of some chemicals in laboratory experiments. There is currently no evidence, however, that a reasonable number of houseplants remove significant quantities of pollutants in homes and offices. Indoor houseplants should not be over-watered because overly damp soil may promote the growth of microorganisms which can affect allergic individuals.

At present, the EPA does not recommend using air cleaners to reduce levels of radon and its decay products. The effectiveness of these devices is uncertain because they only partially remove the radon decay products and do not diminish the amount of radon entering the home. The EPA plans to do additional research on whether air cleaners are, or could become, a reliable means of reducing the health risk from radon. For most indoor air quality problems in the home, source control is the most effective solution.

- Ozone Generators That Are Sold As Air Cleaners (www.epa.gov/indoor-air-quality-iaq/ozone-generators-are-sold-air-cleaners) was prepared by the EPA to provide accurate information regarding the use of ozone-generating devices in indoor occupied spaces.

- "Should You Have the Air Ducts in Your Home Cleaned?" (www.
  epa.gov/indoor-air-quality-iaq/should-you-have-air-ducts-your-
  home-cleaned) was prepared by the EPA to assist consumers in
  answering this often confusing question. The document explains
  what air duct cleaning is, provides guidance to help consumers
  decide whether to have the service performed in their home,
  and provides helpful information for choosing a duct cleaner,
  determining if duct cleaning was done properly, and how to
  prevent contamination of air ducts.

Section 43.2

A Look at Source-Specific Controls

This section includes text excerpted from "The Inside Story:
A Guide to Indoor Air Quality," U.S. Environmental
Protection Agency (EPA), April 27, 2018.

Radon (Rn)

The most common source of indoor radon is uranium in the soil or
rock on which homes are built. As uranium naturally breaks down,
it releases radon gas which is a colorless, odorless, radioactive gas.
Radon gas enters homes through dirt floors, cracks in concrete walls
and floors, floor drains and sumps. When radon becomes trapped in
buildings and concentrations build up indoors, exposure to radon
becomes a concern.

Any home may have a radon problem. This means new and old
homes, well-sealed and drafty homes, and homes with or without
basements.

Sometimes radon enters the home through well water. In a small
number of homes, the building materials can give off radon, too. However, building materials rarely cause radon problems by themselves.

Health Effects of Radon

The predominant health effect associated with exposure to elevated
levels of radon is lung cancer. Research suggests that swallowing

water with high radon levels may pose risks, too, although these are believed to be much lower than those from breathing air containing radon. Major health organizations (like the Centers for Disease Control and Prevention (CDC), the American Lung Association (ALA), and the American Medical Association) agree with estimates that radon causes thousands of preventable lung cancer deaths each year. The EPA estimates that radon causes about 14,000 deaths per year in the United States—however, this number could range from 7,000–30,000 deaths per year. If you smoke and your home has high radon levels, your risk of lung cancer is especially high.

Reducing Exposure to Radon in Homes

Measure Levels of Radon in Your Home

You can't see radon, but it's not hard to find out if you have a radon problem in your home. Testing is easy and should only take a little of your time. There are many kinds of inexpensive, do-it-yourself radon test kits you can get through the mail and in hardware stores and other retail outlets. The EPA recommends that consumers use test kits that are state-certified or have met the requirements of some national radon proficiency program.

If you prefer, or if you are buying or selling a home, you can hire a trained contractor to do the testing for you:

- You should call your state radon office to obtain a list of qualified contractors in your area.

- You can also contact either the National Radon Proficiency Program, or NRPP or the National Radon Safety Board, or NRSB for a list of proficient radon measurement and/or mitigation contractors.

Learn about Radon Reduction Methods

Ways to reduce radon in your home are discussed in the EPA's "Consumer's Guide to Radon Reduction" (www.epa.gov/radon/con- sumers-guide-radon-reduction-how-fix-your-home). There are simple solutions to radon problems in homes. Thousands of homeowners have already fixed radon problems. Lowering high radon levels requires technical knowledge and special skills. You should use a contractor who is trained to fix radon problems.

A trained radon reduction contractor can study the problem in your home and help you pick the correct treatment method.

- Check with your state radon office for names of qualified or state-certified radon-reduction contractors in your area.

Stop Smoking and Discourage Smoking in Your Home

Scientific evidence indicates that smoking combined with radon is an especially serious health risk. Stop smoking and lower your radon level to reduce lung cancer risk.

Treat Radon-Contaminated Well Water

While radon in water is not a problem in homes served by most public water supplies, it has been found in well water. If you've tested the air in your home and found a radon problem, and you have a well, contact a lab certified to measure radiation in water to have your water tested. Radon problems in water can be readily fixed.

- Call your state radon office or the EPA Drinking Water Hotline (800-426-4791) for more information.

Environmental Tobacco Smoke

Environmental Tobacco Smoke (ETS) is the mixture of smoke that comes from the burning end of a cigarette, pipe, or cigar and smoke exhaled by the smoker. It is a complex mixture of over 4,000 compounds, more than 40 of which are known to cause cancer in humans or animals and many of which are strong irritants. ETS is often referred to as "secondhand smoke" and exposure to ETS is often called "passive smoking."

Health Effects of Environmental Tobacco Smoke

In 1992, the EPA completed a major assessment of the respiratory health risks of ETS. The report concludes that exposure to ETS is responsible for approximately 3,000 lung cancer deaths each year in nonsmoking adults and impairs the respiratory health of hundreds of thousands of children.

Infants and young children whose parents smoke in their presence are at increased risk of lower respiratory tract infections (pneumonia and bronchitis) and are more likely to have symptoms of respiratory irritation like cough, excess phlegm, and wheeze. The EPA estimates that passive smoking annually causes between 150,000 and 300,000 lower respiratory tract infections in infants and children under 18 months of age, resulting in between 7,500 and 15,000 hospitalizations each year. These children may also have a buildup of fluid in the middle ear, which can lead to ear infections. Older children who have been exposed to secondhand smoke may have slightly reduced lung function.

Asthmatic children are especially at risk. The EPA estimates that exposure to secondhand smoke increases the number of episodes and severity of symptoms in hundreds of thousands of asthmatic children, and may cause thousands of nonasthmatic children to develop the disease each year. The EPA estimates that between 200,000 and 1,000,000 asthmatic children have their condition made worse by exposure to secondhand smoke each year. Exposure to secondhand smoke causes eye, nose, and throat irritation. It may affect the cardiovascular system and some studies have linked exposure to secondhand smoke with the onset of chest pain.

Reducing Exposure to Environmental Tobacco Smoke

- Don't smoke at home or permit others to do so. Ask smokers to smoke outdoors. The 1986 Surgeon General's report concluded that physical separation of smokers and nonsmokers in a common air space, such as different rooms within the same house, may reduce—but will not eliminate—nonsmokers' exposure to environmental tobacco smoke.

- If smoking indoors cannot be avoided, increase ventilation in the area where smoking takes place. Open windows or use exhaust fans. Ventilation, a common method of reducing exposure to indoor air pollutants, also will reduce but not eliminate exposure to environmental tobacco smoke. Because smoking produces such large amounts of pollutants, natural, or mechanical ventilation techniques do not remove them from the air in your home as quickly as they build up. In addition, the large increases in ventilation it takes to significantly reduce exposure to environmental tobacco smoke can also increase energy costs substantially. Consequently, the most effective way to reduce exposure to environmental tobacco smoke in the home is to eliminate smoking there.

- Do not smoke if children are present, particularly infants and toddlers. Children are particularly susceptible to the effects of passive smoking. Do not allow babysitters or others who work in your home to smoke indoors. Discourage others from smoking around children. Find out about the smoking policies of the day care center providers, schools and other caregivers for your children. The policy should protect children from exposure to ETS.

Biological Contaminants

Biological contaminants include:

- Bacteria

- Molds

- Mildew

- Viruses

- Animal dander and cat saliva

- House dust mites

- Cockroaches

- Pollen

There are many sources of these pollutants. Pollen originate from plants; viruses are transmitted by people and animals; bacteria are carried by people, animals and soil; and plant debris; and household pets are sources of saliva and animal dander. The protein in urine from rats and mice is a potent allergen. When it dries, it can become airborne. Contaminated central air handling systems can become breeding grounds for mold, mildew, and other sources of biological contaminants and can then distribute these contaminants through the home.

By controlling the relative humidity level in a home, the growth of some sources of biologicals can be minimized. A relative humidity of 30–50 percent is generally recommended for homes. Standing water, water-damaged materials, or wet surfaces also serve as a breeding ground for molds, mildews, bacteria, and insects. House dust mites, the source of one of the most powerful biological allergens, grow in damp, warm environments.

Health Effects from Biological Contaminants

Some biological contaminants trigger allergic reactions, including hypersensitivity pneumonitis, allergic rhinitis, and some types of asthma. Infectious illnesses, such as influenza, measles, and chickenpox are transmitted through the air. Molds and mildews release disease-causing toxins. Symptoms of health problems caused by biological pollutants include sneezing, watery eyes, coughing, shortness of breath, dizziness, lethargy, fever, and digestive problems.

Allergic reactions occur only after repeated exposure to a specific biological allergen. However, that reaction may occur immediately upon re-exposure or after multiple exposures over time. As a result, people who have noticed only mild allergic reactions, or no reactions at all, may suddenly find themselves very sensitive to particular allergens.

Some diseases, like humidifier fever, are associated with exposure to toxins from microorganisms that can grow in large building ventilation systems. However, these diseases can also be traced to microorganisms that grow in home heating and cooling systems and humidifiers. Children, elderly people and people with breathing problems, allergies and lung diseases are particularly susceptible to disease-causing biological agents in the indoor air.

Reducing Exposure to Biological Contaminants

- Install and use exhaust fans that are vented to the outdoors in kitchens and bathrooms and vent clothes dryers outdoors. These actions can eliminate much of the moisture that builds up from everyday activities. There are exhaust fans on the market that produce little noise, an important consideration for some people. Another benefit to using kitchen and bathroom exhaust fans is that they can reduce levels of organic pollutants that vaporize from hot water used in showers and dishwashers.

- Ventilate the attic and crawl spaces to prevent moisture buildup. Keeping humidity levels in these areas below 50 percent can prevent water condensation on building materials.

- If using cool mist or ultrasonic humidifiers, clean appliances according to manufacturer's instructions and refill with fresh water daily. Because these humidifiers can become breeding grounds for biological contaminants, they have the potential for causing diseases such as hypersensitivity pneumonitis and humidifier fever. Evaporation trays in air conditioners, dehumidifiers and refrigerators should also be cleaned frequently.

- Thoroughly clean and dry water-damaged carpets and building materials (within 24 hours if possible) or consider removal and replacement. Water-damaged carpets and building materials can harbor mold and bacteria. It is very difficult to completely rid such materials of biological contaminants.

- Keep the house clean. House dust mites, pollen, animal dander, and other allergy-causing agents can be reduced, although not eliminated, through regular cleaning. People who are allergic to these pollutants should use allergen-proof mattress encasement, wash bedding in hot (130°F) water and avoid room furnishings that accumulate dust, especially if they cannot be washed in hot water. Allergic individuals should also leave the house while it is being vacuumed because vacuuming can actually increase airborne levels of mite allergens and other biological contaminants. Using central vacuum systems that are vented to the outdoors or vacuums with high efficiency filters may also be of help.

- Take steps to minimize biological pollutants in basements. Clean and disinfect the basement floor drain regularly. Do not finish a basement below ground level unless all water leaks are patched and outdoor ventilation and adequate heat to prevent condensation are provided. Operate a dehumidifier in the basement if needed to keep relative humidity levels between 30–50 percent.

Stoves, Heaters, Fireplaces, and Chimneys

In addition to environmental tobacco smoke, other sources of combustion products are:

- Unvented kerosene and gas space heaters
- Wood stoves
- Fireplaces
- Gas stoves

The major pollutants released are:

- Carbon monoxide (CO)
- Nitrogen dioxide (NO_2)
- Particles

Unvented kerosene heaters may also generate acid aerosols. Combustion gases and particles also come from chimneys and flues that are improperly installed or maintained and cracked furnace heat exchangers. Pollutants from fireplaces and woodstoves with no dedicated outdoor air supply can be "back-drafted" from the chimney into the living space, particularly in weatherized homes.

Health Effects of Combustion Products

Carbon monoxide (CO) is a colorless, odorless gas that interferes with the delivery of oxygen throughout the body. At high concentrations it can cause unconsciousness and death. Lower concentrations can cause a range of symptoms, including:

- Headaches
- Dizziness
- Weakness
- Nausea
- Confusion
- Disorientation
- Fatigue in healthy people
- Episodes of increased chest pain in people with chronic heart disease

The symptoms of carbon monoxide poisoning are sometimes confused with the flu or food poisoning. Fetuses, infants, elderly people, and people with anemia or with a history of heart or respiratory disease can be especially sensitive to carbon monoxide exposures.

Nitrogen dioxide (NO_2) is a reddish-brown, irritating odor gas that irritates the mucous membranes in the eye, nose and throat, and causes shortness of breath after exposure to high concentrations. There is evidence that high concentrations or continued exposure to low levels of nitrogen dioxide increases the risk of respiratory infection; there is also evidence from animal studies that repeated exposures to elevated nitrogen dioxide levels may lead, or contribute, to the development of lung disease such as emphysema. People at particular risk from exposure to nitrogen dioxide include children and individuals with asthma and other respiratory diseases.

Particles, released when fuels are incompletely burned, can lodge in the lungs and irritate or damage lung tissue. A number of pollutants, including radon and benzo(a)pyrene, both of which can cause cancer, attach to small particles that are inhaled and then carried deep into the lung.

Reducing Exposure to Combustion Products in Homes

- Take special precautions when operating fuel-burning unvented space heaters. Consider potential effects of indoor air pollution if you use an unvented kerosene or gas space heater. Follow the manufacturer's directions, especially instructions on the proper fuel and keeping the heater properly adjusted. A persistent yellow-tipped flame is generally an indicator of maladjustment and increased pollutant emissions. While a space heater is in use, open a door from the room where the heater is located to the rest of the house and open a window slightly.

- Install and use exhaust fans over gas cooking stoves and ranges and keep the burners properly adjusted. Using a stove hood with a fan vented to the outdoors greatly reduces exposure to pollutants during cooking. Improper adjustment, often indicated by a persistent yellow-tipped flame, causes increased pollutant emissions. Ask your gas company to adjust the burner so that the flame tip is blue. If you purchase a new gas stove or range, consider buying one with pilotless ignition because it does not have a pilot light that burns continuously. Never use a gas stove to heat your home. Always make certain the flue in your gas fireplace is open when the fireplace is in use.

- Keep wood stove emissions to a minimum. Choose properly sized new stoves that are certified as meeting EPA emission standards. Make certain that doors in old wood stoves are tight-fitting. Use aged or cured (dried) wood only and follow the manufacturer's directions for starting, stoking, and putting out the fire in woodstoves. Chemicals are used to pressure-treat wood; such wood should never be burned indoors. (Because some old gaskets in wood stove doors contain asbestos, when replacing gaskets refer to the instructions in the Consumer Product Safety Commission (CPSC), the American Lung Association (ALA) and the EPA, to avoid creating an asbestos problem. New gaskets are made of fiberglass.)

- Have central air handling systems, including furnaces, flues and chimneys, inspected annually and promptly repair cracks or damaged parts. Blocked, leaking, or damaged chimneys or flues release harmful combustion gases and particles and even fatal concentrations of carbon monoxide. Strictly follow all service and maintenance procedures recommended by the manufacturer, including those that tell you how frequently to change the filter.

If manufacturer's instructions are not readily available, change filters once every month or two during periods of use. Proper maintenance is important even for new furnaces because they can also corrode and leak combustion gases, including carbon monoxide.

Section 43.3

Household Products

This section includes text excerpted from "The Inside Story: A Guide to Indoor Air Quality," U.S. Environmental Protection Agency (EPA), April 27, 2018.

Organic chemicals are widely used as ingredients in household products. Paints, varnishes and wax all contain organic solvents, as do many cleaning, disinfecting, cosmetic, degreasing, and hobby products. Fuels are made up of organic chemicals. All of these products can release organic compounds while you are using them, and, to some degree, when they are stored.

The U.S. Environmental Protection Agency's (EPA) Total Exposure Assessment Methodology (TEAM) studies found levels of about a dozen common organic pollutants to be two to five times higher inside homes than outside, regardless of whether the homes were located in rural or highly industrial areas. Additional TEAM studies indicate that while people are using products containing organic chemicals, they can expose themselves and others to very high pollutant levels and elevated concentrations can persist in the air long after the activity is completed.

Health Effects of Household Products

The ability of organic chemicals to cause health effects varies greatly, from those that are highly toxic, to those with no known health effect. As with other pollutants, the extent and nature of the health effect will depend on many factors including level of exposure and length of time exposed. Eye and respiratory tract irritation, headaches, dizziness, visual disorders, and memory impairment are among the immediate symptoms that some people have experienced soon after exposure to some organics. At present, not much is known about what health effects occur from the levels of organics usually found in homes. Many organic compounds are known to cause cancer in animals; some are suspected of causing, or are known to cause, cancer in humans.

Reducing Exposure to Household Chemicals

- Follow label instructions carefully. Potentially hazardous products often have warnings aimed at reducing exposure of the user. For example, if a label says to use the product in a well-ventilated area, go outdoors or in areas equipped with an exhaust fan to use it. Otherwise, open up windows to provide the maximum amount of outdoor air possible.

- Throw away partially full containers of old or unneeded chemicals safely. Because gases can leak even from closed containers, this single step could help lower concentrations of organic chemicals in your home. (Be sure that materials you decide to keep are stored not only in a well-ventilated area but are also safely out of reach of children.) Do not simply toss these unwanted products in the garbage can. Find out if your local government or any organization in your community sponsors special days for the collection of toxic household wastes. If such days are available, use them to dispose of the unwanted containers safely. If no such collection days are available, think about organizing one.

- Buy limited quantities. If you use products only occasionally or seasonally, such as paints, paint strippers, and kerosene for space heaters or gasoline for lawn mowers, buy only as much as you will use right away.

- Keep exposure to emissions from products containing methylene chloride to a minimum. Consumer products that contain methylene chloride include paint strippers, adhesive removers, and aerosol spray paints. Methylene chloride is known to cause cancer in animals. Also, methylene chloride is converted to carbon monoxide in the body and can cause symptoms associated with exposure to carbon monoxide. Carefully read the labels containing health hazard information and cautions on the proper use of these products. Use products that contain methylene chloride outdoors when possible; use indoors only if the area is well ventilated.

- Keep exposure to benzene to a minimum. Benzene is a known human carcinogen. The main indoor sources of this chemical are environmental tobacco smoke, stored fuels and paint supplies and automobile emissions in attached garages. Actions that will reduce benzene exposure include eliminating smoking within the home, providing for maximum ventilation during painting and discarding paint supplies and special fuels that will not be used immediately.

- Keep exposure to perchloroethylene emissions from newly dry-cleaned materials to a minimum. Perchloroethylene is the chemical most widely used in dry cleaning. In laboratory studies, it has been shown to cause cancer in animals. Studies indicate that people breathe low levels of this chemical both in homes where dry-cleaned goods are stored and as they wear dry-cleaned clothing. Dry cleaners recapture the perchloroethylene during the dry-cleaning process so they can save money by reusing it, and they remove more of the chemical during the pressing and finishing processes. Some dry cleaners, however, do not remove as much perchloroethylene as possible all of the time. Taking steps to minimize your exposure to this chemical is prudent. If dry-cleaned goods have a strong chemical odor when you pick them up, do not accept them until they have been properly dried. If goods with a chemical odor are returned to you on subsequent visits, try a different dry cleaner.

Formaldehyde

Formaldehyde is an important chemical used widely by industry to manufacture building materials and numerous household products. It is also a by-product of combustion and certain other natural processes. Thus, it may be present in substantial concentrations both indoors and outdoors.

Sources of formaldehyde in the home include building materials, smoking, household products and the use of unvented, fuel-burning appliances, like gas stoves or kerosene space heaters. Formaldehyde, by itself or in combination with other chemicals, serves a number of purposes in manufactured products. For example, it is used to add permanent-press qualities to clothing and draperies, as a component of glues and adhesives and as a preservative in some paints and coating products.

441

In homes, the most significant sources of formaldehyde are likely to be pressed wood products made using adhesives that contain urea-formaldehyde (UF) resins. Pressed wood products made for indoor use include: particle board (used as subflooring and shelving and in cabinetry and furniture); hardwood plywood paneling (used for decorative wall covering and used in cabinets and furniture); and medium density fiberboard (used for drawer fronts, cabinets and furniture tops). Medium density fiberboard contains a higher resin-to-wood ratio than any other UF pressed wood product and is generally recognized as being the highest formaldehyde-emitting pressed wood product.

Other pressed wood products, such as softwood plywood and flake or oriented strandboard, are produced for exterior construction use and contain the dark, or red/black-colored phenol-formaldehyde (PF) resin. Although formaldehyde is present in both types of resins, pressed woods that contain PF resin generally emit formaldehyde at considerably lower rates than those containing UF resin.

Since 1985, the U.S. Department of Housing and Urban Development (HUD) has permitted only the use of plywood and particleboard that conform to specified formaldehyde emission limits in the construction of prefabricated and mobile homes. In the past, some of these homes had elevated levels of formaldehyde because of the large amount of high-emitting pressed wood products used in their construction and because of their relatively small interior space.

The rate at which products like pressed wood or textiles release formaldehyde can change. Formaldehyde emissions will generally decrease as products age. When the products are new, high indoor temperatures or humidity can cause increased release of formaldehyde from these products.

During the 1970s, many homeowners had urea-formaldehyde foam insulation (UFFI) installed in the wall cavities of their homes as an energy conservation measure. However, many of these homes were found to have relatively high indoor concentrations of formaldehyde soon after the UFFI installation. Few homes are now being insulated with this product. Studies show that formaldehyde emissions from UFFI decline with time; therefore, homes in which UFFI was installed many years ago are unlikely to have high levels of formaldehyde now.

Health Effects of Formaldehyde

Formaldehyde, a colorless, pungent-smelling gas, can cause watery eyes, burning sensations in the eyes and throat, nausea and difficulty in breathing in some humans exposed at elevated levels (above 0.1

parts per million). High concentrations may trigger attacks in people with asthma. There is evidence that some people can develop a sensitivity to formaldehyde. It has also been shown to cause cancer in animals and may cause cancer in humans.

Reducing Exposure to Formaldehyde in Homes

Ask about the formaldehyde content of pressed wood products, including building materials, cabinetry, and furniture before you purchase them.

If you experience adverse reactions to formaldehyde, you may want to avoid the use of pressed wood products and other formaldehyde-emitting goods. Even if you do not experience such reactions, you may wish to reduce your exposure as much as possible by purchasing exterior-grade products, which emit less formaldehyde.

- For further information on formaldehyde and consumer products, call the EPA Toxic Substance Control Act (TSCA) assistance line (202-554-1404).

Some studies suggest that coating pressed wood products with polyurethane may reduce formaldehyde emissions for some period of time. To be effective, any such coating must cover all surfaces and edges and remain intact. Increase the ventilation and carefully follow the manufacturer instructions while applying these coatings. (If you are sensitive to formaldehyde, check the label contents before purchasing coating products to avoid buying products that contain formaldehyde, as they will emit the chemical for a short time after application.) Maintain moderate temperature and humidity levels and provide adequate ventilation. The rate at which formaldehyde is released is accelerated by heat and may also depend somewhat on the humidity level. Therefore, the use of dehumidifiers and air conditioning to control humidity and to maintain a moderate temperature can help reduce formaldehyde emissions. (Drain and clean dehumidifier collection trays frequently so that they do not become a breeding ground for microorganisms.) Increasing the rate of ventilation in your home will also help in reducing formaldehyde levels.

Pesticides

According to a survey, 75 percent of U.S. households used at least one pesticide product indoors during the past year. Products used most often are insecticides and disinfectants. Another study suggests that

80 percent of most people's exposure to pesticides occurs indoors and that measurable levels of up to a dozen pesticides have been found in the air inside homes. The amount of pesticides found in homes appears to be greater than can be explained by recent pesticide use in those households; other possible sources include contaminated soil or dust that floats or is tracked in from outside, stored pesticide containers, and household surfaces that collect and then release the pesticides. Pesticides used in and around the home include products to control insects (insecticides), termites (termiticides), rodents (rodenticides), fungi (fungicides), and microbes (disinfectants).

They are sold as:

- Sprays

- Liquids

- Sticks

- Powders

- Crystals

- Balls

- Foggers

In 1990, the American Association of Poison Control Centers (AAPCC) reported that some 79,000 children were involved in common household pesticide poisonings or exposures. In households with children under five years old, almost one-half stored at least one pesticide product within reach of children.

The EPA registers pesticides for use and requires manufacturers to put information on the label about when and how to use the pesticide. It is important to remember that the "-cide" in pesticides means "to kill." These products can be dangerous if not used properly.

In addition to the active ingredient, pesticides are also made up of ingredients that are used to carry the active agent. These carrier agents are called "inerts" in pesticides because they are not toxic to the targeted pest; nevertheless, some inerts are capable of causing health problems.

Health Effects from Pesticides

Both the active and inert ingredients in pesticides can be organic compounds; therefore, both could add to the levels of airborne organics inside homes. As with other household products, there is insufficient understanding at present about what pesticide concentrations are necessary to produce these effects.

Exposure to high levels of cyclodiene pesticides, commonly associated with misapplication, has produced various symptoms, including:

- Headaches

- Dizziness

- Muscle twitching

- Weakness

- Tingling sensations

- Nausea

In addition, the EPA is concerned that cyclodienes might cause long-term damage to the liver and the central nervous system, as well as an increased risk of cancer.

There is no further sale or commercial use permitted for the following cyclodiene or related pesticides:

- Chlordane

- Aldrin

- Dieldrin

- Heptachlor*

The only exception is the use of heptachlor by utility companies to control fire ants in underground cable boxes.

Reducing Exposure to Pesticides in Homes

- Read the label and follow the directions. It is illegal to use any pesticide in any manner inconsistent with the directions on its label. Unless you have had special training and are certified, never use a pesticide that is restricted to use by state-certified pest control operators. Such pesticides are simply too dangerous for application by a noncertified person. Use only the pesticides approved for use by the general public and then only in recommended amounts; increasing the amount does not offer more protection against pests and can be harmful to you and your plants and pets.

- Ventilate the area well after pesticide use. Mix or dilute pesticides outdoors or in a well-ventilated area and only in the amounts that will be immediately needed. If possible, take plants and pets outside when applying pesticides to them.

• Use nonchemical methods of pest control when possible. Since pesticides can be found far from the site of their original application, it is prudent to reduce the use of chemical pesticides outdoors as well as indoors. Depending on the site and pest to be controlled, one or more of the following steps can be effective: use of biological pesticides, such as *Bacillus thuringiensis*, for the control of gypsy moths; selection of disease-resistant plants; and frequent washing of indoor plants and pets. Termite damage can be reduced or prevented by making certain that wooden building materials do not come into direct contact with the soil and by storing firewood away from the home. By appropriately fertilizing, watering and aerating lawns, the need for chemical pesticide treatments of lawns can be dramatically reduced.

• If you decide to use a pest control company, choose one carefully. Ask for an inspection of your home and get a written control program for evaluation before you sign a contract. The control program should list specific names of pests to be controlled and chemicals to be used; it should also reflect any of your safety concerns. Insist on a proven record of competence and customer satisfaction.

• Dispose of unwanted pesticides safely. If you have unused or partially used pesticide containers you want to get rid of, dispose of them according to the directions on the label or on special household hazardous waste collection days. If there are no such collection days in your community, work with others to organize them.

• Keep exposure to moth repellents to a minimum. One pesticide often found in the home is paradichlorobenzene, a commonly used active ingredient in moth repellents. This chemical is known to cause cancer in animals, but substantial scientific uncertainty exists over the effects, if any, of long-term human exposure to paradichlorobenzene. The EPA requires that products containing paradichlorobenzene bear warnings such as "avoid breathing vapors" to warn users of potential short-term toxic effects. Where possible, paradichlorobenzene, and items to be protected against moths, should be placed in trunks or other containers that can be stored in areas that are separately ventilated from the home, such as attics and detached garages.

446

Paradichlorobenzene is also the key active ingredient in many air fresheners (in fact, some labels for moth repellents recommend that these same products be used as air fresheners or deodorants). Proper ventilation and basic household cleanliness will go a long way toward preventing unpleasant odors.

Asbestos

Asbestos is a mineral fiber that has been used commonly in a variety of building construction materials for insulation and as a fire-retardant. The EPA and CPSC have banned several asbestos products. Manufacturers have also voluntarily limited uses of asbestos. Nowadays, asbestos is most commonly found in older homes, in pipe and furnace insulation materials, asbestos shingles, millboard, textured paints, and other coating materials, and floor tiles.

Elevated concentrations of airborne asbestos can occur after asbestos-containing materials are disturbed by cutting, sanding, or other remodeling activities. Improper attempts to remove these materials can release asbestos fibers into the air in homes, increasing asbestos levels and endangering people living in those homes.

Health Effects of Asbestos

The most dangerous asbestos fibers are too small to be visible. After they are inhaled, they can remain and accumulate in the lungs. Asbestos can cause:

- Lung cancer

- Mesothelioma (a cancer of the chest and abdominal linings)

- Asbestosis (irreversible lung scarring that can be fatal)

Symptoms of these diseases do not show up until many years after exposure began. Most people with asbestos-related diseases were exposed to elevated concentrations on the job; some developed disease from exposure to clothing and equipment brought home from job sites.

Reducing Exposure to Asbestos in Homes

If you think your home may have asbestos, don't panic! Usually it is best to leave asbestos material that is in good condition alone. Generally, material in good condition will not release asbestos fiber. There is no danger unless fibers are released and inhaled into the lungs.

447

Do not cut, rip, or sand asbestos-containing materials. Leave undamaged materials alone and, to the extent possible, prevent them from being damaged, disturbed, or touched. Periodically inspect for damage or deterioration. Discard damaged or worn asbestos gloves, stove-top pads, or ironing board covers. Check with local health, environmental, or other appropriate officials to find out about proper handling and disposal procedures.

If asbestos material is more than slightly damaged, or if you are going to make changes in your home that might disturb it, repair or removal by a professional is needed. Before you have your house remodeled, find out whether asbestos materials are present.

When you need to remove or clean up asbestos, use a professionally trained contractor. Select a contractor only after careful discussion of the problems in your home and the steps the contractor will take to clean up or remove them. Consider the option of sealing off the materials instead of removing them.

Call the EPA's TSCA assistance line at 202-554-1404 to find out whether your state has a training and certification program for asbestos removal contractors and for information on EPA's asbestos programs.

Toxic Substances Control Act (TSCA) Hotline—Sponsored by the Office of Pollution Prevention and Toxics, the TSCA Hotline provides technical assistance and information about asbestos programs implemented under TSCA, which include:

- the Asbestos School Hazard Abatement Act (ASHAAM)

- the Asbestos Hazard Emergency Response Act (AHERA)

- the Asbestos School Hazard Abatement Reauthorization Act (ASHARA)

The Hotline provides copies of TSCA information, such as Federal Register notices and support documents, to requesters through its Clearinghouse function.

Lead (Pb)

Lead has long been recognized as a harmful environmental pollutant. In late 1991, the Secretary of the Department of Health and Human Services called lead the "number one environmental threat to the health of children in the United States." There are many ways in which humans are exposed to lead:

- Air

- Drinking water

- Food

- Contaminated soil

- Deteriorating paint

- Dust

Airborne lead enters the body when an individual breathes or swallows lead particles or dust once it has settled. Before it was known how harmful lead could be, it was used in paint, gasoline, water pipes and many other products.

Old lead-based paint is the most significant source of lead exposure in the United States. Harmful exposures to lead can be created when lead-based paint is improperly removed from surfaces by dry scraping, sanding, or open-flame burning. High concentrations of airborne lead particles in homes can also result from lead dust from outdoor sources, including contaminated soil tracked inside and use of lead in certain indoor activities such as soldering and stained-glass making.

Health Effects of Exposure to Lead

Lead affects practically all systems within the body. At high levels it can cause convulsions, coma, and even death. Lower levels of lead can adversely affect the brain, central nervous system, blood cells, and kidneys.

The effects of lead exposure on fetuses and young children can be severe. They include:

- Delays in physical and mental development

- Lower intelligence quotient (IQ) levels

- Shortened attention spans

- Increased behavioral problems

Fetuses, infants and children are more vulnerable to lead exposure than adults since lead is more easily absorbed into growing bodies, and the tissues of small children are more sensitive to the damaging effects of lead. Children may have higher exposures since they are more likely to get lead dust on their hands and then put their fingers or other lead-contaminated objects into their mouths.

Get your child tested for lead exposure. To find out where to do this, call your doctor or local health clinic.

Ways to Reduce Exposure to Lead

- Keep areas where children play as dust-free and clean as possible. Mop floors and wipe window ledges and chewable surfaces such as cribs with either a general all-purpose cleaner or a cleaner made specifically for lead. Wash toys and stuffed animals regularly. Make sure that children wash their hands before meals, nap time and bedtime.

- Reduce the risk from lead-based paint. Most homes built before 1960 contain heavily leaded paint. Some homes built in 1978 may also contain lead paint. This paint could be on window frames, walls, the outside of homes, or other surfaces. Do not burn painted wood since it may contain lead.

- Leave lead-based paint undisturbed if it is in good condition—do not sand or burn off paint that may contain lead. Lead paint in good condition is usually not a problem except in places where painted surfaces rub against each other and create dust (for example, opening a window).

- Do not remove lead paint yourself. Individuals have been poisoned by scraping or sanding lead paint because these activities generate large amounts of lead dust. Consult your state health or housing department for suggestions on which private laboratories or public agencies may be able to help test your home for lead in paint. Home test kits cannot detect small amounts of lead under some conditions. Hire a person with special training for correcting lead paint problems to remove lead-based paint. Occupants, especially children and pregnant women, should leave the building until all work is finished and clean-up is done.

For additional information dealing with lead-based paint abatement contact the U.S. Department of Housing and Urban Development (HUD) for the following two documents: Comprehensive and Workable Plan for the Abatement of Lead-Based Paint in Privately Owned Housing: Report to Congress and Lead-Based Paint: Interim Guidelines for Hazard Identification and Abatement in Public and Indian Housing.

- Do not bring lead dust into the home. If you work in construction, demolition, painting, with batteries, in a radiator repair shop or lead factory, or your hobby involves lead, you may unknowingly bring lead into your home on your hands or clothes. You may also be tracking in lead from soil around your home. Soil very close to homes may be contaminated from lead paint on the outside of the building. Soil by roads and highways may be contaminated from years of exhaust fumes from cars and trucks that used leaded gas. Use door mats to wipe your feet before entering the home. If you work with lead in your job or a hobby, change your clothes before you go home and wash these clothes separately. Encourage your children to play in sand and grassy areas instead of dirt which sticks to fingers and toys. Try to keep your children from eating dirt, and make sure they wash their hands when they come inside.

- Find out about lead in drinking water. Most well and city water does not usually contain lead. Water usually picks up lead inside the home from household plumbing that is made with lead materials. The only way to know if there is lead in drinking water is to have it tested. Contact the local health department or the water supplier to find out how to get the water tested. Send for the EPA pamphlet, "Lead and Your Drinking Water," for more information about what you can do if you have lead in your drinking water. Call the EPA's Safe Drinking Water Hotline (800-426-4791) for more information.

- Eat right. A child who gets enough iron and calcium will absorb less lead. Foods rich in iron include eggs, red meats, and beans. Dairy products are high in calcium. Do not store food or liquid in lead crystal glassware or imported or old pottery. If you reuse old plastic bags to store or carry food, keep the printing on the outside of the bag.

Section 43.4

What about Carpets?

This section includes text excerpted from "The Inside Story:
A Guide to Indoor Air Quality," U.S. Environmental
Protection Agency (EPA), April 27, 2018.

In the past few years, a number of consumers have associated a variety of symptoms with the installation of new carpet. Scientists have not been able to determine whether the chemicals emitted by new carpets are responsible. If you are installing new carpet, you may wish to take the following steps:

- Talk to your carpet retailer. Ask for information on emissions from carpet.

- Ask the retailer to unroll and air out the carpet in a well-ventilated area before installation.

- Ask for low-emitting adhesives if adhesives are needed.

- Consider leaving the premises during and immediately after carpet installation. You may wish to schedule the installation when most family members or office workers are out.

- Be sure the retailer requires the installer to follow the Carpet and Rug Institute's installation guidelines.

- Open doors and windows. Increasing the amount of fresh air in the home will reduce exposure to most chemicals released from carpet. During and after installation, use window fans, room air conditioners, or other mechanical ventilation equipment you may have installed in your house, to exhaust fumes to the outdoors. Keep them running for 48–72 hours after the new carpet is installed.

- Contact your carpet retailer if objectionable odors persist.

- Follow the manufacturer's instructions for proper carpet maintenance.

Section 43.5

When Building a New Home

This section includes text excerpted from "The Inside Story:
A Guide to Indoor Air Quality," U.S. Environmental
Protection Agency (EPA), April 27, 2018.

Building a new home provides the opportunity for preventing indoor air problems. However, it can result in exposure to higher levels of indoor air contaminants if careful attention is not given to potential pollution sources and the air exchange rate.

Express your concerns about indoor air quality to your architect or builder and enlist his or her cooperation in taking measures to provide good indoor air quality. Talk both about purchasing building materials and furnishings that are low-emitting and about providing an adequate amount of ventilation.

The American Society of Heating, Refrigerating and Air-Conditioning Engineers (ASHRAE) recommends a ventilation rate of 0.35 ach (air changes per hour) for new homes, and some new homes are built to even tighter specifications. Particular care should be given in such homes to preventing the buildup of indoor air pollutants to high levels.

Here are a few important actions that can make a difference:

- Use radon-resistant construction techniques.

- Obtain a copy of the EPA booklet, "Model Standards and Techniques for Control of Radon in New Residential Buildings," from your state radon office or health agency, your state homebuilders' association, or your EPA regional office.

- Choose building materials and furnishings that will keep indoor air pollution to a minimum.

There are many actions a homeowner can take to select products that will prevent indoor air problems from occurring—a couple of them are mentioned here. First, use exterior-grade pressed wood products made with phenol-formaldehyde resin in floors, cabinetry, and wall surfaces. Or, as an alternative, consider using solid wood products. Secondly, if you plan to install wall-to-wall carpet on concrete in contact with the ground, especially concrete in basements, make sure that an effective moisture barrier is installed prior to installing the carpet. Do not permanently adhere carpet to concrete with adhesives so that the carpet can be removed if it becomes wet.

- Provide proper drainage and seal foundations in new construction.

- Air that enters the home through the foundation can contain more moisture than is generated from all occupant activities.

- Become familiar with mechanical ventilation systems and consider installing one.

- Advanced designs of new homes are starting to feature mechanical systems that bring outdoor air into the home. Some of these designs include energy-efficient heat recovery ventilators (also known as air-to-air heat exchangers).

- Ensure that combustion appliances, including furnaces, fireplaces, woodstoves, and heaters, are properly vented and receive enough supply air.

- Combustion gases, including carbon monoxide and particles can be back-drafted from the chimney or flue into the living space if the combustion appliance is not properly vented or does not receive enough supply air. Back-drafting can be a particular problem in weatherized or tightly constructed homes. Installing a dedicated outdoor air supply for the combustion appliance can help prevent backdrafting.

Section 43.6

Do You Suspect Your Office Has an Indoor Air Problem?

This section includes text excerpted from "The Inside Story: A Guide to Indoor Air Quality," U.S. Environmental Protection Agency (EPA), April 27, 2018.

Indoor air quality problems are not limited to homes. In fact, many office buildings have significant air pollution sources. Some of these buildings may be inadequately ventilated. For example, mechanical ventilation systems may not be designed or operated to provide adequate amounts of outdoor air. Finally, people generally have less control over the indoor environment in their offices than they do in their homes. As a result, there has been an increase in the incidence of reported health problems.

Health Effects

A number of well-identified illnesses, such as Legionnaires' disease, asthma, hypersensitivity pneumonitis, and humidifier fever, have been directly traced to specific building problems. These are called building-related illnesses. Most of these diseases can be treated, nevertheless, some pose serious risks.

Sometimes, however, building occupants experience symptoms that do not fit the pattern of any particular illness and are difficult to trace to any specific source. This phenomenon has been labeled sick building syndrome. People may complain of one or more of the following symptoms: dry or burning mucous membranes in the nose, eyes and throat; sneezing; stuffy or runny nose; fatigue or lethargy; headache; dizziness; nausea; irritability and forgetfulness. Poor lighting, noise, vibration, thermal discomfort, and psychological stress may also cause, or contribute to, these symptoms.

There is no single manner in which these health problems appear. In some cases, problems begin as workers enter their offices and diminish as workers leave; other times, symptoms continue until the illness is treated. Sometimes there are outbreaks of illness among many workers in a single building; in other cases, health symptoms show up only in individual workers.

In the opinion of some World Health Organization (WHO) experts, up to 30 percent of new or remodeled commercial buildings may have unusually high rates of health and comfort complaints from occupants that may potentially be related to indoor air quality.

What Causes Problems?

Three major reasons for poor indoor air quality in office buildings are the presence of indoor air pollution sources; poorly designed, maintained, or operated ventilation systems; and uses of the building that were unanticipated or poorly planned for when the building was designed or renovated.

Sources of Office Air Pollution

As with homes, the most important factor influencing indoor air quality is the presence of pollutant sources. Commonly found office pollutants and their sources include:

- Environmental tobacco smoke

- Asbestos from insulating and fire-retardant building supplies

- Formaldehyde from pressed wood products

- Other organics from:

  - Building materials

  - Carpet and other office furnishings, cleaning materials, and activities

  - Restroom air fresheners

  - Paints

  - Adhesives

  - Copying machines

  - Photography

  - Print shops

- Biological contaminants from dirty ventilation systems or water-damaged walls, ceilings, and carpets

- Pesticides from pest management practices.

Ventilation Systems

Mechanical ventilation systems in large buildings are designed and operated not only to heat and cool the air, but also to draw in and circulate outdoor air. If they are poorly designed, operated, or maintained, however, ventilation systems can contribute to indoor air problems in several ways.

For example, problems arise when, in an effort to save energy, ventilation systems are not used to bring in adequate amounts of outdoor air. Inadequate ventilation also occurs if the air supply and return vents within each room are blocked or placed in such a way that outdoor air does not actually reach the breathing zone of building occupants. Improperly located outdoor air intake vents can also bring in air contaminated with automobile and truck exhaust, boiler emissions, fumes from dumpsters, or air vented from restrooms. Finally, ventilation systems can be a source of indoor pollution themselves by spreading biological contaminants that have multiplied in cooling towers, humidifiers, dehumidifiers, air conditioners, or the inside surfaces of ventilation ductwork.

Use of the Building

Indoor air pollutants can be circulated from portions of the building used for specialized purposes, such as restaurants, print shops, and dry-cleaning stores, into offices in the same building. Carbon monoxide (CO) and other components of automobile exhaust can be drawn from underground parking garages through stairwells and elevator shafts into office spaces.

In addition, buildings originally designed for one purpose may end up being converted to use as office space. If not properly modified during building renovations, the room partitions and ventilation system can contribute to indoor air quality problems by restricting air recirculation or by providing an inadequate supply of outdoor air.

What to Do If You Suspect a Problem

If you or others at your office are experiencing health or comfort problems that you suspect may be caused by indoor air pollution, you can do the following:

- Talk with other workers, your supervisor, and union representatives to see if the problems are being experienced by others and urge that a record of reported health complaints be kept by management, if one has not already been established.

- Talk with your own physician and report your problems to the company physician, nurse, or health and safety officer.

- Call your state or local health department or air pollution control agency to talk over the symptoms and possible causes.

- You can encourage building management to follow guidance in the EPA's IAQ Building Education and Assessment Model (I-BEAM). I-BEAM updates and expands EPA's existing Building Air Quality guidance and is designed to be comprehensive state-of-the-art guidance for managing IAQ in commercial buildings. This guidance was designed to be used by building professionals and others interested in indoor air quality

457

in commercial buildings. I-BEAM contains text, animation/visual and interactive/calculation components that can be used to perform a number of diverse tasks.

• Frequently, indoor air quality problems in large commercial buildings cannot be effectively identified or remedied without a comprehensive building investigation. These investigations may start with written questionnaires and telephone consultations in which building investigators assess the history of occupant symptoms and building operation procedures. In some cases, these inquiries may quickly uncover the problem and on-site visits are unnecessary.

• More often, however, investigators will need to come to the building to conduct personal interviews with occupants, to look for possible sources of the problems and to inspect the design and operation of the ventilation system and other building features. Because taking measurements of pollutants at the very low levels often found in office buildings is expensive and may not yield information readily useful in identifying problem sources, investigators may not take many measurements. The process of solving indoor air quality problems that result in health and comfort complaints can be a slow one, involving several trial solutions before successful remedial actions are identified.

• If a professional company is hired to conduct a building investigation, select a company on the basis of its experience in identifying and solving indoor air quality problems in nonindustrial buildings.

• Work with others to establish a smoking policy that eliminates involuntary nonsmoker exposure to environmental tobacco smoke.

• Call the National Institute for Occupational Safety and Health (NIOSH) for information on obtaining a health hazard evaluation of your office 800-35-NIOSH (800-356-4674), or contact the Occupational Safety and Health Administration (OSHA), (202-219-8151).

Chapter 44

Improving Indoor Air Quality and Reducing Environmental Triggers

Understand Indoor Air in Homes, Schools, and Offices

Some pollutants in the air are especially harmful for children, elderly people, and those with health problems.

Most of us spend much of our time indoors. The air that we breathe in our homes, in schools, and in offices can put us at risk for health problems. Some pollutants can be chemicals, gases and living organisms like mold and pests.

Several sources of air pollution are in homes, schools, and offices. Some pollutants cause health problems such as sore eyes, burning in the nose and throat, headaches, or fatigue. Other pollutants cause or worsen allergies, respiratory illnesses (such as asthma), heart disease, cancer, and other serious long-term conditions. Sometimes individual

This chapter contains text excerpted from the following sources: Text beginning with the heading "Understand Indoor Air in Homes, Schools, and Offices" is excerpted from "Care for Your Air: A Guide to Indoor Air Quality," U.S. Environmental Protection Agency (EPA), September 6, 2017; Text beginning with the heading "Take Action to Improve Indoor Air Quality in Schools" is excerpted from "Take Action to Improve Indoor Air Quality in Schools," U.S. Environmental Protection Agency (EPA), March 16, 2018.

pollutants at high concentrations, such as carbon monoxide (CO), cause death.

Learn about Pollutants

Understanding and controlling some of the common pollutants found in homes, schools, and offices may help improve your indoor air and reduce your family's risk of health concerns related to indoor air quality (IAQ).

- Radon
- Secondhand smoke
- Combustion pollutants
- Volatile organic compounds (VOCs)
- Asthma triggers

Radon

Radon is a radioactive gas that is formed in the soil. It can enter indoors through cracks and openings in floors and walls that are in contact with the ground.

- Radon is the leading cause of lung cancer among nonsmokers, and the second leading cause of lung cancer overall.

Secondhand Smoke

Secondhand smoke comes from burning tobacco products. It can cause cancer and serious respiratory illnesses.

- Children are especially vulnerable to secondhand smoke. It can cause or worsen asthma symptoms and is linked to increased risks of ear infections and sudden infant death syndrome (SIDS).

Combustion Pollutants

Combustion Pollutants are gases or particles that come from burning materials. In homes, the major source of combustion pollutants are improperly vented or unvented fuel-burning appliances such as:

- Space heaters
- Wood stoves
- Gas stoves

- Water heaters

- Dryers

- Fireplaces

The types and amounts of pollutants produced depends on the type of appliance, how well the appliance is installed, maintained, and vented and the kind of fuel it uses. Common combustion pollutants include:

- Carbon monoxide which is a colorless, odorless gas that interferes with the delivery of oxygen throughout the body.

- Carbon monoxide causes headaches, dizziness, weakness, nausea, and even death.

- Nitrogen dioxide (NO_2) which is a colorless, odorless gas that causes eye, nose, and throat irritation, shortness of breath, and an increased risk of respiratory infection.

Volatile Organic Compounds

VOCs are emitted by a wide array of products used in homes including:

- Paints and lacquers

- Paint strippers

- Cleaning supplies

- Varnishes and waxes

- Pesticides

- Building materials and furnishings

- Office equipment

- Moth repellents

- Air fresheners

- Dry-cleaned clothing

VOCs evaporate into the air when these products are used or sometimes even when they are stored.

- Volatile organic compounds irritate the eyes, nose and throat, and cause headaches, nausea, and damage to the liver, kidneys, and central nervous system. Some of them can cause cancer.

Asthma Triggers

Asthma triggers are commonly found in homes, schools, and offices and include mold, dust mites, secondhand smoke, and pet dander. A home may have mold growing on a shower curtain, dust mites, pillows, blankets or stuffed animals, secondhand smoke; in the air, and cat and dog hairs; on the carpet or floors. Other common asthma triggers include some foods and pollutants in the air.

- Asthma triggers cause symptoms including coughing, chest tightness, wheezing, and breathing problems. An asthma attack occurs when symptoms keep getting worse or are suddenly very severe. Asthma attacks can be life threatening. However, asthma is controllable with the right medicines and by reducing asthma triggers.

Molds

Molds are living things that produce spores. Molds produce spores that float in the air, land on damp surfaces and grow.

- Inhaling or touching molds can cause hay fever-type symptoms such as sneezing, runny nose, red eyes, and skin rashes. Molds can also trigger asthma attacks.

Improving Your Indoor Air

Take steps to help improve your air quality and reduce your IAQ-related health risks at little or no cost by:

- **Controlling the sources of pollution:** Usually the most effective way to improve indoor air is to eliminate individual sources or reduce their emissions.

- **Ventilating:** Increasing the amount of fresh air brought indoors helps reduce pollutants inside. When weather permits, open windows and doors, or run an air conditioner with the vent control open. Bathroom and kitchen fans that exhaust to the outdoors also increase ventilation and help remove pollutants.

Always ventilate and follow manufacturers' instructions when you use products or appliances that may release pollutants into the indoor air.

- **Changing filters regularly:** Central heaters and air conditioners have filters to trap dust and other pollutants in the air. Make sure to change or clean the filters regularly, following the instructions on the package.

- **Adjusting humidity:** The humidity inside can affect the concentrations of some indoor air pollutants. For example, high humidity keeps the air moist and increases the likelihood of mold.

Keep indoor humidity between 30 and 50 percent. Use a moisture or humidity gauge, available at most hardware stores, to see if the humidity in your home is at a good level. To increase humidity, use a vaporizer or humidifier. To decrease humidity, open the windows if it is not humid outdoors. If it is warm, turn on the air conditioner or adjust the humidity setting on the humidifier.

Take Action to Improve Air Quality in Every Room

Important Tips That Will Help Control Indoor Pollutants

- Test for radon and fix if there is a problem.
- Reduce asthma triggers such as mold and dust mites.
- Do not let people smoke indoors.
- Keep all areas clean and dry. Clean up any mold and get rid of excess water or moisture.
- Always ventilate when using products that can release pollutants into the air; if products must be stored following use, make sure to close tightly.
- Inspect fuel-burning appliances regularly for leaks, and make repairs when necessary.
- Consider installing a carbon monoxide alarm.

Radon

Radon is the second leading cause of lung cancer. Radon gas enters your home through cracks and openings in floors and walls in contact with the ground.

Take Action

- Test your home with a do-it-yourself radon kit. If the test result indicates you should fix, call a qualified radon mitigation specialist.

- Ask your builder about including radon-reducing features in your new home at the time of construction.

Asthma

Asthma is a serious, sometimes life-threatening respiratory disease that affects the quality of life for millions of Americans.

Take Action

Environmental asthma triggers are found around the home and can be eliminated with these simple steps:

- Don't allow smoking in your home or car.
- Dust and clean your home regularly.
- Clean up mold and fix water leaks.
- Wash sheets and blankets weekly in hot water.
- Use allergen-proof mattress and pillow covers.
- Keep pets out of the bedroom and off soft furniture.
- Control pests—close up cracks and crevices and seal leaks; don't leave food out.

Children are especially sensitive to secondhand smoke, which can trigger asthma and other respiratory illnesses.

Secondhand Smoke

Secondhand smoke comes from burning tobacco products such as cigarettes, pipes, and cigars.

Take Action

- To help protect children from secondhand smoke, do not smoke or allow others to smoke inside your home or car

Mold

Mold can lead to allergic reactions, asthma, and other respiratory ailments. Mold can grow anywhere there is moisture in a house.

Take Action

- The key to mold control is moisture control.

- If mold is a problem in your home, you should clean up the mold promptly and fix the water problem.

- It is important to dry water-damaged areas and items within 24–48 hours to prevent mold growth.

Volatile Organic Compounds

VOCs cause eye, nose, and throat irritation, headaches, nausea, and can damage the liver, kidney, and central nervous system. Volatile organic compounds are chemicals that evaporate at room temperature. VOCs are released from products into the home both during use and while stored.

Take Action

- Read and follow all directions and warnings on common household products.

- Make sure there is plenty of fresh air and ventilation (e.g., opening windows and using extra fans) when painting, remodeling or using other products that may release VOCs.

- Never mix products, such as household cleaners, unless directed to do so on the label.

- Store household products that contain chemicals according to manufacturers' instructions.

- Keep all products away from children!

Combustion Pollutants

- Carbon monoxide causes headaches, dizziness, disorientation, nausea, and fatigue, and high levels can be fatal. Nitrogen dioxide causes eyes, nose and throat irritation, impairs lung function, and increases respiratory infections.

Sources include:

- Indoor use of furnaces

- Gas stoves

- Unvented kerosene and gas space heaters

- Leaking chimneys

- Tobacco products

Take Action

- Ventilate rooms where fuel-burning appliances are used.

- Use appliances that vent to the outside whenever possible.

- Ensure that all fuel-burning appliances are properly installed, used, adjusted, and maintained.

Remodeling Old Homes and Building New Homes

While remodeling or improving the energy efficiency of your home, steps should be taken to minimize pollution from sources inside the home, either from new materials or from disturbing materials already in the home. In addition, residents should be alert to signs of inadequate ventilation, such as stuffy air, moisture condensation on cold surfaces, or mold and mildew growth.

When building new homes, homebuyers today are increasingly concerned about the IAQ of their homes. Pollutants like mold, radon, carbon monoxide, and toxic chemicals have received greater attention than ever as poor IAQ has been linked to a host of health problems. To address these concerns, builders can employ a variety of construction practices and technologies to decrease the risk of poor IAQ in their new homes using the criteria from the U.S. Environmental Protection Agency's (EPA) Indoor airPLUS (www.epa.gov/indoorairplus) as a guide.

To help ensure that you will have good IAQ in your new or remodeled home:

- Ask about including radon-reducing features.

- Provide proper drainage and seal foundations in new construction.

- Consider installing a mechanical ventilation system. Mechanical ventilation systems introduce fresh air using ducts and fans, instead of relying on holes or cracks in the walls and windows.

- When installing new appliances (like furnaces) make sure they are installed properly with a good vent or flue.

Schools

With nearly 56 million people, or 20 percent of the U.S. population, spending their days inside elementary and secondary schools, IAQ problems can be a significant concern. All types of schools—whether new or old, big or small, elementary or high school—can experience IAQ problems. School districts are increasingly experiencing budget shortfalls and many are in poor condition, leading to a host of IAQ problems.

- The EPA's voluntary Indoor Air Quality Tools for Schools Program (www.epa.gov/iaq-schools) provides district-based guidance to schools about best practices, industry guidelines, and practical management actions to help school personnel identify, solve, and prevent IAQ problems.

- Children may be more sensitive to pollution, and children with asthma are especially sensitive. Asthma is responsible for millions of missed school days each year. Parents' and caregivers' involvement helps daycare facilities become aware of asthma triggers and the need to reduce them.

Office Buildings

Many office buildings have poor IAQ because of pollution sources and poorly designed, maintained, or operated ventilation systems.

- Office workers help to improve the indoor air in their buildings by paying attention to environmental conditions including ventilation, temperature, and the presence of odors. Report any problems to facility managers immediately.

- To improve IAQ, be careful not to block air vents or grilles, keep your space clean and dry, and do not bring in products that may pollute the indoor air.

Take Action to Improve Indoor Air Quality in Schools

In 2014, the National Center for Education Statistics (NCES) surveyed a sample of school districts and estimated that the average age of the nation's main school buildings was 55 years old—putting the average date of construction for our nation's schools at 1959. Additionally, nearly one-fourth of the nation's schools have one or more buildings in need of extensive repair or replacement and nearly half have been reported to have problems related to indoor air quality (IAQ).

The health and comfort of students and teachers are among the many factors that contribute to learning and productivity in the classroom, which in turn affect performance and achievement. The EPA's IAQ Tools for Schools Action Kit (www.epa.gov/iaq-schools/

indoor-air-quality-tools-schools-action-kit) will help ensure good indoor air quality in your school. Providing a healthy, comfortable environment is an investment in your students and staff. Failure to respond promptly and effectively to poor indoor air quality in schools can lead to severe consequences. These may include an increase in short- and long-term health problems costly repairs, potential liability problems, and greater risk that schools will need to close and temporarily relocate staff and students.

What Actions Can You Take to Improve Your School's Indoor Air Quality?

- Access the EPA's IAQ Tools for Schools Action Kit (www.epa. gov/iaq-schools/indoor-air-quality-tools-schools-action-kit). This Action Kit provides guidance and tools to help resolve current IAQ problems, prevent future IAQ problems and maintain good indoor air quality in your school.

- Educate staff, students, and parents about the importance of good IAQ and their role in making the school environment as healthy as possible.

- Utilize the EPA's IAQ Design Tools for Schools (www.epa.gov/ iaq-schools/indoor-air-quality-design-tools-schools) web-based guidance or Protecting IAQ During School Energy Efficiency Retrofit Projects with Energy Savings Plus Health guidelines (www.epa.gov/iaq-schools/protecting-iaq-during-school-energy-efficiency-retrofit-projects-energy-savings-plus) to help school districts, architects, and facility planners design and construct the next generation of high performance schools.

Chapter 45

Guide to Air Cleaners in the Home

The most effective ways to improve your indoor air are to reduce or remove the sources of pollutants and to ventilate with clean outdoor air. In addition, research shows that filtration can be an effective supplement to source control and ventilation. Using a portable air cleaner and/or upgrading the air filter in your furnace or central heating, ventilation, and air-conditioning (HVAC) system can help to improve indoor air quality. Portable air cleaners, also known as air purifiers or air sanitizers, are designed to filter the air in a single room or area. Central furnace or HVAC filters are designed to filter air throughout a home. Portable air cleaners and HVAC filters can reduce indoor air pollution; however, they cannot remove all pollutants from the air.

Portable Air Cleaners and Furnace or Heating, Ventilation, and Air-Conditioning Filters in the Home

Indoor air contains pollutants that can affect human health. Some of these pollutants come from outdoors, and others come from indoor

---

This chapter contains text excerpted from the following sources: Text in this chapter begins with excerpts from "Air Cleaners and Air Filters in the Home," U.S. Environmental Protection Agency (EPA), July 31, 2018; Text beginning with the heading "Portable Air Cleaners and Furnace or HVAC Filters in the Home" is excerpted from "Guide to Air Cleaners in the Home," U.S. Environmental Protection Agency (EPA), July 2018.

sources and activities, such as cooking, cleaning, secondhand smoke, building materials, consumer products, and home furnishings. These indoor air pollutants can be particles or gases, including volatile organic compounds (VOCs). Common contaminants that can be found indoors include particulate matter (including $PM_{2.5}$ (fine) and PM_{10} (coarse)), formaldehyde, mold, and pollen. Indoor air quality will vary from home to home and over the course of a day within a home. Since most people spend about 90 percent of their time indoors, mostly in their homes, much of their exposures to airborne pollutants will happen in the home.

The most effective ways to improve your indoor air are to reduce or remove the sources of pollutants and to ventilate with clean outdoor air. In addition, research shows that filtration can be an effective supplement to source control and ventilation. Using a portable air cleaner and/or upgrading the air filter in your furnace or central heating, ventilation, and air-conditioning (HVAC) system can help to improve indoor air quality. Portable air cleaners, also known as air purifiers or air sanitizers, are designed to filter the air in a single room or area. Central furnace or HVAC filters are designed to filter air throughout a home. Portable air cleaners and HVAC filters can reduce indoor air pollution; however, they cannot remove all pollutants from the air.

Tips for Selecting a Portable Air Cleaner, Furnace Filter, or Heating, Ventilation, and Air-Conditioning Filter

When selecting a portable air cleaner, furnace filter, or HVAC filter, keep in mind:

- No air cleaner or filter will eliminate all of the air pollutants in your home. Note that most filters are designed to filter either particles or gases. So in order to filter both particles and gases, many air cleaners contain two filters, one for particles and another for gases (in some cases including gases that have odors). Other air cleaners only have one filter, usually for particles. In addition, some air cleaners or filters are targeted to specific types of gases or VOCs. Consult the specific product packaging or labeling for more information.

- All filters need regular replacement. If a filter is dirty and overloaded, it won't work well.

Portable Air Cleaners

To filter particles, choose a portable air cleaner that has a clean air delivery rate (CADR) that is large enough for the size of the room or area in which you will use it. The higher the CADR, the more particles the air cleaner can filter and the larger the area it can serve. Most air cleaner packaging will tell you the largest size area or room it should be used in. Portable air cleaners often achieve a high CADR by using a high-efficiency particulate air (HEPA) filter.

To filter gases, choose a portable air cleaner with an activated carbon filter or other filter designed to remove gases. Note that there are no widely used performance rating systems for portable air cleaners or filters designed to remove gases. The CADR rating system is for particles only. Activated carbon filters can be effective, provided that there is a large amount of material used in the filter.

A portable air cleaner with a high CADR and an activated carbon filter can filter both particles and gases.

Generally speaking, higher fan speeds and longer run times will increase the amount of air filtered. An air cleaner will filter less air if it is set at a lower speed. More air will pass through the filter at higher fan speeds, so typically filtration will be greater at higher fan speeds. Increasing the amount of time an air cleaner runs will also increase air filtration.

Table 45.1. Portable Air Cleaner Sizing for Particle Removal

Room Area (Square Feet)	100	200	300	400	500	600
Minimum CADR (CFM)	65	130	195	260	325	390

Note this table is for estimation purposes. The CADRs are calculated based on an 8-foot ceiling. If you have higher ceilings, you may want to select a portable air cleaner with a higher CADR.

Furnace and Heating, Ventilation, and Air-Conditioning System Filters

Furnace and HVAC filters work to filter the air only when the system is operating. In most cases, HVAC systems run only when heating or cooling is needed (usually less than 25% of the time during heating and cooling seasons). In order to get more filtration, the system would have to run for longer periods. This may not be desirable or practical in many cases since longer run times increase electricity costs and may also result in less reliable humidity control during the cooling season.

471

Furnace and HVAC filters for homes are usually designed to filter particles. If you decide to upgrade or use a higher efficiency filter, choose a filter with at least a Minimum Efficiency Reporting Value (MERV) 13 rating, or as high a rating as your system fan and filter slot can accommodate. You may need to consult a professional HVAC technician to determine the highest efficiency filter that will work best for your system.

Other devices that do not have filters may also remove particles and gases. They usually fit inside the HVAC ductwork and are more common in large and commercial buildings. The EPA does not certify or recommend specific brands or models of air filters or portable air cleaners.

Air Cleaning and Filtration

Do Portable Air Cleaners and Furnace/Heating, Ventilation, and Air-Conditioning Filters Used in Homes Have the Potential to Improve My Indoor Air Quality?

Yes. Most portable air cleaners and furnace/HVAC filters can filter particles from the air. Some can filter the small particles of greatest health concern ($PM_{2.5}$). There are also air cleaners and filters that can filter both particles and gases. The longer the air cleaner runs, the more air it filters. Note that it is always important to reduce or remove the sources of indoor air pollutants and to ventilate with clean outdoor air. Filtration does not replace the need to control pollutants and ventilate.

Can Portable Air Cleaners and Furnace/Heating, Ventilation, and Air-Conditioning Filters Potentially Have a Positive Impact on Health?

Possibly. Several studies using portable HEPA air cleaners have demonstrated small improvements in cardiovascular and respiratory health. The improvements are typically small and not always noticeable to the individual, although they may be measurable by health professionals.

Chapter 46

Cleaning up Mold in Your Home

Mold Cleanup

Who should do the cleanup depends on a number of factors. One consideration is the size of the mold problem. If the moldy area is less than about 10 square feet (less than roughly a 3 feet by 3 feet patch), in most cases, you can handle the job yourself, follow the Mold Cleanup Tips and Techniques (www.epa.gov/mold/mold-clean-up-your-home#TipsandTechniques). However:

- If there has been a lot of water damage, and/or mold growth covers more than 10 square feet, consult the U.S. Environmental Protection Agency (EPA) guide Mold Remediation in Schools and Commercial Buildings (www.epa.gov/mold/mold-remediation-schools-and-commercial-buildings-guide). Although focused on schools and commercial buildings, this document is applicable to other building types.

- If you choose to hire a contractor (or other professional service provider) to do the cleanup, make sure the contractor has experience cleaning up mold. Check references and ask the contractor to follow the recommendations in the EPA guide

This chapter includes text excerpted from "Mold Cleanup in Your Home," U.S. Environmental Protection Agency (EPA), February 21, 2017.

Mold Remediation in Schools and Commercial Buildings (www.
epa.gov/mold/mold-remediation-schools-and-commercial-
buildings-guide), the guidelines of the American Conference
of Governmental Industrial Hygenists (ACGIH), or other
guidelines from professional or government organizations.

- If you suspect that the heating/ventilation/air conditioning
  (HVAC) system may be contaminated with mold (it is part of an
  identified moisture problem, for instance, or there is mold near
  the intake to the system), consult the EPA guide Should You
  Have the Air Ducts in Your Home Cleaned? (www.epa.gov/indoor-
  air-quality-iaq/publications-about-indoor-air-quality#should-you-
  have) before taking further action. Do not run the HVAC system
  if you know or suspect that it is contaminated with mold—it could
  spread mold throughout the building.

- If the water and/or mold damage was caused by sewage or
  other contaminated water, then call in a professional who
  has experience cleaning and fixing buildings damaged by
  contaminated water.

- If you have health concerns, consult a health professional before
  starting cleanup.

Tips and Techniques

The tips and techniques presented here will help you clean up your
mold problem. Please note that mold may cause staining and cosmetic
damage. It may not be possible to clean an item so that its original
appearance is restored.

- Fix plumbing leaks and other water problems as soon as
  possible. Dry all items completely.

- Scrub mold off hard surfaces with detergent and water, and dry
  completely.

- Absorbent or porous materials, such as ceiling tiles and carpet,
  may have to be thrown away if they become moldy. Mold can
  grow on or fill in the empty spaces and crevices of porous
  materials, so the mold may be difficult or impossible to remove
  completely.

- Do not paint or caulk moldy surfaces. Clean up the mold and dry
  the surfaces before painting. Paint applied over moldy surfaces
  is likely to peel.

- If you are unsure about how to clean an item, or if the item is expensive or of sentimental value, you may wish to consult a specialist. Specialists in furniture repair, restoration, painting, art restoration and conservation, carpet and rug cleaning, water damage, and fire or water restoration are commonly listed in phone books. Be sure to ask for and check references. Look for specialists who are affiliated with professional organizations.

Floods and Flooding

During a flood cleanup, the indoor air quality in your home or office may appear to be the least of your problems. However, failure to remove contaminated materials and to reduce moisture and humidity can present serious long-term health risks. Standing water and wet materials are a breeding ground for microorganisms, such as viruses, bacteria, and mold. They can cause disease, trigger allergic reactions, and continue to damage materials long after the flood.

Chapter 47

Asthma and Physical Activity in School Settings

Help Students Control Their Asthma

Good asthma management is essential for getting control of asthma. In school settings, it means helping students to:

- follow their written asthma action plan;

- have quick and easy access to their asthma medications;

- recognize their asthma triggers (the factors that make asthma worse or cause an asthma attack); and

- avoid or control asthma triggers.

You can also help by modifying physical activities to match students' current asthma status.

Good asthma management offers important benefits, including allowing students who have asthma to participate fully in physical activities and other regular school activities.

This chapter includes text excerpted from "Asthma and Physical Activity in the School," National Heart, Lung, and Blood Institute (NHLBI), April 2012. Reviewed August 2018.

Benefits of Asthma Control

With good asthma management, students with asthma should:

- Be free from troublesome symptoms day and night:
  - No coughing or wheezing
  - No difficulty breathing or chest tightness
  - No nighttime awakening due to asthma
  - Have the best possible lung function
- Be able to participate fully in any activities of their choice
- Not miss work or school because of asthma symptoms
- Need fewer or no urgent care visits or hospitalizations for asthma
- Use medications to control asthma with as few side effects as possible
- Be satisfied with their asthma care

Follow the Asthma Action Plan

Everyone who has asthma should have a written asthma action plan. The student's healthcare provider, together with the student and his or her parent or guardian, develops the student's written asthma action plan.

It should provide instructions for daily management of asthma (including medications and control of triggers) and explain how to recognize and handle worsening asthma symptoms.

Depending on the student's needs, the school may also develop a more extensive individualized health plan (IHP) or individualized education plan (IEP). A copy of the student's asthma action plan should be on file in the school office or health services office, with additional copies provided to the student's teachers and coaches.

You can help a student to follow his or her written asthma action plan in two ways:

1. By monitoring the student's asthma symptoms and/or

2. By having the student use a peak flow meter, which is a small, handheld device that measures how hard and fast the student

can blow air out of the lungs. A drop in peak flow can warn of worsening asthma even before symptoms appear.

Asthma action plans are most commonly divided into three colored zones—green, yellow, and red—like a traffic light. The individual zones correspond with a range of symptoms and/or peak flow numbers determined by the student's healthcare provider and listed on the asthma action plan. As described on the next page, an increase in asthma symptoms, or a drop in peak flow compared with the student's personal best peak flow number, indicates the need for prompt action to prevent or treat an asthma attack.

Asthma Action Plan Contents

Daily management:

- What medication to take daily, including the specific names and dosages of the medications.

- What actions to take to control environmental factors (triggers) that worsen the student's asthma.

Recognizing and handling signs of worsening asthma:

- What signs, symptoms, and peak flow readings (if peak flow monitoring is used) indicate worsening asthma.

- What medications and dosages to take in response to these signs of worsening asthma.

- What symptoms and peak flow readings indicate the need for urgent medical attention.

Administrative issues:

- Emergency telephone numbers for the physician, emergency department, and person or service to transport the student rapidly for medical care.

- Written authorization for students to carry and self-administer asthma medication, when considered appropriate by the healthcare provider and the parent or guardian.

- Written authorization for schools to administer the student's asthma medication.

Ensure Students Have Easy Access to Their Medication

Asthma Medications

Many students who have asthma require both long-term control medications and quick-relief medications. These medications prevent as well as treat symptoms and enable the student to participate safely and fully in physical activities.

Most asthma medications are inhaled as sprays or powders and may be taken using metered-dose inhalers, dry powder inhalers, or nebulizers. A metered-dose inhaler is a pressurized canister that delivers a dose of medication and does not require deep and fast breathing. A dry powder inhaler is another kind of inhaler that does require deep and fast breathing to get the medication into the lungs. A nebulizer is a machine that turns liquid medication into a fine mist. Whichever delivery method is used, it is important for students to take their medications correctly.

Long-term control medications are usually taken daily to control underlying airway inflammation and thereby prevent asthma symptoms. They can significantly reduce a student's need for quick-relief medication. Inhaled corticosteroids are the most effective long-term control medications for asthma. It is important to remember that inhaled corticosteroids are generally safe for long-term use when taken as prescribed. They are not addictive and are not the same as illegal anabolic steroids used by some athletes to build muscles.

Quick-relief medications (also known as short-acting bronchodilators) are taken when needed for rapid, short-term relief of asthma symptoms. They help stop asthma attacks by temporarily relaxing the muscles around the airways. However, they do nothing to treat the underlying airway inflammation that caused the symptoms to flare up. An additional use for quick-relief medications is the prevention of asthma symptoms in students who have exercise-induced asthma. These students may be directed by their healthcare provider to take their quick-relief medication inhaler five minutes before participating in physical activities.

Ensuring Access

Ensuring that students who have asthma have quick and easy access to their quick-relief medication is essential. These students often require medication during school to treat asthma symptoms or to take just before participating in physical activities or exposure to another asthma trigger. If accessing the medication is difficult, inconvenient, or embarrassing, the student may be discouraged and fail to use his or her quick-relief medication as needed. The student's asthma may become unnecessarily worse and his or her activities needlessly limited.

A parent or guardian should provide to the school the student's prescribed asthma medication so that it may be administered by the school nurse or other designated school personnel, according to applicable federal, state, and district laws, regulations, and policies.

Federal legislation relevant to the needs and rights of students who have asthma includes the Americans with Disabilities Act (ADA), Family Educational Rights and Privacy Act of 1974 (FERPA), Individuals with Disabilities Education Act (IDEA), and Section 504 of the Rehabilitation Act of 1973. Additional information about these laws is available from the Office for Civil Rights at the U.S. Department of Education (ED). In addition, all 50 states and the District of Columbia have laws allowing students to carry and self-administer their prescribed quick-relief asthma medications in school settings. Required documentation usually includes having on file at the school a written asthma action plan and/or medication authorization form signed by the student's physician and parent or guardian, and in some jurisdictions, the school nurse.

Recognize Asthma Triggers

Each student who has asthma has one or more triggers that can make his or her condition worse. These triggers increase airway inflammation and/or make the airways constrict, which makes breathing difficult. There are many possible triggers; table three lists the most common ones.

Asthma Triggers

- Allergens
  - Pollen—from trees, plants, and grasses, including freshly cut grass
  - Animal dander from pets with fur or hair
  - Dust and dust mites—in carpeting, mattresses, pillows, and upholstery
  - Cockroach droppings

- Molds
- Irritants
  - Strong smells and chemical sprays, including perfumes, paints, cleaning solutions, chalk dust, talcum powder, new carpet, and pesticide sprays
  - Air pollutants
  - Cigarette and other tobacco smoke
- Other asthma triggers
  - Upper respiratory infections— colds or flu
  - Exercise—running or playing hard—especially in cold weather
  - Strong emotional expressions, such as laughing or crying hard
  - Changes in weather, exposure to cold air

Recognize Worsening Asthma and Take Action

Act Fast When Signs and Symptoms of an Asthma Attack Appear

An asthma attack requires prompt action to stop it from becoming more serious or even life threatening. Recognizing the signs and symptoms of asthma attacks when they appear, and taking appropriate action in response, is crucial. Prompt treatment can help students resume their activities as soon as possible.

The following lists the immediate steps to take during an asthma attack. Depending on the student's response to treatment, physical activity may then be resumed, modified, or halted. Don't delay getting medical help, however, for a student who has severe or persistent breathing difficulty.

Actions for School Staff

Be prepared to respond to signs and symptoms of an asthma attack:

- Identify students who have asthma.
- Review their asthma action plans and know where their medications are kept.
- Know the common signs and symptoms of worsening asthma that require prompt attention:

- Coughing or wheezing

- Difficulty breathing

- Chest pain, tightness, or pressure—reported by the student

- Other signs, such as low peak flow readings as indicated on the student's asthma action plan

- Be alert for any symptoms or complaints. Even mild symptoms can lead rapidly to severe, life-threatening asthma attacks.

- Be familiar with your school's policies and procedures for administering medications and for responding to asthma attacks.

Action Steps for Staff to Manage an Asthma Attack

ACT FAST! Warning signs and symptoms—such as coughing, wheezing, difficulty breathing, chest tightness or pressure, and low or falling peak flow readings—can worsen quickly and even become life-threatening. They require quick action.

1. Quickly assess the situation.

   - Call 911 right away if the student is struggling to breathe, talk, or stay awake; has blue lips or fingernails; or asks for an ambulance.

   - If accessible, use a peak flow meter to measure the student's lung function.

2. Get help, but never leave the student alone. Have an adult accompany the student to the health room or send for help from the school nurse or designee. Do not wait.

3. Stop activity. Help the student stay calm and comfortable.

   - If the asthma attack began after exposure to an allergen or irritant (such as furry animals, fresh cut grass, strong odors, or pollen) remove the student from the allergen or irritant, if possible.

4. Treat symptoms. Help the student locate and use his or her quick relief medication (inhaler) with a spacer or holding chamber (if available).

   - Many students carry their medicine and can self-manage asthma attacks. They should follow the school protocol. Provide support as needed.

5. Call the parent or guardian.

6. Repeat use of quick-relief inhaler in 20 minutes if:

- Symptoms continue or return;

- Student still has trouble breathing; or

- Peak flow reading is below 80 percent of student's personal best peak flow number on asthma action plan

Be Alert to Signs That Asthma May Not Be Well Controlled on an Ongoing Basis

Teachers and coaches who supervise students' physical activities are in a unique position to notice the signs of poorly controlled asthma, either in a student who lacks an asthma diagnosis or in a student who has a treatment plan for asthma. Look for symptoms or other signs—subtle or dramatic—that suggest a student's asthma is not under good long-term, day-to-day control. Students are not always able to recognize for themselves when their asthma is poorly controlled. Because exercise provokes symptoms in most children with poorly controlled asthma, the student who has asthma symptoms with physical activity may need to be evaluated by his or her healthcare provider. Even for a student who has exercise-induced asthma, the frequent use of quick-relief medication during or after exercise may signal the need to return to his or her healthcare provider to add a daily long-term control medication or to increase the dosage.

If at any time you suspect that a student's asthma is not well controlled, do not hesitate to contact the school nurse or the student's parent or guardian to suggest scheduling an office visit with the student's healthcare provider, who may adjust the student's treatment. The student may also need to learn how to follow his or her asthma action plan more carefully and how to take his or her medications correctly.

Teachers and coaches may sometimes wonder if a student's reported symptoms indicate a desire for attention or a desire not to participate in an activity. At other times, it may seem that students are overreacting to minimal symptoms. At all times, it is essential to respect the student's report of his or her own condition. If a student regularly asks to be excused from recess or avoids physical activity, a real physical problem may be present. The student may also need more assistance and support from his or her teacher and coach in order to become an active participant. Consult with the school nurse, parent or guardian, or healthcare provider to find ways to ensure that the student is safe, feels safe, and is encouraged to participate actively.

Avoid or Control Asthma Triggers

Some asthma triggers—like pets with fur or hair—can be avoided. Others—like exercise and other physical activity—are important for good health and should be managed rather than avoided.

Modify Physical Activities to Match Current Asthma Status

Students who follow their asthma action plans and keep their asthma under control can usually participate in a full range of sports and physical activities. Activities that are more intense and sustained, such as long periods of running, basketball, and soccer, are more likely to provoke asthma symptoms. Nevertheless, most students diagnosed with asthma, including exercise-induced asthma, can participate in these activities if their asthma is properly treated. In fact, Olympic athletes who have asthma have demonstrated that vigorous activities are possible with good asthma management.

However, when a student experiences asthma symptoms, or is recovering from a recent asthma attack, physical activities should be temporarily modified in type, length, and/or frequency to help reduce the risk of further symptoms. Work with the student, parents or guardians, healthcare providers, and other school staff to plan appropriate activities for the student until he or she is fully recovered.

Chapter 48

Controlling Seasonal Allergies

Allergic reactions occur when the body wrongly defends itself against something that is not dangerous. A healthy immune system defends against invading bacteria and viruses. During allergic reactions, however, the immune system fights harmless materials, such as pollen or mold, with production of a special class of antibody called immunoglobulin E (IgE).

Treat respiratory allergy with antihistamines, topical nasal steroids, cromolyn sodium, decongestants, or immunotherapy.

Plant Pollen

Ragweed and other weeds, such as curly dock, lambs quarters, pigweed, plantain, sheep sorrel, and sagebrush are prolific producers of pollen allergens. Ragweed season runs from August to November, but pollen levels usually peak by mid-September in many areas in the country. Pollen counts are highest in the morning, and on dry, hot, windy days.

Protecting Yourself

- Between 5:00 and 10:00 in the morning, stay indoors. Save outside activities for late afternoon or after a heavy rain, when pollen levels are lower.

This chapter includes text excerpted from "How to Control Your Seasonal Allergies," MedlinePlus, National Institutes of Health (NIH), 2013. Reviewed August 2018.

- Keep windows in your home and car closed to lower exposure to pollen. Keep cool with air conditioners. Don't use window or attic fans.

- Use a dryer, not a line outside; dry your clothes and avoid collecting pollen on them.

Grass Pollen

Grass pollens are regional as well as seasonal. Their levels also are affected by temperature, time of day, and rain. Only a small percentage of North America's 1,200 grass species cause allergies, including:

- Bermuda grass

- Johnson grass

- Kentucky bluegrass

- Sweet vernal grass

- Timothy grass

- Orchard grass

Protecting Yourself

- Between 5:00 and 10:00 a.m., stay indoors. Save outside activities for late afternoon or after a heavy rain, when pollen levels are lower.

- Keep windows in your home and car closed to lower exposure to pollen. Keep cool with air conditioners. Don't use window or attic fans.

- Use a clothes dryer, not a line outside, to avoid collecting pollen on them.

- Have someone else mow your lawn. If you mow, wear a mask.

Tree Pollen

Trees produce pollen earliest, as soon as January in the south, and as late as May and June in the northeast. They release huge amounts that can be distributed miles away. Fewer than 100 kinds of trees cause allergies. The most common tree allergy is against oak, but others include catalpa, elm, hickory, sycamore, and walnut.

Protecting Yourself

- Follow the same protective strategies related to time of day, closed windows, and clothes dryers noted in "Protecting yourself" under grass pollen.

- Plant species that do not aggravate allergies, such as crape myrtle, dogwood, fig, fir, palm, pear, plum, redbud, and redwood trees, or the female cultivars of ash, box elder, cottonwood, maple, palm, poplar, or willow trees.

Seasonal Allergies: Nuisance or Real Health Threat?

For most people, hay fever is a seasonal problem—something to endure for a few weeks once or twice a year. But for others, such allergies can lead to more serious complications, including sinusitis and asthma.

- Sinusitis is one of the most commonly reported chronic diseases and costs almost $6 billion a year to manage. It is caused by inflammation or infection of the four pairs of cavities behind the nose. Congestion in them can lead to pressure and pain over the eyes, around the nose, or in the cheeks just above the teeth. Chronic sinusitis is associated with persistent inflammation and is often difficult to treat. Extended bouts of hay fever can increase the likelihood of chronic sinusitis. But only half of all people with chronic sinusitis have allergies.

- Asthma is a lung disease that narrows or blocks the airways. This causes wheezing, shortness of breath, coughing, and other breathing difficulties. Asthma attacks can be triggered by viral infections, cold air, exercise, anxiety, allergens, and other factors. Almost 80 percent of people with asthma have allergies, but we do not know to what extent the allergies trigger the breathing problems. However, some people are diagnosed with allergic asthma because the problem is set off primarily by an immune response to one or more specific allergens. Most of the time, the culprit allergens are those found indoors, such as pets, house dust mites, cockroaches, and mold. Increased pollen and mold levels have also been associated with worsening asthma.

Chapter 49

Preventing Allergy Symptoms during Travel

Although traveling abroad can be relaxing and rewarding, the physical demands of travel can be stressful, particularly for travelers with underlying chronic illnesses. With adequate preparation, however, such travelers can have safe and enjoyable trips. General recommendations for advising patients with chronic illnesses include:

- Ensure that any chronic illnesses are well controlled. Patients with an underlying illness should see their healthcare providers to ensure that the management of their illness is optimized.

- Encourage patients to seek pretravel consultation at least four to six weeks before departure to ensure adequate time to respond to immunizations and, in some circumstances, to try medications before travel.

- Advise patients to consider a destination where they have access to care for their condition.

- Ask about previous health-related issues encountered during travel, such as complications during air travel.

This chapter contains text excerpted from the following sources: Text in this chapter begins with excerpts from "Travelers with Chronic Illnesses," Centers for Disease Control and Prevention (CDC), June 13, 2017; Text under the heading "Travel Tips for People with Asthma" is excerpted from "Travel Tips for People with Asthma," Centers for Disease Control and Prevention (CDC), June 13, 2017.

- Advise the traveler about packing a health kit.

- Advise travelers to pack medications and medical supplies (such as pouching for ostomies) in their original containers in carry-on luggage and to carry a copy of their prescriptions. Ensure the traveler has sufficient quantities of medications for the entire trip, plus extra in case of unexpected delays. Since medications should be taken based on elapsed time and not time of day, travelers may need guidance on scheduling when to take medications during and after crossing time zones.

- Advise travelers to check with the U.S. embassy or consulate to clarify medication restrictions in the destination country. Some countries do not allow visitors to bring certain medications into the country, especially narcotics and psychotropic medications.

- Educate travelers regarding drug interactions. Medications (such as warfarin) used to treat chronic medical illnesses may interact with medications prescribed for self-treatment of travelers' diarrhea or malaria chemoprophylaxis. Discuss all medications used, either daily or on an as-needed basis.

- Provide a clinician's letter. The letter should be on office letterhead stationery and should outline existing medical conditions, medications prescribed (including generic names), and any equipment required to manage the condition.

- Suggest supplemental insurance. Three types of insurance policies can be considered:

  1. Trip cancellation in the event of illness

  2. Supplemental insurance so that money paid for healthcare abroad may be reimbursed, since most medical insurance policies do not cover healthcare in other countries

  3. Medical evacuation insurance. Travelers may need extra help in finding supplemental insurance, as some plans will not cover costs for preexisting conditions

- Encourage travelers with underlying medical conditions to consider choosing a medical assistance company that allows them to store their medical history so it can be accessed worldwide.

- Help travelers devise a health plan. This plan should give instructions for managing minor problems or exacerbations of underlying illnesses and should include information about medical facilities available in the destination country.

- Advise travelers to wear a medical alert bracelet or carry medical information on his or her person (various brands of jewelry or tags, even electronic, are available).

- Advise travelers to stay hydrated, wear loose-fitting clothing, and walk and stretch at regular intervals during long-distance travel.

- Consider advising the traveler to use a mobile application to track certain chronic illnesses, such as diabetes, while traveling.

Severe Allergic Reactions

1. Plan for managing allergic reactions while traveling and consider bringing a short course of steroids for possible allergic reactions.

2. Carry injectable epinephrine and antihistamines (H1 and H2 blockers)—always have on person.

3. Many airlines already have policies in place for dealing with peanut allergies.

4. Make sure to carry injectable epinephrine in case of a severe reaction while in flight.

Travel Tips for People with Asthma

Whether traveling across the world or across town, a person with asthma has to be careful to prepare for a new environment.

A clinician's guidance can help patients plan for a symptom-free trip. Patients should prepare an asthma travel kit that includes all the controller and rescue medications needed for the duration of the travel, an updated asthma action plan, and any spacers or asthma-related devices that are used. This kit should be packed in carry-on luggage when traveling by air.

During the office visit, make sure immunizations are up-to-date, including the annual flu shot. Discuss measures to reduce the risk of respiratory infections, including frequent hand washing and use of hand sanitizers. Review the patient's asthma triggers and discuss strategies for avoiding them. Encourage patients to ask for a smoke-free hotel room, or better yet, look for lodging that doesn't permit smoking at all. A patient who has pollen allergies should avoid travel to destinations during peak pollen season. Patients allergic to dust mites can travel with their own dust-impermeable mattress and pillow covers. If travel plans include staying in a home, encourage patients to ask about potential asthma triggers, such as pets or smoke, and, if necessary, consider alternate accommodations.

Patients with asthma should know how to recognize and respond to worsening symptoms. Advise your patients to keep your contact information with them, and to identify a local clinician in the area they will be visiting. This may help to avoid an emergency room visit. Encourage patients to tell travel companions how they can help if asthma symptoms occur.

The goal of good asthma care is to be symptom-free and fully active, including being able to travel.

Chapter 50

Preventing Food Allergies during Pregnancy/Breastfeeding

About four percent of adults and up to eight percent of children have a food allergy. With the rise of food allergies in children, some pregnant, and breastfeeding women may worry about eating certain foods.

What Are Food Allergies?

In a food allergy, your body's defense system, called the immune system, reacts to a certain food or ingredient as if it were harmful.

What Foods Commonly Trigger Allergic Reactions?

The foods that most often cause allergic reactions in adults are the same for women and men. They include:

- Shellfish, such as shrimp, crayfish, lobster, and crab

- Peanuts

- Tree nuts, such as walnuts, cashews, and pecans

- Fish, such as salmon

This chapter includes text excerpted from "Food Allergies," Office on Women's Health (OWH), U.S. Department of Health and Human Services (HHS), March 2, 2018.

- Milk
- Eggs
- Wheat
- Soybeans

What Are the Symptoms of a Food Allergy?

The symptoms of an allergic reaction to a food usually develop within a few minutes to an hour after you eat the food. You may first feel itching in your mouth as you start to eat the food.

Other symptoms include:

- Stuffy, itchy nose
- Sneezing
- Itchy, watery eyes
- Swelling of the lips, face, tongue, throat, or other parts of your body
- Vomiting
- Diarrhea
- Stomach cramps
- Red, itchy skin, or a rash

If you have food allergy symptoms shortly after eating, see your doctor or nurse. If possible, see your doctor while the allergic reaction is happening.

Are Food Allergies Life-Threatening?

They can be. For some people, an allergic reaction to a food is uncomfortable but not serious. But for others, an allergic food reaction can lead to death. A life-threatening reaction caused by an allergy is called anaphylaxis.

For these people, even the smallest amount of exposure—eating a food or even touching someone who is eating the food—can be dangerous. If you have anaphylactic reactions to certain foods, your doctor may give you a prescription for injectable epinephrine. You need to carry this medicine with you at all times so that you or someone you are with can give you an emergency injection if needed.

Symptoms of anaphylaxis include:

- Hoarseness, throat tightness, or a lump in your throat
- Wheezing, chest tightness, or trouble breathing
- Rapid heart rate
- Dizziness, lightheadedness, or fainting
- Tingling in the hands, feet, lips, or scalp
- Cold, clammy, grayish, or bluish skin

Anaphylaxis is a medical emergency. If you or someone you know has any of these symptoms after eating something, call 911 right away.

Are There Other Health Problems That Can Cause the Same Symptoms as a Food Allergy?

Yes, other health problems can have some of the same symptoms as a food allergy. This can make it hard to know for sure whether you have a food allergy.

These health problems include:

- Food poisoning from contaminated food or foods with poisons, such as certain mushrooms
- Lactose intolerance
- Irritable bowel syndrome (IBS)
- Reactions to large amounts of some food additives, such as monosodium glutamate (MSG, a flavor enhancer)

Should I Avoid Peanuts or Other Foods during Pregnancy or While Breastfeeding?

You do not need to avoid foods such as peanuts, milk, or eggs during pregnancy—unless you are allergic to any of these foods.

According to the American Academy of Pediatrics (AAP):

- Avoiding certain foods in pregnancy does not prevent food allergies in children.
- Breastfeeding may prevent or delay food allergies.
- Soy-based infant formula does not appear to prevent food allergy.

- Delaying the introduction of solid foods beyond 4–6 months of age does not prevent food allergies. Some people have also thought that food allergies might be prevented if parents delayed giving their babies certain solid foods (such as fish, eggs, and milk). But current medical research does not support this idea.

- Recent research has shown that eating foods containing peanuts early in life may prevent a peanut allergy. If your infant has severe eczema, an egg allergy, or both, you may be able to give peanut-containing foods as early as 4–6 months of age to help prevent a peanut allergy. Check with your doctor or nurse before feeding your infant foods containing peanuts.

Can a Baby Be Allergic to Breastmilk?

No. But sometimes babies may be allergic to something their mother eats, such as eggs, milk, or cheese. Babies who are highly sensitive usually react to the food within minutes. Babies who are less sensitive may still react to the food within four to 24 hours.

Symptoms may include:

- Diarrhea, vomiting, and/or green stools with mucus and/or blood

- Rash, eczema, dermatitis, hives, or dry skin

- Fussiness during and/or after feedings

- Inconsolable crying for long periods

- Sudden waking with discomfort

- Wheezing or coughing

These symptoms do not mean your baby is allergic to your milk, but rather to something you are eating. Talk with your baby's doctor about any symptoms. If your baby ever has problems breathing, call 911 or go to your nearest emergency room.

Chapter 51

Avoiding Skin Allergies: Choosing Safe Cosmetics

Chapter Contents

Section 51.1

Hypoallergenic Cosmetics

This section includes text excerpted from
"'Hypoallergenic' Cosmetics," U.S. Food and
Drug Administration (FDA), November 3, 2017.

Hypoallergenic cosmetics are products that manufacturers claim produce fewer allergic reactions than other cosmetic products. Consumers with hypersensitive skin, and even those with "normal" skin, may be led to believe that these products will be gentler to their skin than nonhypoallergenic cosmetics.

What Are Hypoallergenic Cosmetics?

There are no federal standards or definitions that govern the use of the term "hypoallergenic." The term means whatever a particular company wants it to mean. Manufacturers of cosmetics labeled as hypoallergenic are not required to submit substantiation of their hypoallergenicity claims to U.S. Food and Drug Administration (FDA).

The term "hypoallergenic" may have considerable market value in promoting cosmetic products to consumers on a retail basis, but dermatologists say it has very little meaning.

Ever since the days when "She's lovely, she's engaged, she uses Ponds" became one of the best known advertising slogans in America, cosmetics manufacturers have pursued consumers with promises of everything from new beauty to a new lifestyle. Indeed, with cosmetics—perhaps more than with any other type of product—promotion is the key to sales success. Recognizing this, manufacturers have used a wide variety of appeals to break into or increase their share in this lucrative market.

For many years, companies have been producing products which they claim are "hypoallergenic" or "safe for sensitive skin" or "allergy tested." These statements imply that the products making the claims are less likely to cause allergic reactions than competing products. But there has been no assurance to consumers that this actually was the case.

For the past four years, the U.S. Food and Drug Administration has been working to clear up this confusion of claims by establishing testing requirements that would determine which products really are "hypoallergenic." But late last year, the U.S. Court of Appeals for the District of Columbia ruled that FDA's regulation defining "hypoallergenic" was invalid. This means there is now no regulation specifically defining or governing the use of the term "hypoallergenic" or similar claims. And because of the lengthy procedural steps required to establish a new regulation, that is likely to be the situation for some time to come.

Where Does That Leave Consumers?

Consumers concerned about allergic reactions from cosmetics should understand one basic fact: there is no such thing as a "nonallergenic" cosmetic—that is, a cosmetic that can be guaranteed never to produce an allergic reaction.

But Are Some Cosmetics Less Likely to Produce Adverse Reactions than Competing Products?

By and large, the basic ingredients in so-called hypoallergenic cosmetics are the same as those used in other cosmetics sold for the same purposes. Years ago, some cosmetics contained harsh ingredients that had a high potential for causing adverse reactions. But these ingredients are no longer used. FDA knows of no scientific studies which show that "hypoallergenic" cosmetics or products making similar claims actually cause fewer adverse reactions than competing conventional products.

The FDA's ill-fated regulation on "hypoallergenic" cosmetics was first issued as a proposal in February 1974. It said that a cosmetic would be permitted to be labeled "hypoallergenic" or make similar claims only if scientific studies on human subjects showed that it caused a significantly lower rate of adverse skin reactions than similar products not making such claims. The manufacturers of cosmetics claiming to be "hypoallergenic" were to be responsible for carrying out the required tests.

Numerous comments on the proposal were received from consumers, consumer groups and cosmetic manufacturers. Some people urged a ban on the use of the term "hypoallergenic" on grounds that most consumers don't have allergies. Others suggested that the term be banned because allergic individuals cannot use "hypoallergenic" products with any assurance of safety. A number of cosmetic manufacturers complained about the requirement for product comparison tests to validate claims of hypoallergenicity. Among other things, they said the tests would pose an undue economic burden on them.

In responding to the comments, the FDA pointed out that the proposed regulation was not intended to solve all problems concerning cosmetic safety. The primary purpose of the regulation, the Agency said, was to clear up confusion about the term "hypoallergenic" and to establish a definition that could be used uniformly by manufacturers and understood by consumers.

The FDA issued its final regulation on "hypoallergenic" cosmetics on June 6, 1975. Although the final regulation did require comparative tests, procedures for carrying out the tests were changed to reduce the costs to the manufacturers.

The new regulation was quickly challenged in the U.S. District Court for the District of Columbia by Almay and Clinique, makers of "hypoallergenic" cosmetics. The two firms charged that the FDA had no authority to issue the regulation, but the court upheld the FDA.

The firms then appealed to the U.S. Court of Appeals for the District of Columbia, which ruled that the regulation was invalid. The appeals court held that the FDA's definition of the term "hypoallergenic" was unreasonable because the Agency had not demonstrated that consumers perceive the term "hypoallergenic" in the way described in the regulation.

As a result of the decision, manufacturers may continue to label and advertise their cosmetics as "hypoallergenic" or make similar claims without any supporting evidence. Consumers will have no assurance that such claims are valid.

However, cosmetics users who know they are allergic to certain ingredients can take steps to protect themselves. The FDA regulations now require the ingredients used in cosmetics to be listed on the product label, so consumers can avoid substances that have caused them problems.

Section 51.2

Cosmetics: Tips for Women

This section includes text excerpted from "Cosmetics:
Tips for Women," U.S. Food and Drug
Administration (FDA), January 19, 2018.

People use cosmetics to enhance their beauty. These products range from lipstick and nail polish to deodorant, perfume, and hairspray. Get the facts before using cosmetics.

General Tips

- Read the label. Follow all directions.
- Wash your hands before you use the product.
- Do not share makeup.
- Keep the containers clean and closed tight when not in use.
- Throw away cosmetics if the color or smell changes.
- Do not use spray cans while you are smoking or near an open flame. It could start a fire.
- Use aerosols or sprays in a place with good airflow.

Eye Make-Up Tips

1. Do not add saliva or water to mascara. You could add germs.

2. Throw away your eye makeup if you get an eye infection

3. Do not use cosmetics near your eyes unless they are meant for your eyes. For example, do not use lip liner on your eyes.

4. Do not dye or tint your eyelashes. The U.S. Food and Drug Administration (FDA) has not approved any color additives for permanent dyeing or tinting of your eyelashes or eyebrows.

5. Hold still! Even a slight scratch with the mascara wand or other applicator can result in a serious infection. Do not apply makeup in the car or on the bus.

Bad Reaction to Cosmetics?

The FDA does not test cosmetics before they are sold in stores. However, the FDA does monitor the safety of cosmetic products. Tell the FDA if you have a rash, redness, burns, or other serious problems after using cosmetics.

What Should You Do?

- Stop using the product.

- Call your healthcare provider to find out how to take care of the problem.

- Report serious problems to the FDA at: www.fda.gov/medwatch/report.htm or 800-332-1088.

Understanding Cosmetic Labels

Read the label including the list of ingredients, warnings, and tips on how to use it safely.

- **Hypoallergenic:** Do not assume that the product will not cause allergic reactions. The FDA does not define what it means to be labeled "hypoallergenic."

- **Organic or natural:** The source of the ingredients does not determine how safe it is. Do not assume that these products are safer than products made with ingredients from other sources. The FDA does not define what it means to be labeled "organic" or "natural."

- **Expiration dates:** Cosmetics are not required to have an expiration date. A cosmetic product may go bad if you store it the wrong way like if it is unsealed or in a place that is too warm or too moist.

Section 51.3

Using Nail Care Products

This section includes text excerpted from "How to Safely Use Nail Care Products," U.S. Food and Drug 9Administration (FDA), December 22, 2017.

Manicures and pedicures can be pretty. The cosmetic products used, such as nail polishes and nail polish removers, also must be safe—and are regulated by the U.S. Food and Drug Administration (FDA).

The FDA also regulates devices used to dry (or "cure") artificial nails or gel nail polish as electronic products because they emit radiation.

You can do your part to stay safe (and look polished, too) by following all labeled directions and paying attention to any warning statements listed on these products.

Cosmetic Nail Care Products: Ingredients and Warnings

Cosmetic ingredients (except most color additives) and products, including nail products, do not need FDA approval before they go on the market.

But these products are required to be safe when used as intended. (Note that nail products intended to treat medical problems are classified as drugs and do require FDA approval.)

Cosmetic nail care products also must include any instructions or warnings needed to use them safely. For example:

- Some nail products can catch fire easily so you should not expose them to flames (such as from a lit cigarette) or heat sources (such as a curling iron).

- Some can injure your eyes, so you should avoid this exposure.

- Some should only be used in areas with good air circulation (ventilation).

- Some ingredients can be harmful if swallowed, so these products should never be consumed by any person or pet.

Also know that retail cosmetics such as those sold in stores or online must list ingredients in the order of decreasing amounts. If you're concerned about certain ingredients, you can check the label and avoid using products with those ingredients.

For example, some nail hardeners and nail polishes may contain formaldehyde, which can cause skin irritation or an allergic reaction. And acrylics, used in some artificial nails and sometimes in nail polishes, can cause allergic reactions.

The Bottom Line

Read the labels of cosmetic products and follow all instructions. And if you go to a salon for a manicure or pedicure, make sure the space has good ventilation.

Note: Nail salon practices are regulated by the states, and not the FDA. If you're a nail salon owner or employee, you can find information on maintaining safe salons on the webpage (www.osha.gov/SLTC/nailsalons/) of the U.S. Department of Labor's (DOL) Occupational Safety and Health Administration (OSHA).

If you have questions about whether certain nail products are right for you, talk to your healthcare provider.

About Nail Drying and Curing Lamps—and Ultra Violet Exposure

Ultraviolet (UV) nail curing lamps are table-top size units used to dry or "cure" acrylic or gel nails and gel nail polish. These devices are used in salons and sold online. They feature lamps or LEDs that emit UV (ultraviolet) radiation. (Nail curing lamps are different than sun lamps, which are sometimes called "tanning beds."

Exposure to UV radiation can cause damage to your skin, especially if you're exposed over time. For example, it can lead to premature wrinkles, age spots, and even skin cancer.

But the FDA views nail curing lamps as low risk when used as directed by the label. For example, a 2013 published study indicated that—even for the worst case lamp that was evaluated—30 minutes of daily exposure to this lamp was below the occupational exposure limits for UV radiation. (Note that these limits only apply to normal, healthy people and not to people who may have a condition that makes them extra sensitive to UV radiation.)

To date, the FDA has not received any reports of burns or skin cancer attributed to these lamps.

That said, if you're concerned about potential risks from UV exposure, you can avoid using these lamps.

You may particularly want to avoid these lamps if you're using certain medications or supplements that make you more sensitive to

UV rays. These medications include some antibiotics, oral contraceptives, and estrogens—and supplements can include St. John's Wort. Also remove cosmetics, fragrances, and skin care products (except sunscreen!) before using these lamps, as some of these products can make you more sensitive to UV rays.

If you have questions about using nail drying or curing lamps, consult a healthcare professional.

And if you do choose to use these devices, you can reduce UV exposure by:

- Wearing UV-absorbing gloves that expose only your nails

- Wearing a broad-spectrum sunscreen with an SPF of 15 or higher. (Since nail treatments can include exposure to water, follow the sunscreen's labeled directions for use in these situations.)

Finally, nail curing lamps usually come with instructions for exposure time. The shorter your exposure, the less risky the exposure, in general. So always follow labeled directions when available. In general, you should not use these devices for more than 10 minutes per hand, per session.

How to Report Problems with Nail Care Products

If you ever have a bad reaction to a cosmetic nail product or nail curing lamp, please consult your healthcare provider and then tell the FDA.

You can call an FDA Consumer Complaint Coordinator (phone numbers for your area are online) or report the problem via MedWatch (www.accessdata.fda.gov/scripts/medwatch/index.cfm?action=reporting.home), the FDA Safety Information and Adverse Event Reporting program.

Part Seven

Additional Help and Information

Chapter 52

Glossary of Terms Related to Allergies and the Immune System

air spaces: All alveolar ducts, alveolar sacs, and alveoli. To be contrasted with airways.

airways: All passageways of the respiratory tract from mouth or nose down to and including respiratory bronchioles. To be contrasted with air spaces.

allergen-specific immunotherapy: It is a type of treatment in which a patient is given increasing doses of an allergen—for example, milk, egg, or peanut allergen—with the goal of inducing immune tolerance (the ability of the immune system to ignore the presence of one or more food protein allergens while remaining responsive to unrelated proteins).

allergen: A substance that causes an allergic reaction.

allergenic: Describes a substance that produces an allergic reaction.

allergic contact dermatitis (ACD): A form of eczema caused by an allergic reaction to food additives or molecules that occur naturally in foods such as mango. The allergic reaction involves immune cells

---

This glossary contains terms excerpted from documents produced by several sources deemed reliable.

but not IgE antibodies. Symptoms include itching, redness, swelling, and small raised areas on the skin that may or may not contain fluid.

allergic proctocolitis (AP): A disorder that occurs in infants who seem healthy but have visible specks or streaks of blood mixed with mucus in their stool. Because there are no laboratory tests to diagnose food-induced AP, a healthcare professional must rely on a medical history showing that certain foods cause symptoms to occur. Many infants have AP while being breast-fed, probably because the mother's milk contains food proteins from her diet that cause an allergic reaction in the infant.

amino acids: Any of the 26 building blocks of proteins.

anaphylaxis: A severe reaction to an allergen that can cause itching, fainting, and in some cases, death.

angioedema: It is swelling due to fluid collecting under the skin, in the abdominal organs, or in the upper airway (nose, back of the throat, voicebox). It often occurs with hives and, if caused by food, is typically IgE-mediated. When the upper airway is involved, swelling in the voicebox is an emergency requiring immediate medical attention. Acute angioedema is a common feature of anaphylaxis.

antibody: A molecule tailor-made by the immune system to lock onto and destroy specific foreign substances such as allergens.

antigen: A substance or molecule that is recognized by the immune system.

artery: A blood vessel that carries blood from the heart to other parts of the body.

assay: A laboratory method of measuring a substance such as immunoglobulin.

asthma: A respiratory disease of the lungs characterized by episodes of inflammation and narrowing of the lower airways in response to asthma triggers, such as infectious agents, stress, pollutants such as cigarette smoke, and common allergens such as cat dander, dust mites, and pollen.

autoimmune disease: A disease that results when the immune system mistakenly attacks the body's own tissues.

B cell: A small white blood cell crucial to the immune defenses. B cells come from bone marrow and develop into blood cells called plasma cells, which are the source of antibodies.

bacteria: Microscopic organisms composed of a single cell. Some cause disease.

basophil: A white blood cell that contributes to inflammatory reactions. Along with mast cells, basophils are responsible for the symptoms of allergy.

blood vessel: An artery, vein, or capillary that carries blood to and from the heart and body tissues.

bloodborne pathogens: Means pathogenic microorganisms that are present in human blood and can cause disease in humans.

bronchitis: A nonneoplastic disorder of structure or function of the bronchi resulting from infectious or noninfectious irritation.

bronchodilator: An agent that causes an increase in the caliber (diameter) of airways.

celiac disease: A disease of the digestive system that damages the small intestine and interferes with absorption of nutritional contents of food.

cells: The smallest units of life; the basic living things that make up tissues.

chemokine: A small protein molecule that activates immune cells, stimulates their migration, and helps direct immune cell traffic throughout the body.

chronic obstructive pulmonary disease (COPD): This term refers to chronic lung disorders that result in blocked air flow in the lungs.

conjunctivitis: Inflammation of the lining of the eyelid, causing red-rimmed, swollen eyes, and crusting of the eyelids.

contact urticaria (hives): It occurs when the skin comes in contact with an allergen. The hives can be local or widespread. They are caused by antibodies interacting with allergen proteins or from the direct release of histamine, a molecule involved in allergy.

corticosteroids: They are a class of drugs similar to the natural hormone cortisone. These drugs are used to treat inflammatory diseases, such as allergies and asthma.

cytokines: Powerful chemical substances secreted by cells that enable the body's cells to communicate with one another.

dendritic cell: An immune cell with highly branched extensions that occurs in lymphoid tissues, engulfs microbes, and stimulates T cells by displaying the foreign antigens of the microbes on their surfaces.

513

deoxyribonucleic acid (DNA): A long molecule found in the cell nucleus. Molecules of DNA carry the cell's genetic information.

eczema: The term for a group of allergic conditions that causes the skin to become inflamed and is characterized by redness, itching, and oozing lesions that become crusty.

elimination diet: Certain foods are removed from a person's diet and a substitute food of the same type, such as another source of protein in place of eggs, is introduced.

enterocolitis: It is an inflammation of the colon and small intestine.

enteropathy: It is a disease of the intestine.

enzyme: A protein produced by living cells that promotes the chemical processes of life without itself being altered.

eosinophil: A white blood cell containing granules filled with chemicals damaging to parasites and enzymes that affect inflammatory reactions.

eosinophilic esophagitis (EoE): A disorder associated with food allergy, but how it is related is unclear. It occurs when types of immune cells called eosinophils collect in the esophagus. Both IgE- and non-IgE-mediated mechanisms appear to be involved in EoE.

epidemiology: A branch of medical science that deals with the incidence, distribution, and control of disease in a population.

epinephrine (adrenaline): A hormone that increases heart rate, tightens the blood vessels, and opens the airways. Epinephrine is the best treatment for anaphylaxis.

epithelium: A membranous cellular tissue that covers a free surface or lines a tube or cavity of an animal body and serves especially to enclose and protect the other parts of the body, to produce secretions and excretions, and to function in assimilation.

esophagus: The passageway through which food moves from the throat to the stomach.

exercise-induced anaphylaxis (EIA): A type of severe, whole-body allergic reaction that occurs during physical activity. Food is the trigger in about one-third of patients who have experienced exercise-induced anaphylaxis. This reaction is likely to recur in patients.

extract: A concentrated liquid preparation containing minute parts of specific foods.

food protein-induced enterocolitis syndrome (FPIES): A non-IgE-mediated disorder that usually occurs in young infants. Symptoms include chronic vomiting, diarrhea, and failure to gain weight or height. When the allergenic food is removed from the infant's diet, symptoms disappear. Milk and soy protein are the most common causes, but some studies report reactions to rice, oat, or other cereal grains. A similar condition also has been reported in adults, most often related to eating crustacean shellfish.

fungus: A member of a class of relatively primitive vegetable organisms. Fungi include mushrooms, yeasts, rusts, molds, and smuts.

gastrointestinal (GI) tract: An area of the body that includes the stomach and intestines.

gene: A unit of genetic material (DNA) inherited from a parent that controls specific characteristics. Genes carry coded directions a cell uses to make specific proteins that perform specific functions.

genome: A full set of genes in a person or any other living thing.

graft-versus-host disease: A life-threatening reaction in which transplanted cells attack the tissues of the recipient.

granule: A grain-like part of a cell.

granulocyte: A phagocytic white blood cell filled with granules. Neutrophils, eosinophils, basophils, and mast cells are examples of granulocytes.

histamine: A chemical released by mast cells and basophils.

house dust mite: Either of two widely distributed mites of the genus Dermatophagoides (*Dermatophagoides pteronyssinus* and *Dermatophagoides pteronyssinus*) that commonly occur in house dust and often induce allergic responses, especially in children.

human immunodeficiency (HIV) virus: The virus that causes AIDS.

human leukocyte antigen: A protein on the surfaces of human cells that identifies the cells as "self" and, like MHC antigens, performs essential roles in immune responses. HLAs are used in laboratory tests to determine whether one person's tissues are compatible with another person's, and could be used in a transplant.

immune response: A reaction of the immune system to foreign substances. Although normal immune responses are designed to protect the body from pathogens, immune dysregulation can damage normal cells and tissues, as in the case of autoimmune diseases.

immune system: A complex network of specialized cells, tissues, and organs that defends the body against attacks by disease-causing organisms.

immunoglobulin: One of a large family of proteins, also known as antibody.

immunosuppressive: Capable of reducing immune responses.

inflammation: An immune system reaction to "foreign" invader such as microbes or allergens. Signs include redness, swelling, pain, or heat.

inflammatory response: Redness, warmth, and swelling produced in response to infection; the result of increased blood flow and an influx of immune cells and their secretions.

innate: An immune system function that is inborn and provides an all-purpose defense against invasion by microbes.

interferon: A protein produced by cells that stimulates antivirus immune responses or alters the physical properties of immune cells.

interleukins: A major group of lymphokines and monokines.

lactase: The enzyme responsible for breaking down lactose in the gut. Lactase is produced by cells lining the small intestine.

lactose intolerance: The inability to digest lactose, a kind of sugar found in milk and other food products. Lactose intolerance is caused by a shortage of the enzyme lactase, which is produced by the cells that line the small intestine.

latex allergy: Workers exposed to latex gloves and other products containing natural rubber latex may develop allergic reactions such as skin rashes; hives; nasal, eye, or sinus symptoms; asthma; and (rarely) shock.

lymphocytes: Small white blood cells that are important parts of the immune system.

macrophage: A large and versatile immune cell that devours invading pathogens and other intruders. Macrophages stimulate other immune cells by presenting them with small pieces of the invaders.

major histocompatibility complex (MHC): A group of genes that controls several aspects of the immune response. MHC genes code for "self" markers on all body cells.

mast cell: A granulocyte found in tissue. The contents of mast cells, along with those of basophils, are responsible for the symptoms of allergy.

memory cells: A subset of T cells and B cells that have been exposed to antigens and can then respond more readily when the immune system encounters those same antigens again.

microbes: Tiny life forms, such as bacteria, viruses, and fungi, which may cause disease.

molecules: The building blocks of a cell. Some examples are proteins, fats, and carbohydrates.

monoclonal antibody: An antibody produced by a single B cell or its identical progeny that is specific for a given antigen.

monocyte: A large phagocytic white blood cell which, when entering tissue, develops into a macrophage.

natural killer (NK) cell: A large granule-containing lymphocyte that recognizes and kills cells lacking self antigens. These cells' target recognition molecules are different from T cells.

neutrophil: A white blood cell that is an abundant and important phagocyte.

organism: An individual living thing.

parasite: A plant or animal that lives, grows, and feeds on or within another living organism.

particle pollution: Particle pollution (also known as "particulate matter") consists of a mixture of solids and liquid droplets. Some particles are emitted directly; others form when pollutants emitted by various sources react in the atmosphere.

pathogen: Any virus, microorganism, or etiologic agent causing disease.

perennial: Describes something that occurs throughout.

phagocytosis: Process by which one cell engulfs another cell or large particle.

plasma cell: A large antibody-producing cell that develops from B cells.

rhinitis: Inflammation of the nasal passages, which can cause a runny nose.

sinuses: Hollow air spaces located within the bones of the skull surrounding the nose.

sinusitis: When sinuses are infected or inflamed.

stem cell: An immature cell from which other cells derive. Bone marrow is rich in the kind of stem cells that become specialized blood cells.

tissues: Groups of similar cells joined to perform the same function.

tolerance: A state of immune nonresponsiveness to a particular antigen or group of antigens.

toll-like receptor: A family of proteins important for first-line immune defenses against microbes.

toxin: An agent produced in plants and bacteria, normally very damaging to cells.

ultraviolet (UV) radiation: A portion of the electromagnetic spectrum with wavelengths shorter than visible light.

upper respiratory tract: Area of the body that includes the nasal passages, mouth, and throat.

vaccine: A preparation that stimulates an immune response that can prevent an infection or create resistance to an infection. Vaccines do not cause disease.

volatile organic compound: Any organic compound that participates in atmospheric photochemical reactions except those designated by EPA as having negligible photochemical reactivity.

Chapter 53

Directory of Organizations That Provide Information about Allergies

Agencies That Provide Information about Allergies
Government Agencies

Center for Food Safety and Applied Nutrition (CFSAN)
Outreach and Information Center, U.S. Food and Drug Administration (FDA)
5001 Campus Dr.
HFS-009
College Park, MD 20740-3835
Toll-Free: 888-SAFEFOOD (888-723-3366)
Website: www.fda.gov/aboutfda/ centersoffices/officeoffoods/cfsan/ contactcfsan/default.htm

Consumer Affairs Branch (CBER)
Office of Communication, Outreach and Development (OCOD), U.S. Food and Drug Administration (FDA)
10903 New Hampshire Ave.
Bldg. 71 Rm. 3103
Silver Spring, MD 20993-0002
Toll-Free: 800-835-4709
Phone: 240-402-8010
Website: www.fda.gov/ aboutfda/centersoffices/ officeofmedicalproductsand tobacco/cber/ucm125684.htm
E-mail: ocod@fda.hhs.gov

Resources in this chapter were compiled from several sources deemed reliable; all contact information was verified and updated in August 2018.

519

National Center for Health Statistics (NCHS)
Division of Health Interview
Statistics
3311 Toledo Rd.
Rm. 2217
Hyattsville, MD 20782-2064
Phone: 301-458-4901
Website: www.cdc.gov/nchs/
nhanes/contact.htm
E-mail: nhis@cdc.gov

Eunice Kennedy Shriver
*National Institute of
Child Health and Human
Development (NICHD)*
P.O. Box 3006
Rockville, MD 20847
Toll-Free: 800-370-2943
Toll-Free TTY: 888-320-6942
Toll-Free Fax: 866-760-5947
Website: www.nichd.nih.gov
E-mail: NICHDInformation
ResourceCenter@mail.nih.gov

Food and Nutrition Service (FNS)
3101 Park Center Dr.
Alexandria, VA 22302
Phone: 703-305-2062
Website: www.fns.usda.gov

FoodSafety.gov
U.S. Department of Health and
Human Services (HHS)
200 Independence Ave. S.W.
Washington, DC 20201
Website: www.foodsafety.gov

Genetic and Rare Diseases Information Center (GARD)
P.O. Box 8126
Gaithersburg, MD 20898-8126
Toll-Free: 888-205-2311
Phone: 301-251-4925
Toll-Free TTY: 888-205-3223
Fax: 301-251-4911
Website: rarediseases.info.nih.
gov/about-gard/contact-gard

LiverTox
Website: livertox.nih.gov
E-mail: LiverTox@nih.gov

National Cancer Institute (NCI)
BG 9609 MSC 9760
9609 Medical Center Dr.
Bethesda, MD 20892-9760
Toll-Free: 800-4-CANCER
(800-422-6237)
Website: www.cancer.gov

National Eye Institute (NEI)
Information Office
31 Center Dr.
MSC 2510
Bethesda, MD 20892-2510
Phone: 301-496-5248
Website: nei.nih.gov
E-mail: 2020@nei.nih.gov

*National Institute
of Arthritis and
Musculoskeletal and Skin
Diseases (NIAMS)*
31 Center Dr. MSC 2350
Bldg. 31 Rm. 4C02
Bethesda, MD 20892-2350
Toll-Free: 877-22-NIAMS
(877-226-4267)
Phone: 301-496-8190
TTY: 301-565-2966
Fax: 301-480-2814
Website: www.niams.nih.gov
E-mail: NIAMSinfo@mail.nih.
gov

*National Institute of
Diabetes and Digestive and
Kidney Diseases (NIDDK)*
National Institutes of Health
(NIH) Office of Communications
and Public Liaison
Bldg. 31 Rm. 9A06
31 Center Dr. MSC 2560
Bethesda, MD 20892-2560
Toll-Free: 800-860-8747
Website: www.niddk.nih.gov
E-mail: healthinfo@niddk.nih.
gov

*National Toxicology
Program (NTP) Center for
Phototoxicology*
P.O. Box 12233 MD K2-03
Research Triangle Park, NC
27709
Phone: 984-287-3209
Website: ntp.niehs.nih.gov

*Occupational Safety and
Health Administration
(OSHA)*
200 Constitution Ave. N.W.
Rm. Number N3626
Washington, DC 20210
Toll-Free: 800-321-OSHA
(800-321-6742)
Toll-Free TTY: 877-889-5627
Website: www.osha.gov

*Office on Women's Health
(OWH)*
U.S. Department of Health and
Human Services (HHS)
200 Independence Ave. S.W.
Rm. 712E
Washington, DC 20201
Toll-Free: 800-994-9662
Website: www.womenshealth.
gov

*Women, Infants, and
Children (WIC) Works
Resource System*
U.S. Department of Agriculture
(USDA), National Agricultural
Library (NAL)
Website: wicworks.fns.usda.gov
E-mail: wicworks@fns.usda.gov

Private Agencies That Provide Information about Allergies

Academy of Nutrition and Dietetics
120 S. Riverside Plaza
Ste. 2190
Chicago, IL 60606-6995
Toll-Free: 800-877-1600
Phone: 312-899-0040
Website: www.eatrightpro.org

AllergenOnline.org
Website: www.allergenonline.com

AllergicChild.com
6660 Delmonico Dr.
Ste. D249
Colorado Springs, CO 80919
Website: home.allergicchild.com

American Academy of Ophthalmology (AAO)
655 Beach St.
San Francisco, CA 94109
Phone: 415-561-8500
Website: www.aao.org

American Gastroenterological Association (AGA)
4930 Del Ray Ave.
Bethesda, MD 20814
Phone: 301-654-2055
Fax: 301-654-5920
Website: www.gastro.org
E-mail: member@gastro.org

Consortium of Food Allergy Research (CoFAR)
Website: www.cofargroup.org

COPD Foundation
1140 Third St. N.E.
Second Fl.
Washington, DC 20002
Toll-Free: 866-731-COPD
(866-731-2673)
Website: www.copdfoundation.org
E-mail: info@copdfoundation.org

Food Allergy Research & Education (FARE)
7901 Jones Branch Dr.
Ste. 240
McLean, VA 22102
Toll-Free: 800-929-4040
Phone: 703-691-3179
Fax: 703-691-2713
Website: fare.foodallergy.org

Gluten Intolerance Group (GIG)
31214 124th Ave. S.E.
Auburn, WA 98092
Phone: 253-833-6655
Fax: 253-833-6675
Website: www.gluten.org
E-mail: customerservice@gluten.org

Immune Tolerance Network (ITN)
Benaroya Research Institute (BRI)
1201 Ninth Ave.
Seattle, WA 98101-2795
Phone: 206-342-6515
Fax: 206-342-6588
Website: www.immunetolerance.
org

Infectious Diseases Society of America (IDSA)
1300 Wilson Blvd.
Ste. 300
Arlington, VA 22209
Phone: 703-299-0200
Fax: 703-299-0204
Website: www.idsociety.org

Institute for Food Safety and Health (IFSH)
6502 S. Archer Rd.
Bedford Park, IL 60501
Phone: 708-563-1576
Website: www.ifsh.iit.edu

International Food Information Council (IFIC) Foundation
1100 Connecticut Ave. N.W.
Ste. 430
Washington, DC 20036
Phone: 202-296-6540
Website: www.foodinsight.org
E-mail: info@foodinsight.org

Kids with Food Allergies (KFA)
Asthma and Allergy Foundation of America (AAFA)
4259 W. Swamp Rd.
Ste. 408
Doylestown, PA 18902
Phone: 215-230-5394
Fax: 215-230-7674
Website: www.
kidswithfoodallergies.org

La Leche League International (LLLI)
110 Horizon Dr.
Ste. 210
Raleigh, NC 27615
Toll-Free: 800-LALECHE
(800-525-3243)
Phone: 919-459-2167
Fax: 919-459-2075
Website: www.llli.org
E-mail: info@llli.org

SelectWisely
P.O. Box 289
Sparta, NJ 07871
Toll-Free TTY: 888-396-9260
Toll-Free Fax: 888-392-5937
Website: www.selectwisely.com
E-mail: info@selectwisely.com

Chapter 54

Directory of Websites for People with Food Allergies

Allergy Free
Allergy Free Group provides a simple hair analysis test for those who suspect a food intolerance or environmental allergens. Finding the source of allergy/ intolerance symptoms allows someone to make diet, environment, and lifestyle changes to reduce symptoms.
Website: www.allergyfree.in

Allergy Test
Allergy Test develops and improves hair tests with U.S. Food and Drug Administration (FDA) approval.
Website: allergytest.co

AllergyEats
AllergyEats helps you find restaurants in the United States that will accommodate individuals with food-allergy and food-intolerane.
Website: www.allergyeats.com

Cook IT Allergy Free
Cook IT Allergy Free website provides customized recipes for people with food allergies.
Website: www.cookitallergyfree.com

Resources in this chapter were compiled from several sources deemed reliable; all website information was verified and updated in August 2018.

Food Allergy Fund
Food Allergy Fund is dedicated to funding food allergy research focused on the underlying causes of food allergies and improved treatments for people with food allergies.
Website: foodallergyfund.org

Food Allergy Research & Education (FARE)
FARE works to improve the quality of life and the health of individuals with food allergies, and to provide them hope through the promise of new treatments.
Website: www.foodallergy.org

Gluten Free Passport
Gluten Free Passport helps to eat a diet free from gluten, wheat, dairy, and nuts.
Website: glutenfreepassport.com

Gluten-Free Allergy-Free Marketplace—Celiac Disease Foundation
Gluten-Free Allergy-Free Marketplace offers services for diagnosis, treatment, and a cure for celiac disease and nonceliac gluten/wheat sensitivity through research, education, and advocacy.
Website: celiac.org/marketplace

Kids with Food Allergies
Kids with Food Allergies works to improve the day-to-day lives of families raising children with food allergies.
Website: www.kidswithfoodallergies.org

Parenting Food Allergies
Parenting Food Allergies podcast series is for food allergy parents and caregivers that need a bit of advice and support from someone who understand their struggle.
Website: www.foodallergypodcast.com

SnackSafely.com
SnackSafely.com provides straightforward, actionable information to help improve the lives of the estimated 15 million people in the United States suffering with food allergies.
Website: snacksafely.com

Index

Index

529

macrophage, *continued*
allergy 13
bone marrow 4
defined 516
innate immunity 6
major food allergens, described 44
major histocompatibility complex
  (MHC)
  defined 516
  immune tolerance 13
mast cell
  allergic reaction 112
  bone marrow 4
  defined 517
  idiopathic anaphylaxis 124
  omalizumab 402
mastocytosis, overview 112–6
"Mastocytosis" (GARD) 112n
MCS *see* multiple chemical sensitivity
Medicaid, overview 357–62
"Medicaid and CHIP" (CMS) 357n
medical history
  allergic asthma 71
  allergic tests 351
  aspergillosis 88
  atopic dermatitis (AD) 93
  drug allergy 334
  egg allergy 164
  eosinophilic esophagitis (EoE) 221
  food allergy 132
  lactose intolerance 150
  sulfite sensitivity 212
medical identification, overview 126–7
"Medical Identification Critical for
  People with Life-Threatening
  Allergies" (Omnigraphics) 126n
medications
  allergy, overview 376–92
  anaphylaxis 122
  aspergillosis 88
  asthma 480
  atopic dermatitis (AD) 94
  cold urticaria 111
  conjunctivitis 65
  drug allergic reactions 332
  food journal 242
  gluten 197
  hives 109
  mastocytosis 115

medications, *continued*
  nasal polyps 61
  seafood allergy 171
  seed allergies 207
  sensitivity to the sun 117
  sulfite sensitivity 211
  traveling abroad 491
  see also prescription medications
"Medications and Drug Allergic
  Reactions" (Omnigraphics) 332n
memory cells
  defined 517
  immunization 7
MERV *see* Minimum Efficiency
  Reporting Value
methamphetamine
  defined 383
  pseudoephedrine 383
methylene chloride, toxic air
  pollutants 440
MHC *see* major histocompatibility
  complex
microbes, defined 517
milk allergy, overview 144–58
minimum efficiency reporting value,
  furnace and heating, ventilation, and
  air-conditioning system filters 472
moisturizers, skin care 95
"Mold Cleanup in Your Home"
  (EPA) 473n
"Mold—General Information—Basic
  Facts" (CDC) 274n
molds
  air quality 464
  allergic conjunctivitis 63
  allergies in children 41
  allergy, overview 274–7
  asthma 71, 80, 462
  biological pollutants 29
  cleaning up 473
  health effects 31
  seasonal allergic rhinitis (SAR) 395
  work-related asthma 82
molecules, defined 517
"Monoclonal Antibodies" (NIH) 401n
monoclonal antibody
  defined 517
  described 401
monocyte, defined 517